This report contains the collective views of an international group of experts and does not necessarily represent the decisions or the stated policy of the United Nations Environment Programme, the International Labour Organisation, or the World Health Organization.

Environmental Health Criteria 116

TRIBUTYLTIN COMPOUNDS

Published under the joint sponsorship of the United Nations Environment Programme, the International Labour Organisation, and the World Health Organization

First draft prepared by Dr S. Dobson, Institute of Terrestrial Ecology, United Kingdom, and Dr R. Cabridenc, Institut National de Recherche Chimique Appliquée, France

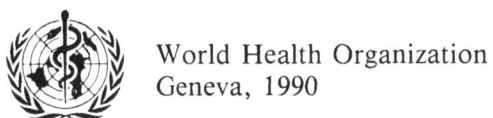

World Health Organization
Geneva, 1990

The **International Programme on Chemical Safety (IPCS)** is a joint venture of the United Nations Environment Programme, the International Labour Organisation, and the World Health Organization. The main objective of the IPCS is to carry out and disseminate evaluations of the effects of chemicals on human health and the quality of the environment. Supporting activities include the development of epidemiological, experimental laboratory, and risk-assessment methods that could produce internationally comparable results, and the development of manpower in the field of toxicology. Other activities carried out by the IPCS include the development of know-how for coping with chemical accidents, coordination of laboratory testing and epidemiological studies, and promotion of research on the mechanisms of the biological action of chemicals.

WHO Library Cataloguing in Publication Data

Tributyltin compounds.

(Environmental health criteria ; 116)

1. Trialkyltin compounds - adverse effects 2. Trialkyltin compounds - toxicity I. Series

ISBN 92 4 157116 0   (NLM Classification: QV 290)
ISSN 0250-863X

©World Health Organization 1990

Publications of the World Health Organization enjoy copyright protection in accordance with the provisions of Protocol 2 of the Universal Copyright Convention. For rights of reproduction or translation of WHO publications, in part or *in toto,* application should be made to the Office of Publications, World Health Organization, Geneva, Switzerland. The World Health Organization welcomes such applications.

The designations employed and the presentation of the material in this publication do not imply the expression of any opinion whatsoever on the part of the Secretariat of the World Health Organization concerning the legal status of any country, territory, city, or area or of its authorities, or concerning the delimitation of its frontiers or boundaries.

The mention of specific companies or of certain manufacturers' products does not imply that they are endorsed or recommended by the World Health Organization in preference to others of a similar nature that are not mentioned. Errors and omissions excepted, the names of proprietary products are distinguished by initial capital letters.

Printed in Finland
DHSS — Vammala — 5000

CONTENTS

ENVIRONMENTAL HEALTH CRITERIA FOR
TRIBUTYLTIN COMPOUNDS

1. SUMMARY 13
   1.1 Physical and chemical properties 13
   1.2 Analytical methods 13
   1.3 Sources of environmental pollution 14
   1.4 Regulations on use 14
   1.5 Environmental concentrations 14
   1.6 Transport and transformation in the environment 15
   1.7 Kinetics and metabolism 16
   1.8 Effects on microorganisms 17
   1.9 Effects on aquatic organisms 17
       1.9.1 Effects on marine and estuarine organisms 17
       1.9.2 Effects on freshwater organisms 19
       1.9.3 Microcosm studies 21
   1.10 Effects on terrestrial organisms 22
   1.11 Effects on organisms in the field 22
   1.12 Toxicity to laboratory mammals 23
       1.12.1 Acute toxicity 23
       1.12.2 Short-term toxicity 23
       1.12.3 Long-term toxicity 26
       1.12.4 Genotoxicity 26
       1.12.5 Reproductive toxicity 26
       1.12.6 Carcinogenicity 27
   1.13 Effects on humans 27

2. IDENTITY, PHYSICAL AND CHEMICAL PROPERTIES, ANALYTICAL METHODS 28

   2.1 Identity of tributyltin compounds 28
   2.2 Physical and chemical properties 28
   2.3 Analytical methods 31
       2.3.1 Measurement of organotin compounds 31
           2.3.1.1 Extraction of tributyltin derivatives 33
           2.3.1.2 Formation of volatile derivatives 33
           2.3.1.3 Separation of organotin derivatives 33
           2.3.1.4 Detection and measurement of different forms of organotin 34

	2.3.2 Interlaboratory calibrations	34
3.	SOURCES OF ENVIRONMENTAL EXPOSURE	36
	3.1 Uses	36
	3.2 Production	37
	3.3 Regulations	38
4.	ENVIRONMENTAL TRANSPORT AND TRANSFORMATION	43
	4.1 Adsorption onto and desorption from particles	43
	4.2 Abiotic degradation	45
	4.2.1 Hydrolytic cleavage of the tin-carbon bond	46
	4.2.2 Photodegradation	47
	4.3 Biodegradation	48
	4.4 Bioaccumulation and elimination	52
5.	ENVIRONMENTAL CONCENTRATIONS	55
	5.1 Sea water and marine sediment	55
	5.2 Fresh water and sediment	61
	5.3 Sewage treatment	64
	5.4 Biota	64
6.	KINETICS AND METABOLISM	70
	6.1 Metabolism of TBT in mammals	70
	6.2 Metabolism of TBTO in other organisms	73
	6.3 General mechanisms of toxicity of TBTO	74
	6.3.1 General toxic mechanisms	74
	6.3.2 Toxic mechanisms in bivalve molluscs	74
7.	EFFECTS ON ORGANISMS IN THE ENVIRONMENT: MICROORGANISMS	76
	7.1 Bacteria and fungi	76
	7.2 Freshwater algae	78
	7.3 Estuarine and marine algae	79
8.	EFFECTS ON ORGANISMS IN THE ENVIRONMENT: AQUATIC ORGANISMS	82
	8.1 Aquatic plants	82

	8.2	Aquatic invertebrates	83
		8.2.1 Trematode parasites of man	83
		8.2.2 Freshwater molluscs	87
		8.2.2.1 Acute toxicity	88
		8.2.2.2 Short- and long-term toxicity	89
		8.2.2.3 Factors affecting toxicity	90
		8.2.3 Marine molluscs	92
		8.2.3.1 Acute toxicity	93
		8.2.3.2 Short- and long-term toxicity	93
		8.2.3.3 Reproductive effects	97
		8.2.3.4 Effects on growth	98
		8.2.3.5 Shell thickening	101
		8.2.3.6 Imposex	101
		8.2.3.7 Genotoxicity	106
		8.2.4 Crustaceans	106
		8.2.4.1 Acute effects	106
		8.2.4.2 Short- and long-term toxicity	107
		8.2.4.3 Reproductive effects	110
		8.2.4.4 Limb regeneration	111
		8.2.4.5 Behavioural effects	111
		8.2.5 Other aquatic invertebrates	112
		8.2.5.1 Acute effects	112
		8.2.5.2 Limb regeneration	113
	8.3	Fish	114
		8.3.1 Acute effects	114
		8.3.2 Short- and long-term toxicity	115
		8.3.3 Embryotoxicity	121
		8.3.4 Behavioural effects	122
	8.4	Amphibians	123
	8.5	Multispecies studies	124
9.	EFFECTS ON ORGANISMS IN THE ENVIRONMENT: TERRESTRIAL ORGANISMS		129
	9.1	Microcosm studies	129
	9.2	Terrestrial insects	129
	9.3	Terrestrial mammals	130
10.	EFFECTS ON ORGANISMS IN THE ENVIRONMENT: FIELD OBSERVATIONS		132
	10.1	Effects on bivalves	132
	10.2	Effects on gastropods: imposex	138
	10.3	Effects on farmed fish	142

10.4	Effects of TBT-contaminated sediment	143
10.5	Effects of freshwater molluscicides	144
10.6	Effects from spills	146
10.7	The use of indicator species for monitoring the environment	146

11. EFFECTS ON EXPERIMENTAL ANIMALS AND *IN VITRO* TEST SYSTEMS — 148

- 11.1 Single exposure — 148
  - 11.1.1 Oral and parenteral administration — 148
  - 11.1.2 Dermal administration — 152
  - 11.1.3 Administration by inhalation — 153
  - 11.1.4 Irritation and sensitization — 154
    - 11.1.4.1 Skin irritation — 154
    - 11.1.4.2 Eye irritation — 156
    - 11.1.4.3 Skin sensitization — 157
  - 11.1.5 *In vitro* studies — 157
- 11.2 Short-term toxicity — 160
  - 11.2.1 Oral dosing: general body effects — 163
  - 11.2.2 Inhalation studies — 164
  - 11.2.3 Histopathological effects — 165
  - 11.2.4 Haematological and biochemical effects — 166
  - 11.2.5 Effects on lymphoid organs and immune function — 167
  - 11.2.6 Mechanism of immunotoxicity — 178
  - 11.2.7 Effects on the endocrine system — 179
- 11.3 Long-term toxicity — 180
- 11.4 Genotoxicity — 181
- 11.5 Reproductive toxicity — 184
  - 11.5.1 *In vivo* — 184
  - 11.5.2 *In vitro* — 187
- 11.6 Carcinogenicity — 188

12. EFFECTS ON HUMANS — 189

- 12.1 Ingestion — 189
- 12.2 Inhalation — 189
- 12.3 Dermal exposure — 189
- 12.4 Miscellaneous effects — 192

13. EVALUATION OF HUMAN HEALTH RISKS AND EFFECTS ON THE ENVIRONMENT — 193

- 13.1 Evaluation of human health risks — 193

13.2 Evaluation of effects on the environment	194
14. RECOMMENDATIONS	196
14.1 Recommendations for protecting human and environmental health	196
14.2 Research needs	196
REFERENCES	198
RESUME	227
EVALUATION DES RISQUES POUR LA SANTE HUMAINE ET EFFETS SUR L'ENVIRONNEMENT	245
RECOMMANDATIONS	249
RESUMEN	251
EVALUACION DE LOS RIESGOS PARA LA SALUD HUMANA Y DE LOS EFECTOS SOBRE EL MEDIO AMBIENTE	268
RECOMENDACIONES	272

WHO TASK GROUP ON TRIBUTYLTIN COMPOUNDS

Members

Dr C. Alzieu, French Institute for Research on Exploitation of the Sea, Nantes, France

Dr I.J. Boyer, Division of Toxicological Review and Evaluation, Food & Drug Administration, Washington, DC, USA

Dr A.H. El-Sabae, Faculty of Agriculture, Alexandria University, Alexandria, Egypt

Dr B. Gilbert, Company for the Development of Technology Transfer (CODETEC), Cidade Universitaria, Campinas, Brazil

Dr Y. Hayashi, Biological Safety Research Centre, National Institute of Hygienic Sciences, Setagaya-ku, Tokyo, Japan

Dr R. Koch, Institute for Geography & Geoecology, Academy of Sciences, German Democratic Republic (*Chairman*)

Dr E.I. Krajnc, National Institute for Public Health and Environmental Hygiene, Bilthoven, Netherlands

Dr H. Schweinfurth, Schering AG, Chemical Industry, Bergkamen, Federal Republic of Germany

Mr D. Spatz, Office of Pesticide Programs, US Environmental Protection Agency, Washington, DC, USA

Dr A.R.D. Stebbing, Natural Environment Research Council, Plymouth Marine Laboratory, Plymouth, United Kingdom

Dr J.H.M. Temmink, Department of Toxicology, Agricultural University, Wageningen, Netherlands

Dr J.E. Thain, Ministry of Agriculture, Fisheries and Food, Fisheries Laboratory, Burnham-on-Crouch, United Kingdom

Prof P.N. Viswanathan, Ecotoxicology Section, Industrial Toxicology Research Centre, Lucknow, India

Observers

Mr J. Chadwick, Health and Safety Executive, Bootle, United Kingdom

Dr R.J. Fielder, Department of Health, London, United Kingdom

Dr R. Lange, Schering AG, Department of Experimental Toxicology, Berlin, Federal Republic of Germany

Secretariat

Dr S. Dobson, Institute of Terrestrial Ecology, Monks Wood Experimental Station, Abbots Ripton, Huntingdon, United Kingdom (*Rapporteur*)

Dr M. Gilbert, International Programme on Chemical Safety, World Health Organization, Geneva, Switzerland (*Secretary*)

Mr P.D. Howe, Institute of Terrestrial Ecology, Monks Wood Experimental Station, Abbots Ripton, Huntingdon, United Kingdom

NOTE TO READERS OF THE CRITERIA DOCUMENTS

Every effort has been made to present information in the criteria documents as accurately as possible without unduly delaying their publication. In the interest of all users of the environmental health criteria documents, readers are kindly requested to communicate any errors that may have occurred to the Manager of the International Programme on Chemical Safety, World Health Organization, Geneva, Switzerland, in order that they may be included in corrigenda, which will appear in subsequent volumes.

* * *

A detailed data profile and a legal file can be obtained from the International Register of Potentially Toxic Chemicals, Palais des Nations, 1211 Geneva 10, Switzerland (Telephone No. 7988400 or 7985850).

ENVIRONMENTAL HEALTH CRITERIA FOR TRIBUTYLTIN COMPOUNDS

A WHO Task Group meeting on Environmental Health Criteria for tributyltin compounds was held at the Institute of Terrestrial Ecology (ITE), Monks Wood, United Kingdom, from 11 to 15 September 1989. Dr M. Roberts, Director, ITE, welcomed the participants on behalf of the host institution and Dr M. Gilbert opened the meeting on behalf of the three cooperating organizations of the IPCS (ILO, UNEP, WHO). The Task Group reviewed and revised the draft criteria document and made an evaluation of the risks for human health and the environment from exposure to tributyltin compounds.

The first draft of this document was prepared by Dr S. Dobson (ITE) and Dr R. Cabridenc (Institut National de Recherche Chimique Appliquée, France). Dr M. Gilbert and Dr P.G. Jenkins, both members of the IPCS Central Unit, were responsible for the technical development and editing, respectively.

ABBREVIATIONS

AA	atomic absorption
BCF	bioconcentration factor
DBT	dibutyltin
EC_{50}	median effective concentration
EEC	European Economic Community
EQT	environmental quality target
FAA	flameless atomic absorption
FMLP	formyl methionyl leucyl phenylalanine
FPD	flame photometric detector
GC	gas chromatography
GLC	gas-liquid chromatography
HPLC	high-performance liquid chromatography
IC_{50}	median inhibitory concentration
ip	intraperitoneal
IU	international unit
iv	intravenous
LC_{50}	median lethal concentration
LDH	lactate dehydrogenase
LT_{50}	median lethal time
MBT	monobutyltin
MIC	minimal inhibitory concentration
MS	mass spectrometry
ND	not detectable
NOEL	no-observed-effect level
OECD	Organization for Economic Cooperation and Development
PALS	periarteriolar lymphocyte sheath
sc	subcutaneous
T_4	thyroxine
TBT	tributyltin
TBTO	tributyltin oxide
TLC	thin-layer chromatography
TLV	threshold limit value

1. SUMMARY

1.1 Physical and chemical properties

Tributyltin (TBT) compounds are organic derivatives of tetravalent tin. They are characterized by the presence of covalent bonds between carbon atoms and a tin atom and have the general formula $(n-C_4H_9)_3$ Sn-X (where X is an anion). The purity of commercial tributyltin oxide (TBTO) is generally above 96%; the principal impurities are dibutyltin derivatives and, to a lesser extent, tetrabutyltin and other trialkyltin compounds. TBTO is a colourless liquid with a characteristic odour and a relative density of 1.17 to 1.18. The solubility in water is low, varying between <1.0 and >100 mg/litre according to the pH, temperature, and anions present in the water (which determine speciation). In sea water and under normal conditions, TBT exists as three species (hydroxide, chloride, and carbonate), which remain in equilibrium. At pH values less than 7.0, the predominate forms are $Bu_3SnOH_2^+$ and Bu_3SnCl, at pH 8, they are Bu_3SnCl, Bu_3SnOH, and $Bu_3SnCO_3^-$, and at pH values above 10, Bu_3SnOH and $Bu_3SnCO_3^-$ predominate.

The octanol/water partition coefficient (log P_{ow}) lies between 3.19 and 3.84 for distilled water and is 3.54 for sea water. TBTO adsorbs strongly to particulate matter, the reported adsorption coefficients ranging between 110 and 55 000. Vapour pressure is low but published values show considerable variation. There was no loss of TBTO from a solution of 1 mg/litre over 62 days, but 20% of the water was lost by evaporation.

1.2 Analytical methods

Several methods are used for measuring tributyltin derivatives in water, sediment, or biota. Atomic absorption spectrometry (AA) is the most common. AA spectrometry with a flame allows a detection limit of 0.1 mg/litre. Flameless AA, using atomization in an electric furnace with graphite, is more sensitive and allows detection limits of between 0.1 and 1.0 µg/litre water. There are

Summary

several different methods of extraction and for forming volatile derivatives. Separation of these derivatives is commonly done using "purge and trap" or gas chromatography. The detection limits are 0.5 and 5.0 µg/kg for sediment and biota.

1.3 Sources of environmental pollution

Tributyltin compounds have been registered as molluscicides, as antifoulants on boats, ships, quays, buoys, crab pots, fish nets, and cages, as wood preservatives, as slimicides on masonry, as disinfectants, and as biocides for cooling systems, power station cooling towers, pulp and paper mills, breweries, leather processing, and textile mills. TBT in antifouling paints was first marketed in a form that allowed free release of the compound. More recently, controlled-release paints, in which the TBT is incorporated in a co-polymer matrix, have become available. Rubber matrices have also been developed to give long-term slow release and lasting effectiveness for antifouling paints and molluscicides. TBT is not used in agriculture because of high phytotoxicity.

1.4 Regulations on use

Many countries have restricted the use of TBT antifouling paints as a result of effects on shellfish. The regulations vary in detail from country to country, but most ban the use of TBT paints on boats of 25 metres length or less. Some countries have excluded boats with aluminium hulls from this ban. In addition, some regulations restrict the TBT content of paints or the leaching rate of TBT from paints (to 4 or 5 $\mu g/cm^2$ per day, long-term).

1.5 Environmental concentrations

High levels of TBT in water, sediment, and biota have been found close to pleasure boating activity, especially in or near marinas, boat yards, and dry docks, fish nets and cages treated with antifouling paints, and cooling systems. The degree of tidal flushing and the turbidity of the water influence TBT concentrations.

TBT levels have been found to reach 1.58 µg/litre in sea water and estuaries, 7.1 µg/litre in fresh water, 26 300 µg/kg in coastal sediments, 3700 µg/kg in freshwater sediments, 6.39 mg/kg in bivalves, 1.92 mg/kg in gastropods, and 11 mg/kg in fish. However, these maximum concentrations of TBT should not be taken as representative, because a number of factors may give rise to anomalously high values (e.g., paint particles in water and sediment samples). It has been found that measured TBT concentrations in the surface microlayer of both fresh water and sea water are up to two orders of magnitude above those measured just below the surface. However, it should be noted that recorded levels of TBT in surface microlayers may be highly affected by the method of sampling.

Older data may not be comparable with newer data because of improvements in the analytical methods available for measuring TBT in water, sediment, and tissue.

1.6 Transport and transformation in the environment

As a result of its low water solubility and lipophilic character, TBT adsorbs readily onto particles. Between 10% and 95% of TBTO introduced into water is estimated to undergo particulate adsorption. Progressive disappearance of adsorbed TBT is not due to desorption but to degradation. The degree of adsorption depends on the salinity, nature and size of particles in suspension, amount of suspended matter, temperature, and the presence of dissolved organic matter.

The degradation of TBTO involves the splitting of the carbon-tin-bond. This can result from various mechanisms occurring simultaneously in the environment, including physico-chemical mechanisms (hydrolysis and photodegradation) and biological mechanisms (degradation by microorganisms and metabolism by higher organisms). Whereas the hydrolysis of organotin compounds occurs under conditions of extreme pH, it is barely evident under normal environmental conditions. Photodegradation occurs during laboratory exposure of solutions to UV light at 300 nm (and to a lesser extent at 350 nm). Under natural conditions, photolysis is limited by the wavelength range of sunlight and by the limited penetration of UV light into water. The presence of photosensitizing substances can accelerate photodegradation. Biodegradation depends on environmental conditions such as temperature, oxygenation, pH, level of mineral elements, the presence of easily biodegradable organic substances for co-metabolism, and the nature of the microflora and its capacity for adaptation. It also depends on the TBTO concentration being lower than the lethal or inhibitory threshold for the bacteria. As with abiotic degradation, biotic breakdown of TBT is a progressive oxidative debutylization founded on the splitting of the carbon-tin bond. Dibutyl derivatives are formed, which are more readily degraded than tributyltin. Monobutyltins are mineralized slowly. Anaerobic degradation does occur but there is a lack of agreement as to its importance. Some workers consider that anaerobic degradation is slow, others that it is more rapid than aerobic degradation. Species of bacteria, algae, and wood-degrading fungi have been identified that can degrade TBTO. Estimates of the half-life of TBT in the environment vary widely.

TBT bioaccumulates in organisms because of its solubility in fat. Bioconcentration factors of up to 7000 have been reported in laboratory investigations with molluscs and fish, and higher values have been reported in field studies. Uptake from food is more important than uptake directly from the water. Higher concentration factors in microorganisms (between 100 and 30 000) may reflect adsorption rather than uptake into cells. There is no indication that TBT is transferred to terrestrial organisms via food chains.

1.7 Kinetics and metabolism

Tributyltin is absorbed from the gut (20-50% depending on the vehicle) and via the skin of mammals (approximately 10%). It can be transferred across the blood-brain barrier and from the placenta to the fetus. Absorbed material is rapidly and widely distributed among tissues (principally the liver and kidney).

TBT metabolism in mammals is rapid; metabolites are detectable in blood within 3 h of TBT administration. In *in vitro* studies, it has been shown that TBT is a substrate for mixed-function oxidases, but these enzymes are inhibited by very high concentrations of TBT.

The rate of TBT loss differs with different tissues, and estimates for biological half-lives in mammals range from 23 to about 30 days.

TBT metabolism also occurs in lower organisms, but it is slower, particularly in molluscs, than in mammals. The capacity for bioaccumulation is, therefore, much greater than in mammals.

TBT compounds inhibit oxidative phosphorylation and alter mitochondrial structure and function. TBT interferes with calcification of the shell of oysters *(Crassostrea* species).

1.8 Effects on microorganisms

TBT is toxic to microorganisms and has been used commercially as a bactericide and algicide. The concentrations that produce toxic effects vary considerably according to the species. TBT is more toxic to gram-positive bacteria (minimal inhibitory concentration (MIC) between 0.2 and 0.8 mg/litre) than to gram-negative bacteria (MIC: 3 mg/litre). The TBT acetate MIC for fungi is 0.5-1 mg/litre and the TBTO MIC for the green alga *Chlorella pyrenoidosa* is 0.5 mg/litre. The primary productivity of a natural community of freshwater algae was reduced by 50% at a TBTO concentration of 3 µg per litre. Recently established no-observed-effect level (NOEL) values for two species of algae are 18 and 32 µg per litre. Toxicity to marine microorganisms is similarly variable between species and between studies; NOEL values are difficult to set but lie below 0.1 µg/litre for some species. Algicidal concentrations range from <1.5 µg per litre to >1000 µg/litre for different species.

1.9 Effects on aquatic organisms

1.9.1 *Effects on marine and estuarine organisms*

A summary diagram relating lethal and sublethal effects to measured marine and estuarine TBT concentrations is presented in Fig. 1. Concentrations exceeding those producing acute lethal effects have been found in many different worldwide locations, particularly associated with pleasure boating activity.

Summary

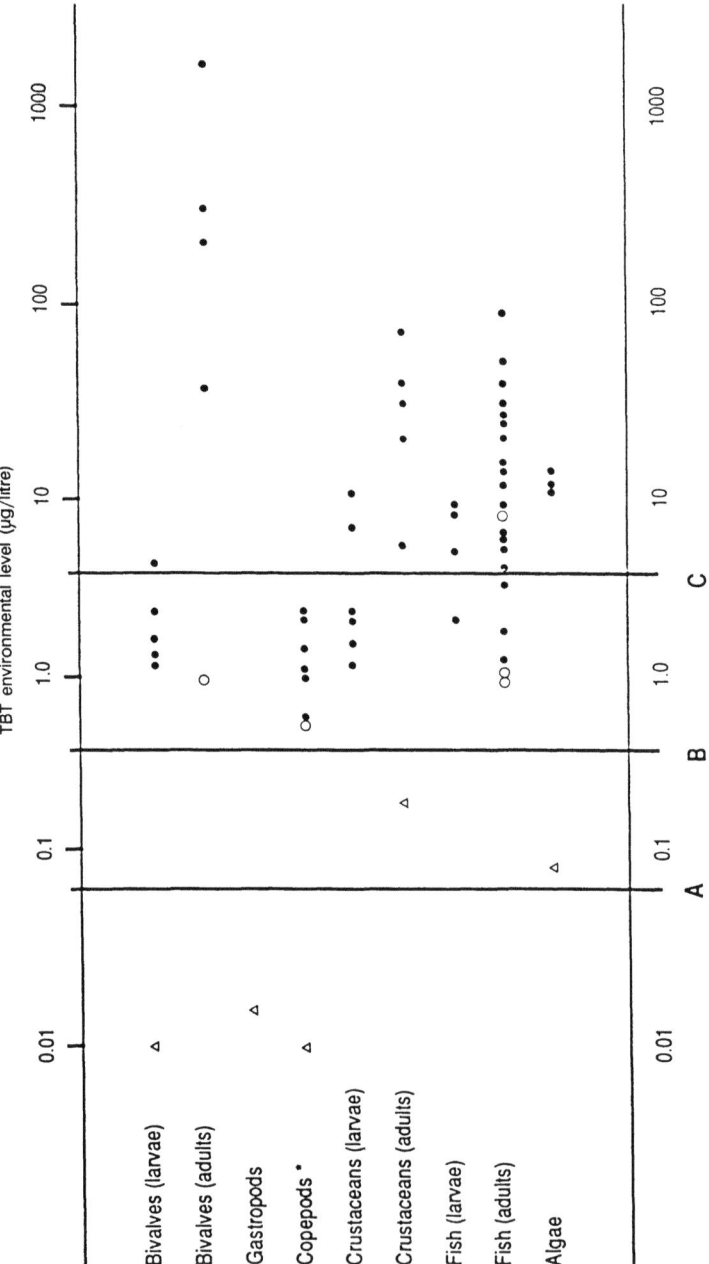

Fig.1. Toxicity of tributyltin to marine organisms

● LC_{50} following exposure for 96 h or less; ○ LC_{50} following exposure for more than 96 h; △ the lowest concentration causing a sublethal effect;
* copepods displayed separately because of greater sensitivity than other crustaceans; A = highest measured concentration in the open sea;
B = highest measured concentration in open estuary; C = highest measured concentration in marinas.

The development of the motile spores of a green macroalga was the stage most sensitive to TBT (5-day EC_{50}: 0.001 µg/litre). There was reduced growth of a marine angiosperm at TBT concentrations of 1 mg/kg sediment but no effect at 0.1 mg/kg.

Tributyltin is highly toxic to marine molluscs. It has been shown experimentally to affect shell deposition of growing oysters, gonadal development and gender of adult oysters, settlement, growth, and mortality of larval oysters and other bivalves, and to cause imposex (the development of male characteristics) in female gastropods. The NOEL for spat of the most sensitive oyster species (*Crassostrea gigas*) has been reported to be about 20 ng/litre. TBT causes deformation of the shell of adult oysters in a dose-related manner. No effect on shell morphology was observed experimentally at TBT concentrations of 2 ng/litre. The NOEL for the development of imposex in female dogwhelks is below 1.5 ng/litre. Larval forms are generally more sensitive than adults; in the case of oysters this difference is particularly marked.

Copepods are more sensitive than other crustacean groups to the acute lethal effects of TBT, LC_{50} values for exposure periods up to 96 h ranging from 0.6 to 2.2 µg/litre. These values are comparable to those of the more sensitive larvae of other crustacean groups. TBT reduces reproductive performance, neonate survival, and juvenile growth rate in crustaceans. The NOEL for reproduction in the mysid shrimp *Acanthomysis sculpta* has been suggested to be 0.09 µg/litre. There was no avoidance of TBT by the grass shrimp at concentrations up to 30 µg/litre.

The toxicity of tributyltin to marine fish is highly variable, 96-h LC_{50} values ranging between 1.5 and 36 µg/litre. Larval stages are more sensitive than adults (Fig. 1). There are indications that marine fish avoid TBTO concentrations of 1 µg/litre or more.

1.9.2 Effects on freshwater organisms

A summary diagram relating lethal and sublethal effects to measured TBT concentrations in fresh water is presented in Fig. 2. Concentrations exceeding those producing sublethal effects have been found, particularly associated with pleasure boating activity.

Summary

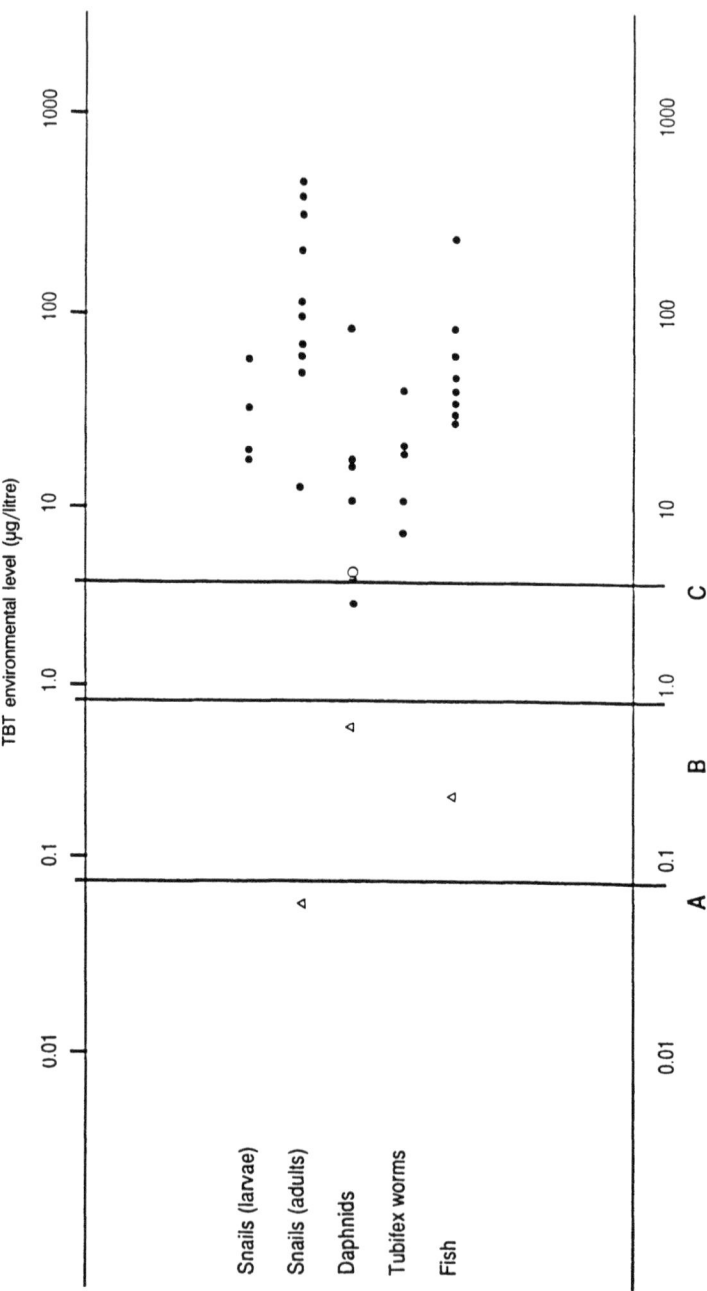

Fig. 2. Toxicity of tributyltin to fresh-water organisms

● LC_{50} following exposure for 96 h or less; ○ LC_{50} following exposure for more than 96 h; △ the lowest concentration causing a sublethal effect;
A = highest measured concentration upstream from marina; B = highest measured concentration downstream from marinas; C = highest measured concentration in marinas.

Fresh-water angiosperms were killed by a TBTO concentration of 0.5 mg/litre, and growth was inhibited at 0.06 mg/litre or more.

Data on fresh-water invertebrate species are few, relating to just three species other than target organisms. Different salts of TBT yield 48-h LC_{50} values for *Daphnia* of 2.3-70 µg/litre and for *Tubifex* of 5.5-33 µg/litre. The NOEL for *Daphnia* has been estimated to be 0.5 µg per litre, based on reversal of normal response to light. The 24-h LC_{50} for the Asiatic clam has been reported to be 2100 µg/litre, and for target snail adults in schistosomiasis control the corresponding values are 30-400 µg/litre.

Tributyltin has been shown to be toxic to schistosome larvae in the aquatic stages; the LC_{50} (TBT fluoride) was calculated to be 16.8 µg/litre for a 1-h exposure. The TBT dose causing 99% to 100% suppression of cercarial infectivity of mice was between 2 and 6 µg/litre.

The sensitivity of snails to TBT decreases with age, but eggs are more resistant than both young and adults. Egg laying is significantly effected at a TBTO concentration of 0.001 µg/litre.

The acute toxicity of TBT to freshwater fish in LC_{50} tests up to 168 h ranges from 13 to 240 µg per litre. The NOEL for the guppy was estimated to be 0.01 µg per litre, based on histopathological effects.

No effect on survival was found when eggs and larvae of the frog *Rana temporaria* were exposed to TBT concentrations of 3 µg/litre or less, but at 30 µg/litre significant mortality was observed.

1.9.3 Microcosm studies

Microcosm studies modelling marine ecosystems have been conducted with introduced organisms and in conditions where inflowing sea water allowed colonization by other organisms. Results showed decreases in both numbers of individuals and in species diversity at TBTO concentrations in water between 0.06 and 3 µg/litre.

Results from freshwater model ecosystems suggest that doses which kill freshwater snails also affect other species, including fish.

Summary

1.10 Effects on terrestrial organisms

The exposure of terrestrial organisms to TBT results primarily from its use as a wood preservative. TBTO is toxic to bees housed in hives made from TBT-treated wood. TBT was toxic to bats in a single study, but this result was not statistically significant owing to high control mortality. TBT compounds are toxic to insects exposed topically or via feeding on treated wood. The acute toxicity of TBT to wild mice is moderate; estimated dietary LC_{50} values, based on consumption of treated seeds used in repellency tests, range from 37 to 240 mg/kg per day.

1.11 Effects on organisms in the field

Field observations have related high concentrations of tributyltin to mortality and settlement failure of larval bivalves, reduced growth, shell thickening and other malformations in developing oysters, imposex in mud snails, and imposex (concurrent with population decline) in the dogwhelk. Complete failure of oyster fisheries was identified initially in France and afterwards in other countries and related to water concentrations of TBT. The effects were most marked in areas close to pleasure boat marinas. Controlling the use of TBT antifouling paints on small boats has resulted in recovery of oyster reproduction and growth. However, water concentrations of TBT are still high enough in some areas to affect marine gastropods.

Both shell growth and chambering in Pacific oysters and imposex in dogwhelks have been used as biological indicators of TBT contamination.

There have been few studies of the effects on organisms of TBT in sediment, but there are indications that the TBT is available to burrowing organisms and can cause mortality in the field.

Gross toxic effects and histopathological changes have been reported in farmed marine fish exposed to TBT by the use of antifouling paints on retaining nets.

The use of TBT as a molluscicide against the freshwater snails that carry schistosomiasis (bilharzia) has been proposed. Some field trials have been conducted which show that it is difficult to apply TBT without damaging non-target organisms.

1.12 Toxicity to laboratory mammals

1.12.1 Acute toxicity

Tributyltin is moderately to highly toxic to laboratory mammals, acute oral LD_{50} values ranging from 94 to 234 mg/kg body weight for the rat and from 44 to 230 mg/kg body weight for the mouse. The acute toxicity to the guinea-pig and the rabbit fall within the same range. The variation comes from the "anion" component of the tributyltin salt. These compounds exhibit greater lethal potential when administered parenterally, as opposed to orally, probably due to only partial absorption from the gut.

Other effects of acute exposure may include alterations in blood lipid levels, the endocrine system, liver, and spleen, and transient deficits in brain development. The toxicological significance of these effects, reported after high single doses of the compound, is questionable and the cause of death remains unknown.

The acute toxicity via the dermal route is low, the LD_{50} being >9000 mg/kg body weight for the rabbit. "Nose only" inhalation LD_{50} (4 h) for the rat is 77 mg/m^3 (65 mg/m^3 when only inhalable particles are considered). TBT vapour/air mixtures produce no observable toxic effects, even at saturation. However, TBT is very hazardous as an inhaled aerosol, producing lung irritation and oedema.

TBT is severely irritating to the skin and an extreme irritant to the eye. TBTO is not a skin sensitizer.

1.12.2 Short-term toxicity

TBT compounds have been studied most extensively in the rat (all the data in this section refer to the rat unless otherwise indicated).

At dietary doses of 320 mg/kg (approximately 25 mg/kg body weight), high mortality rates were observed when the exposure time exceeded 4 weeks. No deaths were noted at 100 mg/kg diet (10 mg/kg body weight) or after daily

Summary

administration of 12 mg/kg body weight by gavage. In rats dosed during early post-natal life, 3 mg/kg body weight resulted in increased deaths. The main symptoms at lethal doses were loss of appetite, weakness, and emaciation.

Borderline effects on rat growth were observed at 50 mg/kg diet (6 mg/kg body weight) and 6 mg/kg body weight (gavage studies). Mice are less sensitive, effects being observed at 150 to 200 mg/kg diet (22 to 29 mg/kg body weight).

Structural effects on endocrine organs, mainly the pituitary and thyroid, have been noted in both short- and long-term studies. Changes in circulating hormone concentrations and altered response to physiological stimuli (pituitary trophic hormones) were observed in short-term tests, but after long-term exposure most of these changes appeared to be absent. The mechanism of action is not known.

Exposure to TBTO aerosol at 2.8 mg/m^3 produced high mortality, respiratory distress, inflammatory reaction within the respiratory tract and histopathological changes of lymphatic organs. However, exposure to the highest attainable vapour concentration (0.16 mg/m^3) at room temperature produced no effects.

Toxic effects on the liver and bile ducts have been reported in three mammalian species. Hepatocellular necrosis and inflammatory changes in the bile duct were observed in rats fed TBTO at a dietary level of 320 mg/kg (approximately 25 mg/kg body weight) for 4 weeks and in mice fed 80 mg/kg diet (approximately 12 mg/kg body weight) for 90 days. Vacuolization of periportal hepatocytes was noted in dogs fed a dose of 10 mg/kg body weight for 8 to 9 weeks. These changes were occasionally accompanied by increased liver weight and increased serum activities of liver enzymes.

Decreases in haemoglobin concentration and erythrocyte volume in rats, resulting from dosing with 80 mg/kg diet (8 mg/kg body weight), indicate an effect on haemoglobin synthesis, leading to microcytic hypochromic anaemia. The decrease in splenic haemosiderin levels suggests alterations in iron status. Anaemia has also been observed in mice.

The formation of erythrocyte rosettes in mesenteric lymph nodes has been observed in certain short-term investigations but not in long-term studies. The biological significance of this finding (possibly transient) is unclear.

The characteristic toxic effect of TBTO is on the immune system; due to effects on the thymus, the cell-mediated function is impaired. The mechanism of action is unknown, but may involve the metabolic conversion to dibutyltin compounds. Non-specific resistance is also affected.

General effects on the immune system (e.g., on the weight and morphology of lymphoid tissues, peripheral lymphocyte counts, and total serum immunoglobulin concentrations) have been reported in several different studies with TBTO using rats and dogs, but not mice, at overtly toxic dose levels (effects in mice have been seen with tributyltin chloride at 150 mg/kg). Only the rat exhibits general effects on the immune system without other overt signs of toxicity and is clearly the most sensitive species. The NOEL in short-term rat studies was 5 mg/kg diet (0.6 mg/kg body weight). In studies with tributyltin chloride, analogous effects on the thymus were seen. These were readily reversible when dosing ceased. TBTO has been shown to compromise specific immune function in rat *in vivo* host resistance studies. Decreased clearance of *Listeria monocytogenes* was seen after exposure to a dietary level of 50 mg/kg (the NOEL being 5 mg/kg per day), and decreased resistance to *Trichinella spiralis* was seen at 50 and 5 mg/kg diet, but not at 0.5 mg/kg diet (2.5, 0.25, and 0.025 mg/kg per day body weight, respectively). Similar effects were seen in aged animals, but these were less pronounced.

With present knowledge, the effects on host resistance are probably of most relevance in assessing the potential hazard to man, but there is insufficient experience in these test systems to fully assess their significance. However, some data on the significance of the *T. spiralis* model are provided by findings in athymic nude rats after the standard challenge. In these studies, the complete absence of thymus-dependent immunity resulted in a 10- to 20-fold increase in muscle larvae counts; by contrast,

Summary

exposure to TBTO concentrations of 5 and 50 mg/kg diet resulted in a 2-fold and a 4-fold increase, respectively.

Although some data are now available from studies on the effects of tributyltin compounds on the developing immune system, there is no information on host resistance.

It would be prudent to base assessment of the potential hazard to humans on data from the most sensitive species. Effects on host resistance to *T. spiralis* have been seen at dietary levels as low as 5 mg/kg (equivalent to 0.25 mg/kg per day body weight), the NOEL being 0.5 mg/kg (equivalent to 0.025 mg/kg per day). However, the interpretation of the significance of these data for human risk assessment is controversial. In all other studies a concentration of 5 mg/kg per day in the diet (equivalent to 0.5 mg/kg body weight, based on the short-term studies) was the NOEL with respect to general, as well as specific, effects on the immune system.

1.12.3 Long-term toxicity

A long-term study in rats indicates a marginal effect of TBT on general toxicological parameters (of limited toxicological significance) at a level of 5 mg/kg diet (0.25 mg/kg body weight).

1.12.4 Genotoxicity

The genotoxicity of TBTO has been the subject of extensive investigations. Negative results were obtained in the vast majority of studies, and there is no convincing evidence that TBTO has any mutagenic potential.

1.12.5 Reproductive toxicity

The potential embryotoxicity of TBTO has been evaluated in three mammalian species (mouse, rat, and rabbit) after oral dosing of the mother. The main malformation noted in rat and mouse fetuses was cleft palate, but this occurred at dosages overtly toxic to the mothers. These results are not considered to be indicative of teratogenic effects of TBTO at doses below those producing maternal toxicity. The lowest NOEL, with regard to embryotoxicity and fetotoxicity for all three species, was 1.0 mg/kg body weight.

1.12.6 Carcinogenicity

One carcinogenicity study has been carried out on rats, in which neoplastic changes were observed in endocrine organs at 50 mg/kg diet. The pituitary tumours reported at 0.5 mg/kg diet were considered as having no biological significance since there was no dose-response relationship. These tumour types usually appear in high and variable background incidences, and their significance is, therefore, questionable. A carcinogenicity study on mice is in progress.

1.13 Effects on humans

Occupational exposure of workers to tributyltin has been found to result in irritation of the upper respiratory tract. TBT as an aerosol poses a hazard to humans. TBTO is a skin and eye irritant and severe dermatitis has been reported after direct contact with the skin. The potential problem is made worse by the lack of an immediate response to the skin.

2. IDENTITY, PHYSICAL AND CHEMICAL PROPERTIES, ANALYTICAL METHODS

2.1 Identity of tributyltin compounds

Tributyltins compounds are organic derivatives of tin (Sn^{IV}) characterized by the presence of covalent bonds between three carbon atoms and a tin atom. They conform to the following general formula $(n\text{-}C_4H_9)_3$ Sn-X, where X is an anion or a group linked covalently through a heteroatom.

The nature of X influences the physico-chemical properties, notably the relative solubility in water and non-polar solvents and the vapour pressure.

These compounds differ from inorganic tin both in behaviour and effects. An important member of the group is tributyltin oxide (TBTO; RTECS number, JN8750000). Commercial TBTO has a purity generally above 96%. Principle impurities are dibutyltin derivatives and, to a lesser extent, tetrabutyl or dibutylalkyl tin compounds.

Other industrially important tributyltin derivatives include tributyltin fluoride, tributyltin methacrylate (monomer or copolymer), tributyltin benzoate, tributyltin linoleate, tributyltin naphthenate, and tributyltin phosphate.

2.2 Physical and chemical properties

TBTO is flammable but does not form explosive mixtures with air. It is a mild oxidizing agent. It reacts quantitatively at room temperature with bromide or iodine with cleavage of the Sn-O bond (a reaction that may be used for quantitative analysis) (Bahr & Pawlenko, 1978).

In the presence of oxygen, light or heat, slow breakdown occurs with the formation of tetra-n-butyltin, di-n-butyltin oxide, and eventually tin (IV) oxide by dealkylation (Evans & Karpel, 1985). This degradation may be inhibited by the addition of 0.1-1.0% of stabilizers (such as lactic or citric acids).

It has been suggested (Maguire et al., 1984; Laughlin et al., 1986a) that TBTO in aqueous solution dissociates with the formation of a hydrated tributyltin cation, which can undergo reaction with anions present. Data are not available on the equilibrium constants for these reactions.

Laughlin et al. (1986a) showed that TBTO can react with normal constituents of the sea water in the following ways:

$Bu_3\text{-Sn-O-Sn-}Bu_3 + HO \rightarrow 2Bu_3\text{-Sn-OH}$

$Bu_3\text{-Sn-OH-}H^+ \rightarrow Bu_3SnOH_2^+$

$Bu_3\text{-Sn-OH} + CO_3^{2-} \rightarrow Bu_3SnCO_3^- + OH^-$

$Bu_3\text{-Sn-}OH_2^+ + Cl^- \rightarrow Bu_3\text{-Sn-Cl} + H_2O$

The predominant forms are $Bu_3SnOH_2^+$ and Bu_3SnCl at pH < 7, Bu_3SnCl, Bu_3SnOH, and $Bu_3SnCO_3^-$ at pH 8, and Bu_3SnOH and $Bu_3SnCO_3^-$ at pH > 10.

Under normal conditions in sea water, it is considered that the three species (hydroxide, chloride, and carbonate) remain in equilibrium.

The physical and chemical properties of some commercially available tributyltin compounds are listed in Table 1.

Varying data on the solubility of TBTO in water, which ranges from < 1.0 to > 100 mg/litre at different temperatures and pH values, may be related to the presence of different anionic species as described above.

In the same way as described in the reaction between TBTO and water, the TBT group can be transferred to other oxygen-, nitrogen-, and sulfur-containing groups. Thus, anaerobically in sediments, TBTO can be transformed to TBT sulfide. With amino acids, or their derivatives such as proteins, reaction can occur on the nitrogen and sulfur atoms, and, with wood, it has been suggested that the TBT group may react with hydroxylic groups (Blunden et al., 1984) or form tributyltin carbonate (Smith et al., 1977). Thus adsorption on to particulate matter could involve chemical reaction as well as physical adsorption or solution. TBTO adsorbs strongly to particulate matter, the reported adsorption coefficients ranging between 110 and 55 000.

Table 1. Identity and physical and chemical properties of tributyltin compounds

	Oxide (TBTO)	Benzoate (TBTB)	Chloride (TBTCl)	Fluoride (TBTF)	Linoleate (TBTL)	Methacrylate (TBTM)	Naphthenate (TBTN)
IUPAC name	distannoxane, hexabutyl	stannane, (benzyloxy)tributyl	stannane, tributyl-chloro	stannane, tributyl-fluoro	stannane, tributyl-(1-oxo-9,12-octadecadienyl)oxy-	stannane, tributyl-(2-methyl-1-oxo-2-propyl)oxy-	stannane, tributyl-mono (naphthenoyloxy) derivatives
CAS name	Bis(tributyltin) oxide	Tributyltin benzoate	Tributyltin chloride	Tributyltin fluoride	Tributyltin linoleate	Tributyltin methacrylate	Tributyltin naphthenate
CAS number	56-35-9	4342-36-3	1461-22-9	1983-10-4	24124-25-2	2155-70-6	85409-17-2
Molecular formula	$C_{24}H_{54}OSn_2$	$C_{19}H_{32}O_2Sn$	$C_{12}H_{27}ClSn$	$C_{12}H_{27}FSn$	$C_{30}H_{58}O_2Sn$	$C_{16}H_{32}O_2Sn$	
Relative molecular mass	596	411	325	309	568.7	374.7	≈ 500
Boiling point (°C)	173 (130 Pa)	≈ 135 (30 Pa)	140 (1300 Pa)	> 350 (extrapol)	≈ 140 (50 Pa)	> 300 (extrapol)	≈ 125 (50 Pa)
Melting point (°C)	< −45	20	−16	240	< 0	16	< 0
Relative density (20 °C)	1.17-1.18	≈ 1.2	≈ 1.2	1.25	1.05	1.14	≈ 1.1
Vapour pressure (Pa at 20 °C)	1×10^{-3}	2×10^{-4}			9×10^{-2}	3×10^{-2}	9×10^{-5}
Refractive index (20 °C)	1.4880-1.4895						

TBTO is soluble in lipids and very soluble in a number of organic solvents (ethanol, ether, halogenated hydrocarbons, etc.).

The octanol/water partition coefficient (log P_{ow}) lies between 3.19 and 3.84 for distilled water and is 3.54 for sea water.

As shown in Table 1, the vapour pressures of TBT compounds are low. The work of Maguire et al. (1983) confirmed this directly by showing no loss of TBTO from a 1 mg/litre solution after 62 days; 20% of the water was lost by evaporation.

2.3 Analytical methods

The control levels of contamination of different environmental compartments (water, sediment, biota) and the interpretation of laboratory experimental and field study results regarding levels, fate, biodegradation, and bioaccumulation of tributyltin compounds require sensitive analytical techniques to allow identification and quantification.

2.3.1 Measurement of organotin compounds

These methods, which are summarized in Table 2, have been applied initially to water and later to sediment and biota. They must be sufficiently sensitive and specific to allow monitoring of ng/litre levels, and they need to be able to distinguish between different forms of organic tin derivatives present in the environment, i.e. mono-, di-, tri-, or tetra-butyltins and different species of alkyl moieties (butyl, methyl). They have also to avoid all interference from other metals and other organometallic derivatives.

Generally there are four successive stages to analysis, although some are optional:

- extraction;
- formation of volatile derivatives;
- separation of these derivatives;
- detection, identification, and quantification.

Table 2. Sampling, preparation, and analysis of tributyltin compounds

Medium	Sampling method	Sample volume	Analytical method	Detection limit	Reference
Air	adsorption on Chromosorb, cation exchange resin, or Tenax	50-100 litres	derivatization with RMgX; GC/MS or GC/FPD		Zimmerli & Zimmermann (1980); Muller (1987a)
Water		250 ml	$NaBH_4$ conversion to hydride; separation by fractional distillation; AA	0.1-2 ng/litre	Hodge et al. (1979); Michel (1987); Donard et al. (1986); Braman & Tompkins (1979); Valkirs et al. (1986); Weber et al. (1986)
Water and sediments	extraction with dichloromethane	8 litres (water) or 1 g (sediment dry weight)	derivatization with C_5H_{11} MgBr; GC-FPD or GC-FAA	1 ng/litre (water) or 5 ng/mg (sediment dry weight)	Maguire & Huneault (1981); Maguire & Tkacz (1983, 1985); Maguire et al. (1986)
Water and biota	acidification, extraction with dichloromethane	1 litre	derivatization with CH_3 MgI; GC-MS or AA	10 ng/litre	Meinema et al. (1978); Bjorklund (1987a)
Water, biota, or sediments		200 ml or 16 litres	$NaBH_4$ conversion to hydride; extraction with dichloromethane	5 ng/litre or 0.2 ng/litre	Matthias et al. (1986a,b); Humphrey & Hope (1987)
Water and sediment	adsorption on silica bonded C18	60 litres (water) or 10 g (sediment)	extraction with dichloromethane/tropolone; derivatization with C_5H_7 MgBr; GC-MS	0.07 ng/litre (water) 0.2 mg/kg (sediment)	Humphrey & Hope (1987)
	macroreticular resin adsorption	1 litre	extraction with n-pentane (water) diethylether (sediment); derivatization with CH_3MgCl; GC-MS	< 1 ng/litre (water) 0.5 mg/kg (sediment)	Muller (1984)

.3.1.1 Extraction of tributyltin derivatives

Extraction may be independent of or coincident with the formation of volatile derivatives. It is necessary for sediments and biological tissues and can also be applied in the analysis of water samples.

Following acidification, various organic solvents have been used. The following are most often cited: methylisobutylketone, hexane, ethyl acetate, toluene, methanol, chloroform, dichloromethane, and mixtures of tropolone (2-hydroxy-2,4,6-cycloheptatrienone) with chloroform, benzene, or dichloromethane.

In the case of water, liquid-liquid extraction may be replaced by adsorption onto silica gel bonded with C18 aliphatic chains (Matthias et al., 1986a,b; Humphrey & Hope, 1987).

.3.1.2 Formation of volatile derivatives

Mono-, di-, and tri-butyltins are not sufficiently volatile to assure their separation on gas-phase chromatography; it is, therefore, necessary to prepare more volatile derivatives to allow better separation. Two procedures have been advocated:

- formation of alkyl derivatives (methyl or pentyl) by the use of Grignard's reagent (reactive organomagnesium);
- formation of hydrides with the general structure R_nSnH_{4-n} by reaction with sodium borohydride ($NaBH_4$) (Hodge et al., 1979).

These volatile derivatives can then be extracted using organic solvents, such as dichloromethane, or purged by a stream of hydrogen.

.3.1.3 Separation of organotin derivatives

Less sensitive methods for direct separation of mono-, di-, and tri-butyltins include high performance liquid chromatography (Jewett & Brinckman, 1981) and thin-layer chromatography. The latter method is only qualitative and little used because of its low sensitivity.

2.3.1.4 *Detection and measurement of different forms of organotin*

Volatile derivatives prepared in the laboratory may be separated by two procedures:

- separation as a function of boiling point with collection in a cold trap ("purge and trap" procedure);
- separation by gas chromatography.

After separation by GLC or by the "purge and trap" procedure, it is possible to detect and quantify, at the ng/litre level, different forms of organotin using the following methods:

- a flame photometric detector selective for tin (FPD) is considered satisfactory;
- a flame atomic absorption (AA) spectrometer or flameless atomic absorption (FAA) spectrometer using a graphite furnace (tin is detected at 286.3 nm or 244.6 nm);
- a mass spectrometer (MS); this is useful for precise identification of the substance but has limited sensitivity.

There are several methods available for measuring TBT down to detection limits of 0.2 to 5 ng/litre in water and 5 to 30 µg/kg (in tissues of biota and in sediments). Some of them can be adapted for routine monitoring purposes. It is necessary, however, to have sophisticated equipment and the difficulty of the methods requires experienced laboratories.

His & Robert (1980, 1985) developed a biological assay based on toxic effects on larvae of the Pacific oyster, *Crassostrea gigas*, sensitive only above 20 ng/litre and nonspecific between organotin and other toxic compounds. Colorimetric methods (Sherman & Carlson, 1980) have been based on forming coloured derivatives with phenylfluorone (nonspecific and with a sensitivity around 0.1 to 4 µg tin).

2.3.2 *Interlaboratory calibrations*

Interlaboratory comparison of assay methods have been performed to compare the various proposed methods and to validate their usefulness as standards.

Young et al. (1986) reported the conclusions of a workshop held in the USA to examine the problems posed by the analysis of organotins in water. Nine methods, based on the principles outlined above, were considered as satisfactory, since the range of results fell within + 15% of the mean when the TBT concentration was in the order of ng/litre.

Stephenson et al. (1987) reported the results of interlaboratory calibrations conducted in 1986-1987 and carried out on TBT derivatives in mussel tissues and in sediments. The measurements were made in seven laboratories, each using its own technique and using different extraction conditions, derivative formation, and detection. A first examination of results showed that they did not vary by more than a factor of 3. The results were considered satisfactory.

Blair et al. (1986) took part in an interlaboratory calibration exercise organised by the National Bureau of Standards (NBS) in 1984 in the USA and carried out determinations of TBT in water (at a concentration of 1 μg/litre).

Under the auspices of the OECD, it was decided recently to organize a new worldwide intercalibration to be carried out on:

- water samples containing 10 ng/litre each of mono-, di-, and tri-butyltin;
- samples of dried sediment containing the above compounds at a concentration of 100 μg/kg;
- samples of mussel tissue, frozen or freeze-dried, containing the above compounds at 100 μg/kg.

It seems premature to impose a single analytical method and preferable to allow a certain freedom of choice between methods to allow sufficient sensitivity to be attained. However, control of the competence of laboratories that carry out such difficult and complex analysis is required through new calibration procedures.

3. SOURCES OF ENVIRONMENTAL EXPOSURE

3.1 Uses

Dutch scientists first recognized the biocidal properties of triorganotin compounds in the 1950s; major production and use of these substances dates from this period. It was found that the different triorganotin compounds have different toxicities to different organisms. Tributyltin compounds were found to be the most toxic of the triorganotins to gram-positive bacteria and to fungi. They were also found to have biocidal properties to a wide spectrum of aquatic organisms.

In the early 1960s, both tributyltin oxide (TBTO) and TBT fluoride were tested, mainly in Africa, as molluscicides against several freshwater snail species that are vectors of the disease schistosomiasis, the snails being the intermediate hosts of the trematode parasite. This use led to the introduction of TBT, during the mid 1960s, as an antifouling paint on boats. At the same time TBT compounds were being registered as wood preservatives (the first registration was in 1958).

Tributyltin compounds have been registered as molluscicides, as antifoulants on boats, ships, quays, buoys, crabpots, fish nets, and cages, as wood preservatives, as slimicides on masonry, as disinfectants, and as biocides for cooling systems, power station cooling towers, pulp and paper mills, breweries, leather processing, and textile mills.

When introduced as antifouling paints, TBT paints were of the "free association" type, where the TBT is physically incorporated into the paint matrix. In this form it has a high early release and very short life. Co-polymer paints were introduced later; in these the TBT moiety is chemically bonded to a polymer backbone, e.g., those formed from TBT acrylate or methacrylate and the corresponding acid. The biocide is released by chemical hydrolysis of the organotin ester linkage. Dissolution is slow from ships' hulls and a low level of released TBT can be achieved over a prolonged period. TBT compounds have also been impregnated into neoprene rubber to produce elastomeric antifoulant coatings and slow-release molluscicides. In this form, much of the TBT remains in the matrix of the rubber, though the effectiveness lasts for several years.

TBT compounds have not been suggested for use in agriculture because of their high phytotoxicity.

3.2 Production

The world consumption of tin in 1976 was estimated to be 200 x 10^3 tonnes, of which 28 x 10^3 tonnes was organotin. Approximately 40% of the total was consumed in the USA (Zuckerman et al., 1978). The United Kingdom Department of the Environment (1986) reported that the worldwide use of organotin in 1980 was 30 x 10^3 tonnes. This total was made up as follows:

- PVC stabilizers (dibutyl), approximately 20 x 10^3 tonnes;
- wood preservatives (tributyl), 3-4 x 10^3 tonnes;
- antifouling paints (tributyl), 2-3 x 10^3 tonnes;
- other uses of both di- and tri-butyltin, < 2 x 10^3 tonnes.

The annual world production of TBT compounds is estimated to be 4000 to 5000 tonnes (Organotin Environmental Programme Association (ORTEPA); personal communication to IPCS, 1989).

The total annual use (production and imports) of organotin compounds in Canada was reported by Thompson et al. (1985) to be in excess of 1 x 10^3 tonnes. The total annual production of TBTO in the Federal Republic of Germany is reported to be 2 x 10^3 tonnes, of which 70% is exported. National usage is as follows: 70% antifouling paints; 20% timber protection; 10% textile and leather protection; small amounts are also used as a preservative in dispersion paints and as a disinfecting agent. Annual tin emissions are reported to be less than 300 kg (TWG, 1988a). Annual TBT use in the Netherlands in 1985 was reported to be 1.5 x 10^4 kg for wood preservation and 10 x 10^4 kg for antifouling paints (TWG, 1988c). Organotin antifoulant use in Norway was 13.7 x 10^4 kg in 1986 for the treatment of nets and sea pens at approximately 600 fish farms (Linden, 1987). In Japan, usage was estimated at 1300 tonnes in 1987, of which two-thirds was used for antifouling paints on vessels and one-third for antifouling of nets in fish culture.

A survey of total and retail sales of TBT-containing paints and antifouling preparations for nets was carried out in Finland in 1987. Of a total of 42 000 litres, 37 000 litres were sold retail. The concentration of TBT in the antifouling paints was 4-18%. The previous use of TBT as a slimicide or fungicide (estimated at 2.1 tonnes per year during the period 1968-1970) has been discontinued. The estimated sale of wood preservatives containing TBT was 130 tonnes in 1987; these contained between 0.9 and 1.8% of TBT. Champ & Pugh (1987) reported that about 300 TBT antifouling paints were registered in the USA in 1987, but only about 17 paints are now registered for use (US EPA; personal communication to IPCS, 1989). MAFF/HSE (1988) listed 345 different wood preservative formulations, 24 surface biocides and 215 antifouling paints containing TBT with registration approval for use in the United Kingdom under the Control of Pesticides Regulations. In 1989, the number of antifouling paints containing TBT registered for use in the United Kingdom had fallen to 148, with the number of wood preservatives and surface biocides remaining about the same (337 and 26 registered products, respectively) (MAFF/HSE, 1989).

3.3 Regulations

In 1974, the USA set an occupational limit for organotin compounds in air of 0.1 mg tin/m^3 (time-weighted average). In 1979, the American Conference of Governmental Industrial Hygienists (ACGIH) recommended that the occupational exposure standard for organotin compounds in air should be set at a threshold limit value (time-weighted average) of 0.1 mg tin/m^3 and a short-term TLV at 0.2 mg tin/m^3. The Federal Republic of Germany was recommended, in 1979, to adopt an occupational exposure standard for organotin compounds in air of 0.1 mg tin/m^3, specified as a maximum worksite concentration (MAK). The United Kingdom has also set a recommended occupational exposure limit of 0.1 mg tin/m^3.

A tentative acceptable daily intake (ADI) of 1.6 µg/kg per day has been adopted in Japan.

In December 1979, the Japanese Government banned the use of tributyltin compounds in certain products for household use, e.g., paint, adhesive, wax, shoe polish, and textile products.

Following the effects on the oyster industry in France in the late 1970s, and the subsequent correlation of the effects with TBT usage, the French government banned the use of TBT antifouling paints for an initial trial period of three months, which was later extended. In 1982, paints containing more than 3% TBT by weight were banned on boats of < 25 m in length, although boats with aluminium hulls were excluded. Initially the regulation only covered the Atlantic coast (January 1982) but was later extended (September 1982) to the whole French coastline. All use of organotin compounds in antifouling paints, at any concentration, is now banned in France.

The exception in the regulations for TBT-based antifouling paints that many countries have made for boats with aluminium hulls is based on the fact that the copper-based alternative paints react chemically with the aluminium.

In January 1986, the United Kingdom enforced regulations that prohibited the retail sale and supply of antifouling paints with a total tin concentration greater than 7.5% by weight in co-polymer paints (reduced to 5.5% in January 1987) or 2.5% in other paints. These regulations were meant to control the use on small pleasure craft, ban the sale of "free association" paints containing high levels of organotin and set an upper limit on organotin compounds in co-polymer paints. An ambient water quality target of 20 ng/litre was set. The United Kingdom Department of the Environment took steps to determine the effectiveness of the legislation by setting up a monitoring programme. Based on the results of this monitoring, a total ban on the use of TBT paints on small boats (< 25 m) and fish farming equipment was implemented in July 1987 (Abel et al., 1987). An environmental quality standard (EQS) of 20 ng/litre for fresh water (covering both potable water and protection of sensitive aquatic biota) and 2 ng/litre for sea water has been set (United Kingdom Department of the Environment, 1989).

The paint industry of the Federal Republic of Germany (FRG) issued a renunciation in 1986 on the use of monomeric organotin compounds in antifouling paints and a restriction to 3.8% TBT in co-polymeric paints. The FRG has not, as yet, issued any national ban on TBT marine antifouling paints and is awaiting the outcome of discussions on an EEC directive (TWG, 1988b). Champ & Pugh (1987) reported that both Switzerland and the FRG have banned all uses of TBT in antifouling paints in the freshwater environment.

In 1987, the US EPA reviewed TBT usage, weighing risks to the environment against benefits to users. In the meantime, some individual States have passed their own regulations. Both Virginia and Washington State have banned the use of TBT antifouling paints on boats of < 25 m in length, excepting those with aluminium hulls. Only paints that conform to a leaching rate of 5 μg/cm^2 per day (steady state) can be used on boats longer than 25 m. Both states continued to permit the use of TBT paints, with acceptable leach rates, in 16 oz (0.45 kg) aerosol cans for use on outboard motors and lower units. Maryland instituted similar restrictions but set a lower permissible leaching rate of 1 μg/cm^2 per day (steady state). Since 1985, North Carolina, Oregon, and Michigan have instituted restrictions on TBT use. California, Alaska, New York, and New Jersey had TBT Bills pending in their respective legislatures (Champ & Pugh, 1987). In April 1988, both the US House of Representatives and the Senate passed bills to restrict the use of TBT in antifouling paints. The legislation was signed by the President on 16th June 1988 and came into effect on 16th December 1988. This Act established an interim release rate restriction of 4.0 μg/cm^2 per day (steady state) and a provision prohibiting application of TBT antifouling paints to non-aluminium vessels under 25 m length. Application to larger vessels was restricted to certified applicators only. The outboard motor or lower drive unit of a vessel less than 25 m in length was exempted. A limit on sales, delivery, purchase, and receipt of TBT paints was set in December 1988 and a limit on use in June 1989 for existing stocks of paint.

A voluntary ban on the use of TBT compounds for nets in fish culture was imposed in 1987 by the National

Federation of Fisheries Cooperative Association of Japan. In 1988, the Japanese Ministry of Health and Welfare and the Japanese Ministry of International Trade and Industry "designated" eight TBT compounds (and a further five TBT compounds in 1989) on the basis of persistence, accumulation, and toxicity. "Designated" indicates that no final decision on regulation has yet been taken but that the compounds have a recognized hazard. Following this action, the Japan Paint Manufacturers Association voluntarily reduced the upper limit for TBT in paints to < 10% wet weight for monomers and < 15% wet weight for polymers. There is current action to monitor release rates from paint products as the next step in limiting human exposure.

Maguire (1987) reported that tributyltin for the preservation of fish-farm nets is banned in Canada. In 1987, the Canadian Department of Agriculture served notice that antifouling uses of TBT compounds must conform to the following: a maximum short-term (first 14 days) cumulative release-rate from paint formulations of 168 $\mu g/cm^2$; a long-term average daily release of 4 $\mu g/cm^2$; and a minimum hull length of 19.5 m for the use of TBT antifouling paints on non-aluminium vessels.

In Australia, control measures on the use of TBT-based paints were introduced in the States of New South Wales and Victoria. TBT is prohibited for use on boats with a hull length of less than 25 m, while a leaching rate of 5.0 $\mu g/cm^2$ per day was set for hulls of 25 m or more. Aluminium vessels are not exempt from the ban.

The Republic of Ireland instituted a by-law banning the use of organotin compounds on boats and other aquatic structures in April 1987 (Minchin et al., 1987).

Norway has also prohibited use of TBT in antifouling paints except for boats longer than 25 m and those with aluminium hulls; the regulation became effective from January 1989. There is also prohibition on the sale, manufacture, and import of paints containing TBT without a specific permit from the State Pollution Control authority. An agreement to prohibit use on nets of fish farms has been concluded. Under the Helsinki Convention, the Baltic States have formed an agreement on the banning of TBT paints on small boats and have set up a joint monitoring programme.

The Commission of the European Communities has made a proposal to the Council of Ministers concerning restrictions on the use of antifouling paints that mirrors national restrictions in member states (except that there would be no derogation for boats with aluminium hulls). This proposal is currently being considered by the European Parliament and Council.

4. ENVIRONMENTAL TRANSPORT AND TRANSFORMATION

Summary

Due to its physico-chemical properties, TBT introduced into natural waters will partly adsorb onto particles. The quantitative data show large variation due to differences in experimental conditions such as salinity and concentration and organic content of particulate matter. Once it is adsorbed, decrease in TBT concentration takes place mainly by degradation. It is known that TBT degradation rates in sediment are slower than in the water column, particularly in anaerobic conditions.

Although abiotic degradation occurs, the process remains less important than biological action.

Biodegradation of TBTO in soil and water depends on the environmental conditions and the toxic effect of the available concentrations to the organisms involved. Hydroxylated intermediates are formed during stepwise debutylation. Aerobic and anaerobic organisms both cause biodegradation, but the relative efficiency is not known conclusively. Illumination of the cultures lowers the half-life, indicating the involvement of photosynthetic organisms.

The lipophilic properties of TBTO contribute to bioaccumulation in aquatic organisms, especially molluscs. Laboratory and field studies corroborate this, although it is unclear how adsorption processes complicate the results. Bioaccumulation in all organisms studied is due, at least in part, to bioconcentration from the water phase. Elimination takes place when organisms are no longer exposed to tributyltin compounds.

Whether it is directly discharged into the environment or diffuses progressively (at 1 to 10 $\mu g/cm^2$ per day) from coatings of the hulls of boats or nets, TBTO enters the aquatic environment and is subject to transformation resulting from physico-chemical and biochemical processes. Speciation is outlined in chapter 2.

4.1 Adsorption onto and desorption from particles

The effects of TBTO vary in relation to the state in which the substance is present in the aquatic environment, in particular whether it is available to organisms in estuaries or sea shores. It is important to have information on its distribution in natural waters likely to have large amounts of suspended matter of various types. Several workers (Valkirs et al., 1986; Maguire et al., 1986; Randall et al., 1986; Harris & Cleary, 1987; Stang & Seligman, 1987; Hinga et al., 1987) have conducted studies on adsorption and desorption of TBTO in laboratory experiments, observations in the field, studies conducted in microcosms, and mathematical modelling.

Mathematical models have been developed to estimate the distribution of TBT in enclosed or semi-enclosed harbours (Walton et al., 1986) and estuaries (Harris & Cleary, 1987). Good agreement has been found between measured and estimated concentrations of tin in San Diego harbour, USA (Walton et al., 1986). The authors considered the results useful in predicting levels in ecologically sensitive areas of the bay. The Harris & Cleary (1987) model was based on the estuary of the River Tamar in south-west England. This model, still under development, aimed to reduce inputs in order to allow the model to be used by non-experts and to be applicable to all estuaries. Output for the River Tamar suggested that sediment-bound tin would be distributed up the estuary by tidal influence leading to increased bound tin further from the open sea. This effect would be most marked in the summer. Relative to soluble TBT, this bound fraction does not currently amount to a significant source of tin for organisms. The authors point out, however, that this source may become increasingly important as use of TBT declines and sediment-bound TBT represents the only available source of the compound.

The chemical properties of TBT, particularly its lipophilic character and poor water solubility, are such that, when TBTO is introduced into water, repartition will occur, TBTO leaving the aqueous phase and preferentially adsorbing onto particles (Hinga et al., 1987). Adsorption and desorption are dependant on the nature of the sediment. Little data is available to indicate whether adsorbed TBT is bioavailable.

If this phenomenon is generally evident, its intensity varies considerably as a function of the method of study used and the measurements made. Contradictory results are apparent in the literature.

Reports from different authors using various conditions have estimated that between 10% and 95% of TBTO introduced into water is adsorbed onto particles. There is, however, general agreement that the compound remains strongly adsorbed. It has been stated that sediments remain contaminated for at least 10 months; progressive disappearance of TBTO is not due to desorption but to degradation.

In an *in situ* study of Pearl Harbour sediment, the rate of adsorption of tributyltin derivatives was found to be 0.57 ng TBT/cm^2 per day (Stang & Seligman, 1987). There was, apparently, no desorption of TBTO itself but dibutyltin derivatives formed by degradation desorbed with rates varying between 0.16 and 0.55 ng DBT/cm^2 per day.

Variability in results, more evident in field studies than laboratory studies, is explained by the fact that adsorption depends on many different factors, amongst which are the following:

- salinity;
- nature and size of particles in suspension;
- amount of suspended particles;
- temperature;
- presence of dissolved organic matter.

Uncertainties are also evident in relation to the bioavailability of TBT adsorbed onto sediment. Salazar et al. (1987) considered that the effects of adsorbed TBTO were partially masked, i.e. that the compound was unavailable to organisms. This conclusion could not be verified regarding effects on filtering or burrowing organisms living in the sediment.

It is generally agreed that part of the TBTO accumulates in the surface monolayer of natural waters. This TBTO will also be adsorbed onto organic matter and lipid material present on the surface.

4.2 Abiotic degradation

A number of studies have shown that a degradation pathway for tributyltin compounds exists in the environment, which involves progressive debutylation. It is theoretically completed with the liberation into water of the tin oxide (SnO_2).

$$R_3SnX \rightarrow R_2SnX_2 \rightarrow RSnX_3 \rightarrow SnX_4$$

A number of studies have looked for evidence of such degradation, the cause and mechanisms, and an understanding of the kinetics in different environmental conditions (Chapman & Price, 1972; Brinckman, 1981; Blunden et al., 1984; Maguire & Tkacz, 1985; and Seligman et al., 1986a).

Degradation of TBTO proceeds via splitting of the carbon-tin bond, which can result from various mechanisms occurring simultaneously in the environment. These include physico-chemical mechanisms (hydrolysis and photodegradation) and biological mechanisms (degradation by microorganisms and metabolism by higher organisms). While degradation definitely occurs as a result of these different mechanisms in laboratory studies, it is necessary to assess the relative importance of these different pathways to degradation of TBTO in the field.

4.2.1 Hydrolytic cleavage of the tin-carbon bond

Since hydrolysis of the tin-carbon bond of organotin derivatives occurs only under conditions of extreme pH, it is barely evident under normal environmental conditions.

Studies were carried out in darkness and a sterile medium to assess the importance of hydrolysis in the degradation of TBTO. According to the work of Maguire et al. (1983) and of Maguire & Tkacz (1985), TBTO remains stable for 11 months in distilled or natural water at 20 °C, in the dark, and in a sterile medium. Under various conditions of pH, between 2.9 and 10.3, these authors found no change in TBTO over 63 days. According to Seligman et al. (1986a), slight degradation of TBTO was apparent after 94 days in darkness in the presence of formalin as a sterilizing agent.

It is, therefore, considered that degradation occurs either not at all or only very slowly in normal environmental conditions of pH and temperature, when monitored in the dark and in a sterile medium.

4.2.2 Photodegradation

Photodegradation of TBTO by ultraviolet light is theoretically possible. UV light with a wavelength longer than 290 nm possesses an energy of 300 kJ/mol, whereas the energy required to break the carbon-tin bond is 190-220 kJ/mol. At the same time, TBTO absorbs in the UV region at 300 nm and, less strongly, at 350 nm.

Field and laboratory measurements have shown that this route of degradation can occur and that it forms derivatives of dibutyltin. These seem to be resistant to photolysis, since very little monobutyltin is formed (Blunden & Chapman, 1986). While the phenomenon clearly exists, its importance varies considerably with different environmental conditions. Conditions of illumination, conditions of transmission of light, and the presence of photosensitizing substances (acetone, humic acids, etc.) can considerably accelerate the process.

Results of laboratory studies vary considerably depending on whether experiments are conducted under natural sunlight or UV light of known wavelength. According to Slesinger & Dresser (1978), the half-life of TBTO in sea water subjected to ultraviolet light is 18.5 days. In the presence of a photosensitizing substance, such as acetone, the half-life is 3.5 days. Seligman et al. (1986a) suggested that, under natural conditions, photodegradation is less important than biological action, the development of phytoplankton leading to a partial degradation of TBTO. Their measurements were made at relatively high concentrations of TBTO (744 µg/litre). Under these conditions, light caused no degradation over 144 days. According to Lee et al. (1987), degradation of low concentrations of TBTO (less than 5 ng/litre) in estuary water is increased when the assay is conducted in light. The half-life is between 6 and 12 days, and the presence of significant concentrations of phytoplankton increases the speed of degradation. According to Maguire et al. (1983), photolysis under natural light conditions in distilled or natural water is limited, leading to a TBTO half-life in excess of 89 days. Under experimental conditions of strong UV light, degradation is apparent. At 300 nm the half-life of TBTO is 1.1 days, whereas at 350 nm it is more than 18 days.

In these assays, it is possible to demonstrate the role of humic acids, particularly fulvic acid, which considerably augment the speed of photolysis. Under such conditions, the half-life of TBTO falls to 0.6 days at 300 nm and to 6 days at 350 nm. Under natural conditions in the port of Toronto, Canada, the degradation after 89 days, remained less than 50%.

4.3 Biodegradation

A number of studies have been conducted to verify that microorganisms, notably bacteria, are capable of degrading TBTO. In practice, physico-chemical mechanisms and biological mechanisms of degradation overlap. Evidence for biodegradation constitutes an important element in the assessment of risk. Published studies of observations made in the field or the laboratory have shown definite evidence of biological degradation of TBTO. Biodegradation kinetics depend on environmental conditions such as temperature, oxygenation, pH, the level of mineral elements, the presence of easily biodegradable organic substances, and the nature of the microflora and the possibility of their adaptation. Biodegradation also depends on the concentration of TBTO being lower than the lethal or inhibitory threshold for the bacteria.

Biodegradation is based on the formation of intermediate hydroxylated derivatives, progressive oxidative debutylization following the splitting of the carbon-tin bond. Dibutyl derivatives are formed, which appear to be degraded more rapidly than tributyl derivatives to give monobutyl derivatives; these, conversely, are mineralized slowly. The end product may be butene. The quantities of carbon dioxide formed remain small. The biodegradation of organotin compounds does not seem to involve the formation of methyl derivatives of tin. Such methyl derivatives have been measured in some studies (Braman & Tompkins, 1979; Guard et al., 1981; Hallas et al., 1982; Brinckman et al., 1983), but have been shown to be the result of the transmethylation of inorganic tin by certain marine bacteria (*Pseudomonas*) frequently found in estuaries.

Sheldon (1975) proposed the following scheme for degradation involving microorganisms:

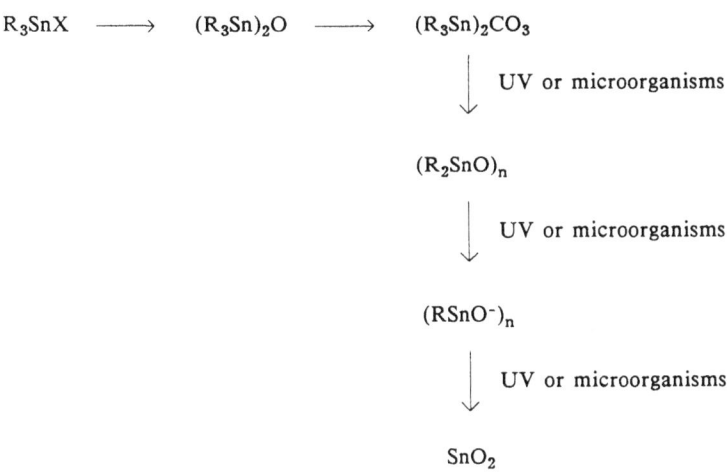

A mechanism of biodegradation also exists under anaerobic conditions (Maguire & Tkacz, 1985). Anaerobic degradation is considered to be very slow by some workers and more rapid than aerobic degradation by others.

Slesinger & Dresser (1978) conducted studies in a Warburg respirometer under aerobic conditions and showed that microflora derived from activated sludge and soil were capable of partially degrading TBTO. The half-life was 70 days, whereas under anaerobic conditions it was 200 days.

Henshaw et al. (1978) showed that pure cultures of certain wood-degrading fungi, such as *Coniophora puteana* and *Coriolus polystictus*, were capable of slowly biodegrading TBTO and transforming it to dibutyl and monobutyl derivatives.

Barug & Vonk (1980) studied the degradation of TBTO in soil but could show no clear evidence for the action of microorganisms. Under their experimental conditions, in sterile or non-sterile medium, the half-life of TBTO varied between 15 and 20 weeks depending on the soil type. Barug (1981) was not able to isolate, from sediment or soils, microorganisms capable of utilizing TBTO as a sole carbon source. By contrast, in the presence of easily biodegradable organic matter, biodegradation of TBTO is apparent with the production of monobutyl derivatives and smaller quantities of dibutyl derivatives. A number of species were found to be capable of conducting such degradation aerobically (bacteria: *Pseudomonas aeruginosa* and *Alcaligenes faecalis*; wood-degrading fungi: *Coniophora puteana, Trametes versicolor*, and *Chaetomium globosum*). Under these conditions, they observed 70% degradation in 3 weeks. However, the breakdown of TBTO is not clearly proved since the authors showed that TBTO accumulates in the cell walls of bacteria and fungi.

Using water containing natural microflora, Olson & Brinckman (1986) found no degradation of TBTO at a concentration of 100 µg/litre and a temperature of 5 °C but did record degradation at 28 °C. Their work also confirmed an acceleration of degradation when the incubations were conducted under light; the authors explained this acceleration by invoking the role played by photosynthetic microorganisms.

Seligman et al. (1986a) also showed evidence for biodegradation; in medium polluted by TBTO at 0.5 µg/litre, the TBTO half-life was 7 days in the dark and 6 days in the light. In water containing 0.03 µg TBTO/litre, the half-life was 19 days in the dark and 9 days in the light. In all cases, dibutyl derivatives were formed and, to a lesser extent, monobutyl derivatives. In studies with ^{14}C-labelled TBTO, the measurement of $^{14}CO_2$ production suggested a half-life of between 50 and 75 days.

Stein & Kuster (1982) demonstrated that TBTO is eliminated from waste water passing through sewage treatment plants by adsorption onto sludge and biodegradation by sludge organisms, provided that concentrations of TBTO remain less than 5 mg/litre (see also section 5.3).

According to Maguire et al. (1984), the green alga *Ankistrodesmus falcatus* was capable of bioaccumulating TBTO (with bioconcentration factors of 3×10^4) when it was cultured in the presence of 20 µg TBTO/litre. When the cultures were transferred to a non-contaminated medium, 50% of the TBTO was transformed to dibutyl derivatives or monobutyl derivatives and even to inorganic tin over the course of 4 weeks. The assays were conducted on axenic cultures of algae. It may be supposed that a biological effect was superimposed on physico-chemical degradation mechanisms.

Maguire & Tkacz (1985) have shown that in sediments there are oligochaetes that are also capable of metabolizing TBTO after it has been accumulated. However, the simultaneous presence of bacteria in the test systems means that a clear conclusion could not be reached.

According to Maguire et al. (1986), degradation can be characterized as follows:

- Loss of TBTO by volatilization is very limited with a half-life of more than 11 months.
- Hydrolysis of TBTO is equally slow with a half-life of 11 months.
- Photodegradation of TBTO plays a more important role but the half-life of photodegradation is longer than 3 months. This route theoretically takes place but, under natural conditions of illumination and the poor penetration of UV light into turbid or coloured water, it is inefficient.
- Aerobic biodegradation plays a role in water and sediment. The half-life varies considerably according to conditions but is in the region of 4 to 5 months.
- Anaerobic degradation plays a role in water and sediment. The half-life varies considerably but is around 1.5 months.

The kinetics of degradation of dibutyl and monobutyl tins are less well known. However, the degradation processes of TBTO always results in the formation of metabolites less toxic than the parent compound.

Hinga et al. (1987) indicated a TBTO half-life of between 5 and 19 days at 22-24 °C in model ecosystems. Thain et al. (1987) suggested half-lives of 6 days in fresh water and 60-90 days at 5 °C in sea water. In water and sediment of the port of Toronto, the half-life varied between 4 and 5 months (Maguire & Tkacz, 1985). In estuarine waters of San Diego Bay, USA, the half-life varied between 7 and 11 days at 12 °C, while in waters of the Skidaway Estuary, it varied between 5 and 9 days at 28 °C (Seligman et al., 1986a). Stang & Seligman (1986) using contaminated sediment from San Diego Bay found that TBT was degraded to monobutyltin. The degradation kinetic was lower than in water, the half-life being approximately 162 days. In studies carried out by J.E. Thain & M.J.

Waldock (Personal communication to IPCS, 1989), naturally contaminated sediments were maintained in the laboratory, under flow-through conditions, at 12 °C. Degradation of sediment-bound TBT was found to be a slow process. In aerobic layers the half-life of TBT was between 4 and 5 months, but in deeper anaerobic layers a half-life value was not obtained within 500 days.

4.4 Bioaccumulation and elimination

The lipophilic properties of TBTO and its moderately high octanol-water partition coefficient (log P_{ow} > 3) contribute to bioaccumulation in living organisms.

Evidence for such mechanisms and an evaluation of their importance is highly relevant for hazard assessment, both for the environment and for humans, since some of the organisms exposed to TBTO are human food items, e.g., bivalve molluscs, crustaceans, and fish. Alzieu et al. (1980) showed that in contaminated areas tin levels in the flesh of oysters were 100 times higher than concentrations in the water.

Laboratory experiments have been conducted under different conditions to demonstrate such bioaccumulation, and have shown that bioconcentration factors vary considerably between species.

In estuarine bacteria, Blair et al. (1982) found bioconcentration factors varying between 100 and 30 000 in species resistant to concentrations of 20 mg TBTO/litre. As was indicated earlier, such bioconcentration might result either from adsorption to the surface of the organisms or from true bioaccumulation into the cells. In phytoplankton, Maguire et al. (1984) reported a bioconcentration factor of 30 000 in the green alga *Ankistrodesmus falcatus* exposed for 1 week to concentrations of 20 µg TBTO/litre. In the diatom *Isochrysis galbano*, Laughlin et al. (1986b) reported a bioconcentration factor of 5500.

Studies on the possibility of bioaccumulation and biomagnification in molluscs, particularly bivalve molluscs, are prominent in the literature because of human consumption of oysters and mussels. Alzieu et al. (1982) showed that TBTO accumulated in oysters, maintained in tanks with panels of antifouling paint based on TBTO, to levels of

25 mg/kg (dry weight) of tissue and that this resulted in problems of cavitation of the shell. Waldock et al. (1983), in studies of the Pacific oyster *Crassostrea gigas* exposed for 22 days to TBTO concentrations of 0.15 µg/litre and 1.25 µg/litre, reported bioconcentration factors of 6000 and 2000, respectively. In European oysters *(Ostrea edulis)* exposed to the same concentrations, they found concentration factors of 1500 and 1000, respectively. In both cases, after transfer of the oysters to clean water there was a 50% fall in TBTO levels due to loss or degradation. Laughlin et al. (1986b) reported bioconcentration factors between 1000 and 7000 for mussels *(Mytilus edulis)* exposed for between 3 and 7 weeks to TBTO concentrations of 23, 45, 63, 141, and 670 ng/litre. For the higher concentrations, a plateau in uptake was reached within 2 weeks, but for lower concentrations, no plateau was reached within the 7-week experiment. The authors considered that the mussel would be a good indicator organism for monitoring marine pollution. Cheng & Jensen (1989) transferred mussels *(Mytilus edulis)* from an unpolluted area into net bags suspended in a marina in Denmark. They monitored tin uptake and water concentrations of tin over a period of 51 days. Accumulation was found to increase exponentially with time for both total tin and organic tin. Bioconcentration factors of 5000 to 60 000, much higher than those from laboratory experiments, were reported. Transfer of the mussels to the laboratory after exposure resulted in a half-time for loss of organic and total tin of 40 and 25 days, respectively. Laughlin et al. (1986b) showed that bioaccumulation of TBTO by mussels was not significantly affected by the presence of humic acids or kaolin but that the presence of mucins secreted by bacteria did limit bioaccumulation. It was also shown that bioaccumulation by mussels was greater if the phytoplankton used as a food organism *(Isochrysis galbana)* was also contaminated with TBT. Contamination via food organisms was more important than via the water.

When feeding crabs with the brine shrimp *(Artemia salina)* containing concentrations of TBTO of 6200 µg/kg wet weight, Evans & Laughlin (1984) found a concentration factor of 4400. Allen et al. (1980) reported limited bioaccumulation (< 50) in a 1-week study using freshwater gastropods *(Biomphalaria glabrata)*. In crustaceans, particularly the crab *Rhithropanopeus harisii*, accumulation of TBTO from a water concentration of 0.28 µg/litre produced a moderate bioconcentration factor of 60 over 4 days.

Bioaccumulation of TBTO is equally evident in fish. After exposure of the sheepshead minnow *(Cyprinodon variegatus)* for 58 days to concentrations of TBTO varying between 0.96 and 2.07 µg/litre, Ward et al. (1981) reported a whole body concentration factor of 2600. After returning the fish to clean water, loss of TBTO was rapid over the first 7 days then slower. After 20 days, the authors reported a loss of 74% from the muscle and 80% from the viscera. Detection of dibutyltin, monobutyltin, and inorganic tin suggested possible metabolism. Bressa et al. (1984) exposed the mullet *Liza aurata* for 2 months to concentrations of 5 µg TBTO/litre and reported bioconcentration factors of 20 to 30 in the liver and kidneys but no residues in the muscle. After transfer to clean water, concentrations of tin fell in all organs. Short & Thrower (1986) studied bioaccumulation in salmon *(Oncorhynchus tshawytscha)* exposed for 96 h to concentrations of 1.49 µg/litre and obtained concentration factors of 4300 in the liver, 1300 in the brain, and 200 in muscle. Tsuda et al. (1987) showed that TBTO was accumulated by carp *(Cyprinus carpio)* exposed for 14 days to concentrations varying between 1.8 and 2.4 ng/litre. Over 10 days they found a plateau in uptake and a concentration factor of 1000; metabolism was evident. Tsuda et al. (1986) reported concentration factors ranging between 360 and 3400 for round crucian carp *(Carassius carassius grandoculis)* tissues exposed to tributyltin chloride for 7 days.

5. ENVIRONMENTAL CONCENTRATIONS

Summary

Levels of TBT in water, sediment, and biota are elevated within the proximity of marinas, commercial harbours, cooling systems, and fish nets and cages treated with TBT-based antifoulant paints.

TBT levels have been found to reach 1.58 µg/litre in sea water and estuaries, 7.1 µg/litre in fresh water, 26 300 µg/kg in coastal sediments, 3700 µg/kg in fresh water sediments, 6.39 mg/kg in bivalves, 1.92 mg/kg in gastropods, and 11 mg/kg in fish. However, these maximum concentrations of TBT should not be taken as representative, because a number of factors may give rise to anomalously high values (e.g., paint particles in water and sediment samples).

It has been found that measured TBT concentrations in the surface microlayer of both sea water and fresh water are up to two orders of magnitude above those measured just below the surface. However, it should be noted that the recorded levels of TBT in surface microlayers may be highly affected by the method of sampling.

Older data may not be comparable to newer data because of improvements in the analytical methods available for measuring TBT in water, sediment, and tissue.

5.1 Sea water and marine sediment

The concentrations of TBT in sea water and sediment are shown in Tables 3 and 5, respectively. Many papers have reported an association between increased levels of TBT in water, sediment, and biota and proximity to pleasure boating activity (especially marinas) and the use of antifouling paints on fish nets and cages. The degree of tidal flushing and turbidity of water also influence TBT concentrations in particular locations.

Alzieu et al. (1986) monitored tin and organotin concentrations in both water and oyster tissue from Arcachon Bay, France, between 1982 and 1985. They found that levels in oyster tissue decreased by 5 to 10 times over this

Environmental Concentrations

Table 3. Concentrations of tributyltin in estuarine and sea water

Location	Year	Sample depth[a] (metres)	Concentration (μg/litre)	Form[b]	Detection limit (μg/litre)	Reference
Denmark						
Coastal waters	1986	0.1-0.2	< 0.04	tin	0.04	Jensen & Cheng (1987)
Marinas	1986		< 0.04-1.05	tin	0.04	Jensen & Cheng (1987)
Harbour areas			0.63-2.64	OT_o		ICES (1987)
Finland						
Harbours	1988	0.2	0.02-0.2	TBT	0.01	Yla-Mononen (1988)
France						
Bay of Arcachon	1982		0.1-0.3	OT		Alzieu & Heral (1984)
	1984		0.7-1.2	tin	0.15	Alzieu et al. (1986)
			< 0.15-0.5	OT	0.1	Alzieu et al. (1986)
	1985		0.3-1.0	tin	0.15	Alzieu et al. (1986)
			< 0.15	OT	0.1	Alzieu et al. (1986)
Anse de Camaret, Brest	1987	(1)	< 0.002-0.004	TBT	0.002	Alzieu et al. (1989)
Auray river estuary	1986-1987	(1)	0.009-0.069	TBT	0.002	Alzieu et al. (1989)
La Rochelle	1986-1987	(1)	0.02-0.119	TBT	0.002	Alzieu et al. (1989)
Oleron Island	1986-1987	(1)	0.039-1.5	TBT	0.002	Alzieu et al. (1989)
Arcachon Bay	1986-1987	(1)	< 0.002-0.089	TBT	0.002	Alzieu et al. (1989)
Norway						
Oslo fjord			< 0.01	TBT_t	0.01	NIVA (1986)
Sweden						
Coastal waters			ND-0.04	TBT_t		Bjorklund (1987b)
United Kingdom						
Essex coast	1982	0.1-0.2	< 0.03-0.9	TBT_t	0.03	Waldock & Miller (1983)
South-west coast	1984		< 0.04-0.35	OT	0.04	Cleary & Stebbing (1985)
South-west coast	1986	surface water	0.12-5.34	OT	0.04	Cleary & Stebbing (1987)
South-west coast	1986	0.5	< 0.04-1.44	OT	0.04	Cleary & Stebbing (1987)
South-west coast	1986	bottom	< 0.04-2.6	OT	0.04	Cleary & Stebbing (1987)
South-west coast	1985		< 0.02-0.68	TBT	0.02	Ebdon et al. (1988)
Poole harbour	1986		0.002-0.646	TBT_t		Langston et al. (1987)
Essex coast	1986	0.1	< 0.001-0.831	TBT	0.001	Waldock et al. (1987b)
South coast	1986	0.1	< 0.001-1.52	TBT	0.001	Waldock et al. (1987b)
South-west coast	1986	0.1	< 0.001-1.27	TBT	0.001	Waldock et al. (1987b)
South Wales coast	1986	0.1	< 0.001-0.29	TBT	0.001	Waldock et al. (1987b)
North Wales coast	1986	0.1	< 0.001-0.012	TBT	0.001	Waldock et al. (1987b)

Table 3 (contd).

Location	Year	Sample depth[a] (metres)	Concentration (μg/litre)	Form[b]	Detection limit (μg/litre)	Reference
USA						
Chesapeake Bay	1985	surface microlayer	ND-1.171	TBT	0.008-0.01	Hall et al. (1986)
Chesapeake Bay (South)	1986	0.15	ND-0.1	TBT	0.001	Huggett et al. (1986)
San Diego Bay	1986	> 0.5	0.005-0.235	TBT	0.005	Seligman et al. (1986b)
Californian coast	1986		< 0.002-0.6	TBT	0.001-0.002	Stallard et al. (1987)
San Diego Bay	1983-1985	0.3-0.6	< 0.01-0.93	TBT	0.01	Valkirs et al. (1986)
San Diego Bay	1983-1985	(0.1)	< 0.01-0.55	TBT	0.01	Valkirs et al. (1986)
USA harbours & estuaries		(0.5)	< 0.005-0.35	TBT	0.005	Grovhoug et al. (1986)
Coos Bay, Oregon		surface water	0.007-0.014	TBT		Wolniakowski et al. (1987)

[a] Figures in parentheses indicate distance from water bottom.
[b] TBT = sample analysed for TBT and expressed as TBT.
   TBT_t = sample analysed for TBT and expressed as tin.
   tin = total tin expressed as tin.
   OT = total organic tin expressed as tin.
   OT_o = total organic tin expressed as TBTO.

sampling period following French Government restrictions on the use of TBT in antifouling paints. Alzieu et al. (1989) monitored TBT water levels at various locations on the French Atlantic coast in 1986 and 1987 (Table 3), and found that concentrations generally ranged between < 0.002 and 0.1 μg TBT/litre with the exception of a marina on Oleron Island, which had levels of up to 1.5 μg/litre. Levels were highest both in marinas and in the autumn, presumably when boats were being hosed off ready for the winter. The authors concluded that levels of TBT had generally decreased since the restrictions on TBT antifouling paints, but in certain marinas levels were significantly higher, suggesting continued use of TBT paints in contravention of restrictions.

Waldock & Miller (1983) measured TBT levels in water samples collected monthly during 1982 at Burnham-on-Crouch on the east coast of the United Kingdom. They found a rise in TBT levels in May, at a time when boats were being freshly painted with TBT antifouling paints. There was a second rise in TBT water concentrations in August, at a time when boats were repainted for the major sailing event of the year. Analysis of water samples from several areas on the Essex coast showed that the highest levels (up to 2.25 µg TBTO/litre) were associated with the highest density of pleasure craft. The authors also reported that a site used by a large number of boats (on the south coast of the United Kingdom but situated on an open coastal site and with less turbid water) had relatively low TBT levels in the sea water (< 0.08 µg TBTO/litre in early August).

Waldock et al. (1987b) analysed water samples from nine sites around the United Kingdom coast during 1986 following restrictions placed on the tin content of antifouling paints containing TBT in January 1986. They sampled from an enclosed bay, an open coastal site, and seven estuarine sites. Within these general areas, locations were found which reflected the incoming water from a river, an area fished for shellfish, and a harbour or marina. Half of the 250 samples taken during 1986 were found to equal or to be above the United Kingdom environmental quality target level (EQT; 20 ng/litre). Levels were barely above the detection limits at the sites upstream of boats. Harbours and marinas showed the highest levels with tidal flushing being an important factor in determining amounts of TBT detected. A marina in Plymouth, which has poor flushing, had TBT concentrations consistently greater than 1 µg/litre from May to September, whereas a marina in the estuary of the River Dart, with good flushing, had levels of less than 0.2 µg/litre. Six of the nine sites exceeded the EQT by 3 to 4 times; these were all sites used regularly by yachts. The other three sites not used by yachts all showed low but often detectable levels with just one sample exceeding the EQT. The authors also found increased levels of TBT close to areas where boats were hosed down. Other reports confirmed that the distribution of TBT in water was associated with the proximity to intense boating activity (Cleary & Stebbing, 1985; Ebdon et al., 1988). Langston et al. (1987) reported that sediments, likewise, contained more TBT (up to

520 µg tin/kg) near marinas than at the harbour mouth (20 µg tin/kg) in Poole harbour, United Kingdom. There was poor flushing in the harbour and sediment was not distributed; this was reflected in the water levels, which were 0.002 to 0.139 µg tin/litre in the general harbour area and 0.234 to 0.646 µg/litre in the marina.

Cleary & Stebbing (1987) surveyed vertical water profiles in south-west England at sites already investigated two years before. They did not find a systematic decline in concentrations between the two surveys. The concentrations in the surface microlayer were 1.9 to 26.9 times higher than those at 0.5 m below the surface (see Table 3).

Waldock et al. (1988) analysed water samples collected in 1987 from commercial harbours and anchorages in the United Kingdom. Significant concentrations were found; several samples taken in the immediate vicinity of ships had levels exceeding 0.05 µg TBT/litre. However, the highest concentrations were found near to centres of yachting activity, with over 0.6 µg/litre being found at one site. The highest concentration found close to commercial vessels in harbours was 0.078 µg/litre, but this was within 2 m of an oil tanker. A concentration of 0.25 µg per litre was recorded outside a shipyard where a 3000-tonne vessel was being hosed down on the foreshore, and a concentration of 0.137 µg/litre was measured in surface water close to a vessel at anchor in the River Fal. In general, however, few samples taken in close proximity to commercial ships exceeded 0.02 µg/litre.

Bacci & Gaggi (1989) monitored TBT and its degradation products in harbours, marinas, and the open sea from the northern Tyrrhenian Sea, Italy. Concentrations of up to 3.93 µg TBT/litre were measured in the various harbours and marinas, but no organotin compounds were detected in samples from the open sea. However, considering the detection limits of the analytical technique used (0.02 µg per litre for both TBT and DBT), levels higher than the NOEL (i.e. 0.01 µg/litre, UNEP, 1989) cannot be excluded. From these preliminary results, it appears that, under unfavourable meteorological conditions (e.g., moderate southerly winds), significant quantities of TBT and related compounds could contaminate open sea sites for a few days per year.

The highest levels of TBT around the coasts of the USA and Denmark were also associated with marinas or harbours used by small pleasure craft, with TBT levels generally showing a falling trend from the inner part to the entrance (Grovhoug et al., 1986; Seligman et al., 1986b; Jensen & Cheng, 1987). Stallard et al. (1987) analysed both water and sediment from the Californian coast. Highest TBT levels, up to 0.6 µg/litre water and 23 µg/kg sediment, were found near marinas. Levels were lower in other coastal areas and were lowest out in the open sea. Valkirs et al. (1986) measured TBT in surface water (at a depth of 0.3 to 0.6 m) and found that, over the period 1983-1985, TBT levels had increased in San Diego Bay, USA. Seligman et al. (1989) measured TBT in the waters of several harbours in the USA. Of the samples collected, 75% contained TBT levels below the detection limit (< 5 ng per litre). The highest concentrations were found in yacht harbours and near to vessel repair facilities, with significant levels being found near dry docks. The authors also found a high degree of variability in TBT concentrations depending on the tidal movement, the season, and intermittent point source discharges.

Hall et al. (1988a) measured TBT biweekly for a 4-month period (June-September 1986) in the Port Annapolis marina, Mears marina, Back Creek, and the Severn River area of northern Chesapeake Bay, USA. Maximum concentrations of TBT were reported at both Port Annapolis marina (1.8 µg tin/litre) and Mears marina (1.17 µg tin per litre) during early June, followed by significant reductions during late summer and early autumn. The day of the week (Thursday-Monday) on which samples were taken during the daily experiments was not found to significantly affect TBT concentrations. Peak concentrations were found to occur during a rising tide.

Balls (1987) reported that TBT levels in water were initially (immediately after fish cages were treated with antifoulants) 1 µg/litre (as tin) within fish cages, falling to 0.1 µg/litre after 2 weeks and 0.005 µg per litre after 5 months. Initial concentrations were 0.1 µg tin/litre at a distance of 20 m from the cages, with concentrations in the main body of the sea loch being < 0.028 µg/litre.

5.2 Fresh water and sediment

Analysis for TBT compounds in the Great Lakes, N. America, has revealed levels often comparable, and in many cases higher (200 times higher in one sample), than those measured in estuaries (Maguire et al., 1982; Maguire, 1984; Maguire et al., 1985; Maguire et al., 1986; Maguire & Tkacz, 1987). Levels of TBT in water were found to be greater in the surface microlayer than in the subsurface samples. For example, water samples from Ontario lakes and rivers showed surface levels of 0.15 to 60.7 µg tin/litre compared to subsurface levels of between 0.01 and 2.91 µg per litre (Maguire et al., 1982). TBT was found in the Great Lakes and in rivers at levels up to those causing effects on trout in the laboratory; Maguire & Tkacz (1987) reported a level of 66.8 µg tin/litre in the surface microlayer. In the United Kingdom, samples of fresh water from near boatyards contained up to 3.2 µg TBT/litre (Waldock 1989). In Lake Zurich and Swiss rivers, levels were found to be much lower, i.e. up to 0.015 µg/litre (Muller, 1987b). Kalbfus (1988) analysed water samples from marinas on Lake Constance in 1987 and 1988 and found that TBT levels rose to a peak in May which corresponded to the boating activity on the lake. For example, at Goren, TBT levels rose from 0.13 µg/litre in April to 0.58 µg/litre in May, but by July the levels had fallen again to 0.028 µg/litre. At the same time TBT levels in sediment rose from 830 µg/kg in May to 2700 µg/kg in June and then to 3700 µg/kg in July. Similarly, when samples were taken on Wannsee in Berlin, levels were found to be 0.02 µg/litre when there were no boats on the water, but at Tegel, Berlin, TBT levels were 0.25 µg per litre when most of the boats were in the water. A coastal marina at Kiel, on the Baltic, showed levels of 0.35 µg per litre in April when only half of the moorings were occupied.

Shiff et al. (1975) monitored water and mud samples 6.5 months after the application of controlled-release BioMet SRM pellets (rubber formulation containing TBTO) in Zimbabwe. The pellets were applied at a rate of 20 g/m^2 for the control of freshwater snails, intermediate hosts of the schistosomiasis parasite. Highest levels of organotin were found in the mud immediately under the pellets

Environmental Concentrations

Table 4. Concentrations of tributyltin in fresh water

Location	Year	Sample depth (metres)	Concentration (μg/litre)	Form[a]	Detection limit (μg/litre)	Reference
Canada						
Ontario lakes & rivers			0.01-2.91	TBT_t	0.01	Maguire et al. (1982)
Ontario lakes & rivers		surface microlayer	0.15-60.7	TBT_t	0.01	Maguire et al. (1982)
St Clair River, Ontario		surface microlayer	ND-0.03	TBT_t	0.01	Maguire et al. (1985)
Canadian waterways		0.5	< 0.01-2.34	TBT_t	0.01	Maguire et al. (1986)
Ontario waterways		surface microlayer	1.9-473	TBT_t	1.0	Maguire & Tkacz (1987)
Ontario waterways		0.5	< 0.01-1.72	TBT_t	0.01	Maguire & Tkacz (1987)
Quebec waterways		surface microlayer	5.5 & 15.2	TBT_t	1.0	Maguire & Tkacz (1987)
Quebec waterways		0.5	< 0.01-0.03	TBT_t	0.01	Maguire & Tkacz (1987)
British Columbian coast			up to 0.078	TBT		Humphrey & Hope (1987)
Federal Republic of Germany						
Lake Constance marinas	1987-1988		up to 0.58	TBT		Kalbfus (1988)
Switzerland						
Lake Zurich & rivers	1985	surface water	0.007-0.015	TBT_c	0.001	Muller (1987b)
Harbours	1983-1984		0.005-1.636	TBT		[d]
Rivers	1983-1985		0.001-0.016	TBT		[d]
United Kingdom						
Wroxham Broad, Norfolk	1987		up to 0.9[b]	TBT		Waldock et al. (1987a)
River Thames	1987		0.064[c]	TBT		Waldock et al. (1987a)
River Bure	1986-1987	0.1	ND-1.54	TBT	0.001	Waldock (1989)
River Yare	1986-1987	0.1	< 0.001-3.26	TBT	0.001	Waldock (1989)
USA						
New York State waterways		surface microlayer	2.0-23.8	TBT_t	1.0	Maguire & Tkacz (1987)

[a] TBT = sample analysed for TBT and expressed as TBT.
TBT_t = sample analysed for TBT and expressed as tin.
TBT_c = sample analysed for TBT and expressed as tributyltin chloride.
[b] Samples from local boatyards contained up to 1.5 μg/litre.
[c] Samples from marinas contained up to 1.3 μg/litre.
[d] Personal communication from M.D. Muller to IPCS.

Table 5. Concentrations of tributyltin in sediment

Location	Year	Sample depth (metres)	Concentration[a] (µg/kg)	Form[c]	Detection limit (µg/kg)	Reference
Canada						
Ontario lakes & rivers		0.02	30.9-110	TBT	5	Maguire (1984)
Canadian waterways		0.02	< 10-10 780	TBT_t	10	Maguire et al. (1986)
British Columbian coast			up to 17 000	TBT		Humphrey & Hope (1987)
Canada & USA						
Detroit & St Clair rivers		0.02	ND-70	TBT_t	5	Maguire et al. (1985)
Netherlands						
Eems-Dollard			< 25[b]	TBT_t	25	TWG (1988c)
Various locations			< 50-8800	TBT_t	50	TWG (1988c)
Switzerland						
Lake Zurich	1880-[d] 1985	120	ND	TBT_c	0.01	Muller (1987b)
Lake Zurich	1980- 1984	120	280	TBT_c	0.01	Muller (1987b)
Lake Zurich & Boden	1984		2.0-3550	TBT		[e]
United Kingdom						
Poole Harbour, Dorset	1986		20-520	TBT_t		Langston et al. (1987)
USA						
Californian coast	1986	0.1	< 2.0-23	TBT	1.0-2.0	Stallard et al. (1987)
San Diego Bay	1983	0.35	< 2.0-300	TBT		Stang & Seligman (1986)
USA harbours & estuaries			1.4-178	OT		Grovhoug et al. (1986)
Californian coast			15-527	TBT		Stephenson et al. (1987)
Virginian coast		0.02	23-290	TBT		Rice et al. (1987)
Great Bay estuary		0.02	12-44	TBT_t		Weber et al. (1986)

[a] Concentrations given as µg/kg dry weight unless stated otherwise.
[b] Wet weight value.
[c] TBT = sample analysed for TBT and expressed as TBT.
  TBT_t = sample analysed for TBT and expressed as tin.
  TBT_c = sample analysed for TBT and expressed as tributyltin chloride.
  OT = total organic tin expressed as tin.
[d] Museum core from the nineteenth century.
[e] Personal communication from M.D. Muller to IPCS.

(up to 5 mg/kg). Levels in the mud dropped off rapidly further away from the pellets; at 2 cm organotin levels were < 0.6 mg/kg. The organotin level in surface water was < 0.01 mg/litre and in background mud < 0.06 mg/kg.

5.3 Sewage treatment

The mono-, di-, and tri-butyltin content of waste water entering a sewage treatment plant in Switzerland was measured and its fate was monitored through the various processes of settlement, digestion, and filtration of the sewage (Fent, 1989a; Fent et al., 1989). Concentrations of MBT, DBT, and TBT were 170, 152, and 155 ng/litre, respectively, in the incoming raw waste water, averaged over three days of monitoring. About 90% of the organotin was associated with particulate matter, 10% being in solution (Table 6). A substantial amount of the incoming butyltin compounds was lost from the effluent during primary settlement. The removal of particulate matter at this stage took 74% of the incoming organotin. In the secondary effluent, after activated sludge digestion, MBT and DBT were found at levels similar to those in the primary effluent; TBT concentrations were reduced to 6 ng/litre and found only on the particulate matter. In the final effluent from the plant, after filtration, concentrations were 4, 3, and 4 ng/litre for MBT, DBT, and TBT, respectively. Thus, 98% of the butyltin was removed from waste water in the sewage plant. The authors point out that not all treatment plants have filtration; in these cases only 87% would be removed and effluent concentrations of 9-70 ng/litre found. Levels of butyltin in the sewage sludge (which is removed from the plant and used as fertiliser on farm land) were 0.36, 0.38, and 0.34 mg/kg dry weight for MBT, DBT, and TBT, respectively, in the raw sludge and 0.62, 1.23, and 1.12 mg/kg dry weight in the digested sludge after 35 days of anaerobic conditions. The authors point out that 900 kg/year of butyltin could be added to Swiss soils via sewage sludge. The source of TBT detected in the sludge was not identified or specified in the report.

5.4 Biota

Concentrations of TBT in biota are given in Table 7.

Table 6. Levels of organotin compounds in municipal waste water[a]

Date	MBT water	particles	%	DBT water	particles	%	TBT water	particles	%
23 February 1988	34	216	86	14	113	89	14	178	93
23 February 1988	25	181	88	10	163	94	14	158	92
28 February 1988	28	114	80	11	180	94	27	129	83
Mean	29	170	85	12	152	93	18	155	90

[a] Levels in ng/litre are calculated as ions and corrected for recovery (55-70%); the percentage of organotins associated with particles is also given. From Fent (1989a).

Alzieu (1981) analysed the Pacific oyster *(Crassostrea gigas)* for total tin levels following problems in the French oyster industry in the late 1970s (see section 10.1). He reported that most of the tin accumulated was in the digestive gland and in the gills. Highest residues were found in oysters from the Bay of Arcachon (residues in digestive gland and gill were up to 7.03 and 17.37 mg/kg, respectively), an area with large numbers of small pleasure boats. Tin levels were stated to be influenced by tidal flushing; both the Bay of Arcachon and Marennes Oleron were used by a large number of boats, but residue levels in oysters collected from the latter site had lower tin levels (the Bay of Arcachon has poor tidal flushing compared to Marennes Oleron). Alzieu & Heral (1984) reported that the greatest accumulation of tin was in close proximity to a marina. Oysters transferred to the marina site accumulated a total tin level of 110 mg/kg (dry weight) within 80 days, whereas oysters maintained as controls in a local river or in the laboratory accumulated < 1 mg/kg over the same period. Waldock & Miller (1983) analysed oysters from the Essex coast, United Kingdom, and, although both Pacific and European oysters *(Ostrea edulis)* contained similar residues of total tin, the Pacific oyster residues had a higher percentage of TBT.

There are seasonal differences in the levels of TBT (and DBT) found in mussels *(Mytilus edulis)* in the field. It has been suggested that, while these are predominantly due to changes in boating activity affecting the availability of TBT to the organisms, physiological differences in the animals at different times of year may also partly

Environmental Concentrations

Table 7. Concentrations of tributyltin in biota

Organism	Year	Location[a]	Organ[b]	Concentration[c] (mg/kg)	Form[f]	Detection limit (mg/kg)	Reference
Invertebrates							
European oyster (*Ostrea edulis*)		French coast	DG	0.54-7.03	tin		Alzieu (1981)
		French coast	gill	<0.5-17.37	tin		Alzieu (1981)
	1982	Essex coast, UK	DG	<0.23-2.05	TBT_o	0.075	Waldock & Miller (1983)
	1982	Essex coast, UK	rest	<0.4-1.99	TBT_o	0.075	Waldock & Miller (1983)
Pacific oyster (*Crassostrea gigas*)		French coast	DG	<0.5-2.5	tin		Alzieu (1981)
		French coast	gill	<0.5-3.5	tin		Alzieu (1981)
	1982	Essex coast, UK	DG	4.05-8.64	TBT_o	0.075	Waldock & Miller (1983)
	1982	Essex coast, UK	rest	3.5-7.5	TBT_o	0.075	Waldock & Miller (1983)
		Coos Bay, USA		0.05-0.189	TBT		Wolniakowski et al. (1987)
Eastern oyster (*Crassostrea virginica*)		Virginia, USA	WB	0.59-1.57	TBT		Rice et al. (1987)
		USA coast	WB	<0.12-3.9	TBT		Wade et al. (1988)
Common mussel (*Mytilus edulis*)	1985-1987	Japan		ND-0.289	TBT_o	0.05	EAJ (1988)
		USA coast	WB	0.25-3.85	TBT		Wade et al. (1988)
Asiatic mussel	1985-1987	Japan		0.3-0.489	TBT_o	0.05	EAJ 1988
Mussel		Californian coast, USA		0.107-6.39	TBT		Stephenson et al. (1987)
Shellfish		USA coast		0.23-7.35	OT		Grovhoug et al. (1986)
		B.C., Canada		up to 1.8	TBT		Humphrey & Hope (1987)
		Netherlands		<0.025-0.22	TBT_t	0.025	TWG (1988c)
Dogwhelk (*Nucella lapillus*)		Fal estuary, UK		0.023-0.786	TBT_t		Bryan et al. (1987)
		South-west coast, UK		0.036-0.633	TBT_t		Gibbs et al. (1987)
Various snail species	1988	Finnish harbours	SP	0.04-0.19	TBT	0.01	Yla-Mononen (1988)

EHC 116: Tributyltin Compounds

Table 7 (contd).

	Year	Location	Sample	Concentration	Form	Detection limit	Reference
Fish							
Herring (*Clupea harengus*)	1984	Vancouver harbour, Canada	WB	0.24	TBT_t	0.01	Maguire et al. (1986)
Finfish		B.C., Canada	DM	up to 11	TBT		Humphrey & Hope (1987)
Salmon species		USA	MT	ND-0.2^d	TBT		Short & Thrower (1986)
		USA		0.28-0.9^e	TBT		Short & Thrower (1986)
Various fish species	1982-1983	Jordan harbour, Canada	WB	<0.01-0.029	TBT_t	0.01	Maguire et al. (1986)
Various fish species		Japan	MT	ND-0.31^d	TBT_c		Hada (1986)
Various fish species	1985-1987	Japan		ND-1.79^f	TBT_o	0.05	EAJ (1988)
Various fish species		Netherlands		<0.025-0.26	tin	0.025	TWG (1988c)
Various fish species	1988	Finnish harbours	WB	<0.01-0.19	TBT	0.01	Yla-Mononen (1988)
Birds							
Oystercatcher (*Haematopus ostralegus*)	1986	Exe estuary, UK	liver	TR-0.08	TBT_t	0.02	Osborn & Leach (1987)
	1986	Exe estuary, UK	MT	0.01-0.19	TBT_t	0.02	Osborn & Leach (1987)
Grey starling	1985-1987	Japan		ND (< 0.05)^g	TBT_o	0.05	EAJ (1988)
Black-tailed gull	1985-1987	Japan		ND (< 0.05)^g	TBT_o	0.05	EAJ (1988)
Mammals							
Seals			BL	ND	TBT	0.01	^{h}

^{a} UK = United Kingdom; B.C. = British Columbia.
^{b} DG = digestive gland; rest = tissues other than digestive gland; DM = dorsal muscle; MT = muscle tissue; BL = blubber; WB = whole body; SP = soft parts.
^{c} Concentrations measured as mg/kg dry weight unless stated otherwise; TR = trace; ND = not detectable.
^{d} Fish collected from local fish markets.
^{e} Salmon raised in TBT-treated sea pens.
^{f} TBT = sample analysed for TBT and expressed as TBT; TBT_t = sample analysed for TBT and expressed as tributyltin chloride; OT = total organic tin expressed as tin; TBT_c = total tin expressed as tin; TBT_o = sample analysed for TBT and expressed as TBTO.
^{g} Wet weight value.
^{h} Personal communication from M.J. Waldock to IPCS.

explain the results. The relative amounts of TBT and DBT in mussels are thought to reflect the rate of input to the animal. A high ratio of DBT to TBT residues reflects low input rates, and vice versa (Page, 1989).

Gibbs et al. (1987) found highest levels of TBT (0.132-0.633 mg tin/kg dry weight) in dogwhelks from the "enclosed" waters of Plymouth Sound and Torbay, United Kingdom, whereas levels were less than 0.113 mg tin/kg on the North Cornish coast. Bryan et al. (1987) reported residues between 0.374 and 0.786 mg tin/kg (TBT fraction) for dogwhelks from the Fal estuary, in the south-west of England, whereas dogwhelks from around the Isle of Mull, off the Scottish mainland, contained levels of less than 0.03 mg/kg. The Environment Agency of Japan monitored various fish and shellfish species from different areas of Japan between 1985 and 1987. The lowest levels of TBTO (< 0.05 mg/kg wet weight) were found off the open coast of Japan, higher levels being found in bays and estuaries. The highest levels reported were in sea bass from the Seto Inland Sea (up to 1.7 mg/kg). The level of TBTO in the biota did not change significantly during the sampling period (EAJ, 1988).

Since 1987 only vessels of > 25 m have been allowed to use TBT antifouling paints in the United Kingdom (see section 3.3). Bailey & Davies (1988a) analysed dogwhelk and scallop from an area around an oil terminal frequented by large ships at Sullom Voe, Shetland. Elevated tin levels were found in both dogwhelk (up to 0.16 mg tin/kg wet weight) and scallops (up to 0.23 mg/kg in gonadal tissue) within Sullom Voe (especially in areas close to the oil terminal) compared to those collected from the surrounding area (< 0.03 mg/kg).

Increased levels of TBT in biota have been found associated with fish nets and cages. Davies et al. (1987b) found that residues of total tin in dogwhelks were higher near fish cages in Loch Laxford (< 0.01-0.33 mg/kg), a sea loch in Scotland, and in the harbour areas of Loch Crinan (< 0.01-0.17 mg/kg) than outside the sea lochs (< 0.02 mg/kg).

Short & Thrower (1986) found TBT residues of between 0.28 and 0.9 mg tin/kg in salmon *(Oncorhynchus tshawytscha)* maintained in TBT-treated sea pens for 3 to

19 months. The authors also monitored salmon for sale in American fish markets and found TBT residues of up to 0.2 mg/kg. They also found that cooking does not effectively destroy or remove TBT from salmon tissues.

6. KINETICS AND METABOLISM

Summary

Tributyltin is absorbed from the gut (20-50% depending on the vehicle) and via the skin of mammals (about 10%), and can be transferred across the blood-brain barrier and from the placenta to the fetus. Absorbed material is rapidly and widely distributed amongst tissues (principally liver and kidney).

Metabolism in mammals is rapid; metabolites are detectable in blood within 3 h of TBT administration. TBT is a substrate for mixed-function oxidases in vitro, but these enzymes are inhibited by TBT in vitro at very high concentrations. Rate of loss differs with different tissues and estimates for biological half-lives in mammals range from 23 to about 30 days.

Metabolism occurs in lower organisms but is slower, particularly in molluscs. The capacity for bioaccumulation is, therefore, much greater than in mammals.

TBT compounds inhibit oxidative phosphorylation and alter mitochondrial structure and function. TBT interferes with the calcification of the shell of oysters (Crassostrea species).

6.1 Metabolism of TBT in mammals

A number of workers have studied the absorption, metabolism, and elimination of organotin derivatives in various animals species, especially in mammals. Some studies were conducted *in vivo* and others *in vitro* using isolated liver microsomes.

The behaviour of organotin compounds depends partly on their chemical structure and partly on speciation. However, the following statements generally apply:

- The distribution of TBT in organisms is usually rapid. In a number of species (rat, mouse, rabbit, guinea-pig), it is found preferentially in the liver and kidney and, to a lesser extent, in the spleen, fat, lungs, brain, and muscle.
- Excretion is via the bile rather than the urine.
- In tissues, particularly the liver, there is a process of biotransformation characterized by progressive

de-alkylation leading to breakdown to inorganic tin (Cremer, 1957; Bridges et al., 1967).

In an *in vivo* study, Brown et al. (1977) administered ^{113}Sn-labelled TBTO to mice by ip injection. They reported an initial rapid elimination, followed by a slower phase, in the faeces. Part of the radiolabel was retained in the tissues but turn-over occurred, with a biological half-life for elimination of 23 to 29 days.

Evans et al. (1979), under similar conditions, administered ^{14}C-labelled TBTO to mice in the drinking-water, at low doses continuously for up to 30 days. There was absorption from the intestine and accumulation in the liver, spleen, kidney, and fat (and to a lesser degree in muscle, lung, brain, and blood). In a second study, mice were similarly dosed for 31 days. On cessation of dosing with ^{14}C-labelled TBTO, examination of the animals for a further 15 days demonstrated loss of TBTO retained in these tissues; the loss reached 97% in liver, 73% in kidney, and 30% in fat, and the TBTO had disappeared completely from the blood. Studies in metabolism cages indicated that the principal route of loss was via the faeces; limited amounts of labelled CO_2 were exhaled.

Iwai et al. (1980) studied the distribution and accumulation of tributyltin and its metabolites in areas of the brain of rabbits. After a single oral dose of TBT chloride, high concentrations of tributyltin were found in the frontal and temporal lobes and in the cerebellum initially. Thereafter, there was a rapid decrease in TBT residues and an increase in levels of monobutyltin, which persisted for much longer. Persistence occurred preferentially in the grey matter rather than the white matter. The authors' interpretation was that TBT, which passes readily through the blood-brain barrier, is mainly dealkylated in the grey matter and that the metabolic product remains there.

Humpel et al. (1986) administered ^{113}Sn-labelled TBTO orally to rats and found that the absorption varied between 20% and 55% depending on the vehicle used. High residues of tin were found in the liver and kidney (1 to 3 days after dosing) of which only approximately 5% was unchanged TBT. Other tissues showed lower concentrations of the label but the fraction of unchanged TBT was higher. The exact nature of the metabolites could not be identified by the analytical method used (HPLC), but the pattern was indicative of progressive debutylation. Daily administration of TBTO for 14 days resulted in steadily increasing concentrations of label in all tissues. Steady-state levels were estimated to be reached after 3 to 4 weeks. When Snoeij et al. (1987) administered ^{14}C-labelled TBT acetate as a single oral dose to rats, about 20% absorption occurred. The presence of DBT and MBT in plasma (after TLC separation) was demonstrated 3 h and 27 h after dosing.

TBT may cross the placenta to some extent, as was shown by the presence of label in rat fetuses after a single oral dose to the mother at day 18 of pregnancy. The concentration in fetal tissue was comparable to that of the mother's muscle tissue (Humpel et al., 1986).

After administration of neat ^{113}Sn-labelled TBTO to the intact skin of baboons for 7 h, 10 to 15% was estimated to reach the systemic circulation (Humpel et al., 1986).

Metabolism of tributyltin derivatives has been clearly demonstrated in *in vitro* studies. Casida et al. (1971) and Fish et al. (1975, 1976) studied the possible metabolism of TBT acetate using rat hepatic microsomes in the presence of NADPH. They demonstrated hydroxylation by monooxygenases of the principal carbon-hydrogen bonds (*alpha* and *beta* to the tin atom) of 24% (at the *alpha* position) and 50% (at the *beta* position). The hydroxylated *alpha* metabolite is unstable and rapidly splits to form the dibutyl derivative, followed by 1-butanol and then butane. According to Kimmel et al. (1977), the same type of reaction occurs in microsome preparations from mice.

Uhl (1986) dissolved TBTO (9.88 or 5.54 mg) in a mixture of 3 ml cherry brandy and 7 ml ethanol and gave it orally to a volunteer. TBTO and its degradation products were determined in urine by gas chromatography after reaction with methyl magnesium bromide. Only 5.1% to 5.4% of the dose was found in the urine, mainly as dibutyltin metabolites. Butyltin levels in the urine decreased rapidly during the first days after administration. After dermal application of 20 µl (23.4 mg) of undiluted TBTO on the arm of a volunteer, approximately 0.2% of the dose was excreted in the urine, of which about 20% was found to be tributyltin.

6.2 Metabolism of TBTO in other organisms

Lee (1985, 1986) examined the capacity of organisms from various aquatic trophic levels to metabolize TBTO. He used the blue crab *(Callinectes sapidus)*, the brown shrimp *(Penaeus aztecus)*, a fish (the spot, *Leiostomus xanthurus)*, and the Eastern oyster *(Crassostrea virginica)*. The organisms were exposed to ^{14}C-labelled TBTO via the water (6 µg/litre for the crab and shrimp; 2 µg/litre for the fish and the oyster) and via food (shrimp containing about 20 mg/kg) in the case of the crab and fish. In all test species he reported a rapid uptake of ^{14}C-labelled TBTO into various organs. In crabs and shrimps, he observed, after 3 days, the appearance of various metabolites in the hepatopancreas (dibutyl, monobutyl, and polar derivatives). In the fish, the same was seen in the liver. In oysters, the process was much slower and metabolites appear only at low concentrations after 4 days. *In vitro* studies, conducted with liver microsomes from fish and stomach microsomes from crabs, confirmed the presence of a route of metabolism comparable to that in mammals. Within microsomes, a cytochrome-P-450-dependent oxygenase acts in the presence of NADPH and oxygen to allow progressive degradation of TBTO. Such biochemical mechanisms are apparent in a number of species. However, their activity is limited in molluscs, particularly in bivalves; thus the capacity of molluscs to metabolize xenobiotics is generally weak. Tsuda et al. (1988) followed the metabolism of tributyltin oxide in various tissues of the carp *Cyrpinus carpio* over 14 days. In muscle, there was little evidence of metabolites and almost all of the tin present was in the form of tributyltin. In the kidney, liver, and gall bladder, large amounts of monobutyltin were evident. Little dibutyltin was present in any of the tissues, suggesting that further metabolism of the intermediate to the monobutyl form was rapid. Ebdon et al. (1989) could not positively determine whether dibutyltin and monobutyltin present in adult and seed oysters in British estuaries derived from intake of the metabolites or from metabolism within the oysters. However, they observed that peak seasonal levels of the metabolites occurred approximately 1 month after peaks of tributyltin. They concluded that metabolism within the oysters was responsible for the DBT and MBT present. This also suggests that metabolism in oysters is slow.

6.3 General mechanisms of toxicity of TBTO

Different mechanisms of action have been advanced to explain the biological effects and toxicity of TBTO. Some of the mechanisms are present in all living organisms, others only in certain species.

6.3.1 General toxic mechanisms

Several studies (Aldridge, 1958; Aldridge & Street, 1964, 1970) have demonstrated that the trialkyl derivatives of tin, and notably tributyltin compounds, are inhibitors of oxidative phosphorylation in mitochondria and are, therefore, responsible for inhibiting energy transfer. This inhibition results from various phenomena:

- disturbance of synthesis of ATP;
- action on mitochondrial membranes causing swelling and rupture;
- alteration in ion transport across lipid membranes.

Rosenberg et al. (1980, 1981, 1984) and Rosenberg & Drummond (1983) showed TBTO inhibition of cytochrome P-450 activity in cells from various tissues (liver, kidney, small intestine mucosa) after dosing *in vitro* or *in vivo*. Evans et al. (1979) demonstrated inhibition of oxidative phosphorylation due to formation of complexes between trialkyltin derivatives and proteins or certain *alpha* or *beta* amino acids. They most notably form chemical links with nitrogen and sulfur atoms in protein chains (see chapter 2).

6.3.2 Toxic mechanisms in bivalve molluscs

In bivalve molluscs, notably in oysters, one sublethal effect of TBTO involves abnormal calcification. This is shown particularly in *Crassostrea gigas*, the Pacific or Eastern oyster, in areas contaminated with TBTO. The effect is reproducible in experiments where healthy oysters are transferred to contaminated areas, and also reversible in transfers from contaminated to clean areas.

The abnormal calcification leads to distortion of the shells; layers are formed successively of calcium carbonate, flaking and open space (Alzieu et al., 1982), and result partly from interference with synthesis of the organic matter (gel) (which allows calcium deposition) and partly from interference with crystallization of calcium carbonate. Krampitz et al. (1976, 1983) showed that the protein constituents of the interlamellar gel assisting deposition of calcium were deficient in the amino acids necessary for calcium fixation (serine, alanine, glycine, glutamic acid, aspartic acid); these amino acids are complexed by TBTO.

The work on mammals showing effects of TBTO on oxidative phosphorylation (Aldridge & Street, 1971) suggests another possible effect, since ATP plays an important role in the crystallization of calcium carbonate, as shown in the following schematic diagram.

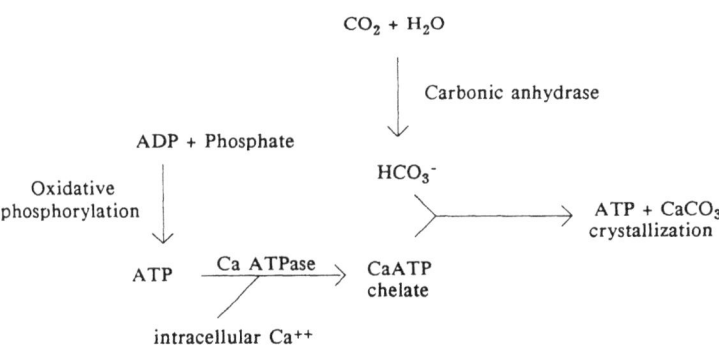

From: Alzieu et al. (1982)

7. EFFECTS ON ORGANISMS IN THE ENVIRONMENT: MICROORGANISMS

Summary

Tributyltin is toxic to microorganisms and is used commercially to control bacteria and fungi. Concentrations producing toxic effects are very variable between species. The primary productivity of a natural community of freshwater microalgae was reduced by 50% at a TBTO concentration of 3 µg/litre. Recently established no-observed-effect-levels for two species are 18 and 32 µg/litre. Toxicity to sea-water microorganisms is similarly variable between species and between studies; no-observed-effect-levels are difficult to set but lie below 0.1 µg per litre for some species. Most toxicity tests with microorganisms use batch cultures, and in these systems concentrations of TBT in solution may decline rapidly. Such tests may, therefore, underestimate true toxicity.

7.1 Bacteria and fungi

Bokranz & Plum (1975) presented data on the effectiveness of TBT compounds against bacteria, algae, and fungi. TBT is more toxic to gram-positive bacteria (such as *Staphylococcus aureus* with a minimal inhibitory concentration of between 0.2 and 0.8 mg/litre in culture) than to gram-negative bacteria (such as *Escherichia coli* with an MIC of 3.1 mg/litre) in serial dilution tests for various TBT compounds. MIC values for four species of fungus in culture (*Botrytis, Penicillium, Aspergillus,* and *Rhizopodium*) varied from 0.5 to 1.0 mg/litre for TBT acetate. Impregnation of textiles with TBTO, TBT sulfide, or TBT fluoride at 0.01%, 0.05%, and 0.2% showed clear inhibition of fungal growth on agar nutrient medium. The TBT compounds were resistant to leaching from the textiles when washed before culture at the two highest concentrations. Fungicidal action was also retained in textiles treated with TBTO and subsequently buried in soil. In tests with three species of fungus, limiting values for complete inhibition of effects on wood were determined. Values for TBTO ranged from 0.058 to 0.704 kg/m^3 without prior leaching of the compound and from 0.055 to 2.178 kg per m^3 after prior leaching. For TBT fluoride, values ranged from 0.055 to 0.88 kg/m^3 without prior leaching and from 0.135 to 0.886 kg/m^3 after leaching.

Soracco & Pope (1983) investigated the action of TBTO on various physiological and biochemical activities of the bacterium *Legionella pneumophila*, the organism causing Legionnaires disease, which commonly lives in the water of cooling systems. The minimal concentration of TBTO having any effect on *Legionella* growth was about 0.02 mg/litre. At concentrations between 0.5 and 1.1 mg/litre, TBTO reduced the growth rate initially and subsequently caused a further reduction in growth rate. At 1.1 mg/litre, growth was almost static, while at higher concentrations TBTO was bactericidal, causing a reduction in the optical density of the cultures. The effect of TBTO on the cultures was dependent on cell density; its effectiveness was reduced at high cell densities. Between 69% and 88% of the added TBTO was found to be associated with the cells rather than in free solution. There was a dose-response relationship between TBTO concentration per unit biomass and the effect on growth. The bacteriostatic concentration of 1.1 mg/litre did not kill the cells; transfer of cells from this culture to fresh nutrient medium established that all cells were still viable. A concentration of 2.24 mg/litre was similarly lacking in bactericidal action and only a dose of 11.2 mg/litre successfully killed cultures. The most marked and immediate effect of TBTO was on intracellular ATP levels and on "energy charge" (the ratio between ATP and AMP in the cell). Three concentrations of TBTO (0.112, 1.12, and 11.2 mg/litre) were tested and produced reductions of intracellular ATP to 45%, 18%, and 15%, respectively, each within 1 min of addition of the TBTO. The effect persisted at the lowest exposure level for at least 3 h. Dramatic and immediate falls were also seen in energy charge. The authors consider this to be the major effect of the TBTO. Concomitant falls in nucleic acid synthesis, synthesis of macromolecules, and CO_2 production were assumed to follow from the basic action. The wide range of concentrations producing graded growth inhibition, compared to the very small additional increase in exposure required to cause cell death, suggested to the authors that there were two separate mechanisms for the growth inhibition and lethality of TBTO.

Argaman et al. (1984) investigated the toxic effect of TBTO on activated sludge from municipal sewage treatment plants. Sludge challenged with a single dose of TBTO was inhibited (Warburg respirometer oxygen consumption measurements) by concentrations of 25 µg/litre or more. However, sludge pre-treated with TBTO at levels of 200 or 1000 µg/litre adapted to the TBTO and no effect was found on the ability of sludge organisms to break down organic materials.

7.2 Freshwater algae

The MIC for cultures of the green alga *Chlorella pyrenoidosa* with TBTO was 0.5 mg/litre (Bokranz & Plum, 1975). Floch et al. (1964) reported a no-observed-effect-level on the growth of a freshwater green alga (desmid) of 0.25 mg TBTO/litre or 0.15 mg TBT acetate/litre over an exposure period of 10 days. No growth occurred at concentrations of 0.5 mg TBTO/litre or 0.3 mg TBT acetate/litre. Deschiens & Floch (1968) reported an LC_{100} value for *Chlorella* over 10 to 20 days of 0.5 mg TBTO/litre.

More recent studies have suggested that aquatic algae are much more sensitive to TBT than earlier reports indicated.

Wong et al. (1982) determined the IC_{50} (concentration required to produce a 50% inhibition) for primary productivity (uptake of ^{14}C-labelled carbonate) and reproduction of pure cultures of algae and for a natural phytoplankton community from Lake Ontario, Canada. The natural community was the most sensitive to TBTO, with an IC_{50} for primary productivity of 3 µg/litre. *Ankistrodesmus falcatus* showed similar patterns for the effect of TBTO on primary productivity and on reproduction (growth), though the latter was slightly more sensitive with an IC_{50} of 5 µg/litre compared to 20 µg/litre for productivity. The green alga *Scenedesmus quadricaudata* and the cyanobacterium (blue-green alga) *Anabaena flos-aquae* gave IC_{50} values for primary productivity of 16 and 13 µg/litre, respectively. RIVM (1989) reported 96-h EC_{50} values for *Chlorella* and *Scenedesmus pannonicus* of 42 and 64 µg TBTO/litre, respectively, and no-observed-effect-levels of 18 and 32 µg/litre, respectively.

7.3 Estuarine and marine algae

Many diatoms are highly resistant to the effects of organometallic compounds. Thomas & Robinson (1987) studied the tolerance of the diatom *Amphora coffeaeformis* to TBT fluoride and found that its growth was unaffected at concentrations of less than 10^{-7} mol/litre when the initial culture cell density was 10×10^4 cells/ml. At the end of the incubation, when the diatom had stopped growing, there was no nitrate left in the medium. There was a significant effect of TBT fluoride at 10^{-7} mol/litre on growth when the diatom was grown in nitrate-deficient medium. Growth was also affected, to a lesser degree, by reducing the silicate in the medium in the presence of TBT fluoride. The authors concluded that TBTO tolerance in the diatom is not due to the exclusion of the organotin but to detoxification mechanisms requiring increased uptake of nitrate. Recovery of the organisms after 24 h exposure supported this theory. After short-term exposure to sublethal, but inhibitory, concentrations of TBT fluoride, *Amphora* recovered within 24 h (Thomas & Robinson, 1986). Uptake of nitrate was inhibited initially but recovered after 24 h.

Salazar (1985) exposed three species of marine phytoplankton *(Gymnodinium splendens, Dunaliella* sp., and *Phaeodactylum tricornutum)* to TBTO concentrations of 1.5, 3, and 6 µg/litre for a period of 72 h. At the lowest concentration, all of the *G. splendens* cells were killed and growth of *Dunliella* sp. was inhibited. The growth of *Dunliella* sp. was completely inhibited at both 3 and 6 µg/litre, whereas no effect on the growth of *P. tricornutum* was observed at any of the test concentrations. Beaumont & Newman (1986) cultured the marine algae *Pavlova lutheri, Dunaliella tertiolecta,* and *Skeletonema costatum* with TBTO at 0.1, 1.0, and 5.0 µg per litre. All algae exposed to 5.0 µg/litre died within 2 days. A comparison of the slope of the growth curve with maximum increase in cell density in the culture showed that all of the algae were significantly inhibited by TBTO at the lowest concentration tested. This concentration was not algicidal. Thain (1983) gave the algistatic concentration for TBTO against *Tetraselmis suecica* as 560 to 1000 µg/litre and against *Skeletonema costatum* as 1.0 to 18 µg/litre, within 5 days of exposure. Corresponding algicidal concentrations were > 1000 µg/litre for *Tetraselmis* and > 18 µg/litre for *Skeletonema*. Walsh et al. (1985) calculated the EC_{50} values for growth inhibition of the marine alga *Skeletonema costatum* by TBT acetate, TBTO, TBT chloride, and TBT fluoride to be 0.36, 0.33, 0.36, and 0.25-0.50 µg/litre, respectively, for a 72-h exposure period. The EC_{50} values for growth inhibition of *Thalassiosira pseudonanna*, another marine species, by TBT acetate and TBTO were 1.28 and 1.03 µg per litre, respectively. The LC_{50} for *Skeletonema* was 14.7, 14.2, 11.5, and 11.9 µg/litre for TBT acetate, TBTO, TBT chloride, and TBT fluoride, respectively. Algae did not adapt to the presence of TBTO after exposure through 12 serial transfers over 12 weeks; EC_{50} values were the same for previously exposed cells as for naive cells. Dojmi Di Delupis et al. (1987) calculated the 8-day EC_{50} for growth inhibition of the marine algal species *Dunaliella tertiolecta* and *Nitzschia* sp., exposed to TBTO, to be 4.53 µg/litre and 1.19 µg/litre, respectively.

His et al. (1986) conducted bioassays to measure the susceptibility of algae that are food organisms for oysters to TBT-containing antifouling paints. Four algal species were used in the studies: *Isochrysis galbana* (Prymnesiophyceae); *Chaetocerus calcitrans* (Bacillariophyceae); *Tetraselmis (Platymonas) suecica* (Prasinophyceae); and *Phaeodactylum tricornutum* (Bacillariophyceae). Cultures were maintained in filtered sea water with a salinity of 27°/$_{oo}$ and at a temperature of 20 °C. TBT exposure was either to pure TBT acetate or as plates painted with "International TBT antifouling" with a surface area of between 0.01 and 1.0 cm^2 in a culture of 2 litres. Culture density was estimated every 3 to 4 days using a Coulter counter. Exposure to the pure TBT acetate at 1 µg/litre had no effect on any of the algal cultures. *Isochrysis* growth was totally inhibited by painted panels of 1.0, 0.25, and 0.125 cm^2 within 2 days of culture. Smaller panels were then used to find the limit of the effect. A 0.02-cm^2 panel was also totally toxic to growth of the alga; panels of 0.01 cm^2 allowed growth comparable to a control culture over the first week of culture but then inhibited growth. By the 21st day of culture, the number of cells was reduced to 1.8 x 10^6 cells per ml, compared to a control density of 3.2×10^6 cells per ml. For *Chaetocerus*, panels of 0.02 cm^2 were toxic to the alga from the beginning of the culture period; numbers of cells were reduced, indicating that not only growth but also viability was affected. With panels of 0.01 cm^2, there was complete inhibition of development over the first 4 days, followed by a decrease in cell numbers from the original value. The two other algal species were less sensitive. *Phaeodactylum* was inhibited by panels of 1.0 and 0.5 cm^2 from the outset of culture. Inhibition also occurred with panels of 0.25 and 0.125 cm^2, but only after several days. *Tetraselmis* grew in the presence of panels of all sizes up to 1.0 cm^2, though at this exposure, growth was reduced. Exposure to panels of 0.5 cm^2 had little effect. The authors also tested the effect on algal growth of fresh water from the river feeding the area of interest and also the effect of river sediment. In both cases, growth of the algae was greater than growth of controls, suggesting a greater availability of nutrients. However, it should be noted that no analysis was made of actual water concentrations of TBT in this study; since the precise exposure levels are unknown, the results are difficult to interpret or evaluate.

8. EFFECTS ON ORGANISMS IN THE ENVIRONMENT: AQUATIC ORGANISMS

8.1 Aquatic plants

Summary

Few studies have been carried out on the effects of TBT on aquatic plants. The lowest effect level was observed for Enteromorpha intestinalis. Motile spores were inhibited from settling by TBTO, the EC_{50} being 1 ng/litre; newly settled spores increased in resistance with time. Results should be interpreted with care because TBT concentrations were not measured and the experimental protocols were incomplete.

Reduction in the growth of freshwater species was observed at concentrations down to 0.06 mg/litre.

Davies et al. (1984) studied the effect of various TBT compounds on spore development in the marine green macro-alga, *Enteromorpha intestinalis*. The 5-day EC_{50} values for newly-settled *Enteromorpha* spores ranged from 0.027 µg/litre (TBT benzoate) to 8.6 µg/litre (TBT acrylate). The authors stated that the toxicity appeared to be influenced by the type of anion. Using TBTO it was found that sensitivity decreased with increasing settlement time; the 5-day EC_{50} values for spore development ranged from 0.22 µg/litre, when exposure began 30 min after settlement, to 10 µg/litre, when exposure began 72 h after settlement. Motile spores were the most sensitive (5-day EC_{50} = 0.001 µg/litre).

The marine angiosperm *Zostera marina* showed reduced growth at TBT concentrations in sediment of 1.0 mg/kg but no effect at 0.1 mg/kg (Personal communication by M.J. Waldock to IPCS, 1989).

Floch et al. (1964) exposed freshwater aquatic plants to TBTO or TBT acetate, at water concentrations between 0.03 and 1.2 mg/litre, for 10 days. The duckweed *Lemna media* and Canadian pondweed *Elodea* sp. both showed some growth at TBTO concentrations of 0.03 mg/litre. Duckweed maintained itself, without significant growth, at concentrations between 0.06 and 0.25 mg/litre, but died at 0.5

mg/litre. *Elodea* showed degeneration between 0.06 and 0.25 mg/litre and died at 0.5 mg/litre. Degeneration of *Elodea* was evident at 0.15 mg TBT acetate/litre; growth occurred at 0.03 mg/litre and death at 0.3 mg/litre. *Lemna* grew in 0.15 mg TBT acetate/litre and died at 1.2 mg/litre; there was maintenance without growth at 0.6 mg/litre.

L.A. Boorman (personal communication to the IPCS, 1989) grew plants of two salt marsh species, *Aster tripolium* and *Limonium vulgare*, in mud with added TBTO. Plants of *Aster* were killed by sediment TBTO levels in excess of 10 µg/kg (dry weight), while *Limonium* was not significantly affected by levels of up to 150 µg/kg.

Chu (1976) found that the aquatic weed *Ceratophyllum* died within 2 months exposure to a controlled release rubber formulation containing 5% TBTO (5 mg/litre); the exposure period being 24 h every 3 to 5 days.

8.2 Aquatic invertebrates

The acute toxicity of tributyltin to aquatic invertebrates is summarized in Tables 8, 9, and 10. Larval stages are considerably more sensitive to TBT than adults; the LC_{50} for the larval Pacific oyster is 1.6 µg per litre, over 48 h, whereas that for adults is 1800 µg per litre (Thain, 1983). Other species show similar differences between life stages. The 96-h LC_{50} values for crustaceans range between 1.0 and 41 µg/litre. There are fewer data on freshwater species; these relate to just three species other than target organisms. Various TBT salts give a range of 48-h LC_{50} values for *Daphnia* of 2.3 to 70 µg/litre and for *Tubifex* of 5.5 to 33 µg per litre. The 24-h LC_{50} for the Asiatic clam is 2100 µg per litre, and that for target snail adults in schistosomiasis control is 30 to 400 µg/litre.

8.2.1 Trematode parasites of man

Some organotin molluscicides have been shown to be toxic to schistosome larvae in the aquatic stages. Ritchie et al. (1974) found that TBTO concentrations of 10 and 100 µg/litre rendered *Schistosoma mansoni* cercariae, the infective stage released from the secondary host (water snails), incapable of progressive movement, following a 5-min exposure. Infectivity of the cercariae to mice was

Effects on Organisms in the Environment: Aquatic Organisms

Table 8. Toxicity of tributyltin to marine invertebrates

Organism	Size/age	Stat/flow[a]	Temperature (°C)	Salinity (°/oo)	pH	TBT salt	Duration (h)	LC_{50}[c] (µg/litre)	Reference
Eastern oyster (Crassostrea virginica)	embryo larva	stat[b]	28		7.1	chloride	48 48	1.3 (0.78-1.38)[d] 3.96 (2.42-4.21)[d]	Roberts (1987)
European oyster (Ostrea edulis)	adult	stat[b]				oxide	48 96	> 300 210	Thain (1983)
Pacific oyster (Crassostrea gigas)	larva adult adult	stat[b]				oxide	48 48 96	1.6 1800 290	Thain (1983)
Mussel (Mytilus edulis)	larva adult adult	stat[b]				oxide	48 48 96	23 300 38	Thain (1983)
Hard clam (Mercenaria mercenaria)	embryo larva	stat[b]	28		7.1	chloride	48 48	1.13 (0.72-1.31)[d] 1.65[d]	Roberts (1987)
Brown shrimp (Crangon crangon)	larva larva adult adult	stat[b]				oxide	48 96 48 96	6.5 1.5 73 41	Thain (1983)
Grass shrimp (Palaemonetes pugio)	sub-adult	flow	19.4-21.3	9.8-12.1	8.15-8.31	oxide chloride	96 96	20[d] > 31[d,f]	Walsh (1986) Bushong et al. (1988)

Table 8 (contd).

Species	Stage	Conditions	Temp	Salinity	pH	Compound	Duration (h)	LC50 (μg/litre)	Reference
Mysid shrimp (*Mysidopsis bahia*)	< 1 day 5 day 10 day	flow	24-26	19-22.3	7.98-8.01	chloride	96	1.1 (0.68-1.4)[d] 2 (1.4-2.6)[d] 2.2 (1.4-2.6)[d]	Goodman et al. (1988)
Shore crab (*Carcinus maenus*)	larva	stat[b]				oxide	48 96	110 10	Thain (1983)
Harpacticoid copepod (*Nitocra spinipes*)	adult	stat	20-22	7	7.8	fluoride oxide	96 96	2 (1-2)[e] 2 (1-3)[e]	Linden et al. (1979)
Copepod (*Eurytemora affinis*)	sub-adult sub-adult sub-adult sub-adult	flow flow stat stat	20 20 19.4-20.3 19.4-20.3	10 10 10.1-11.2 10.1-11.2	8.17-8.32 8.17-8.32	chloride chloride chloride chloride	72 48 48 72	0.6 (0.1-2.0)[d,f] 1.4 (0.8-2.3)[d,f] 2.2 (0.2-7.3)[d,f] 0.6 (0-3.3)[d,f]	Bushong et al. (1987) Hall et al. (1988b)
Copepod (*Acartia tonsa*)	sub-adult adult	flow stat[b]	20 19.5-20.5	10		chloride oxide	48 96	1.1 (0.7-2.2)[d,f] 1.0 (0.8-1.2)[d]	Bushong et al. (1987) U'Ren (1983)
Amphipod (*Gammarus* sp.)	young adult	flow	19.4-21.3	9.8-12.1	8.15-8.31	chloride chloride	96 96	1.3[d,f] 5.3[d,f]	Bushong et al. (1988)

[a] stat = static conditions (water unchanged for the duration of the test unless stated otherwise); flow = flow-through conditions (TBT concentration in water continuously maintained).
[b] Static renewal conditions (water changed periodically).
[c] 95% confidence limits are given in brackets.
[d] Measured concentration.
[e] Nominal concentration.
[f] Concentration expressed as TBT.

Table 9. Toxicity of tributyltin to freshwater invertebrates

Organism	Size/age	Stat/flow[a]	Temperature (°C)	Hardness[c] (mg/litre)	pH	TBT salt	Duration (h)	LC_{50}[d] (μg/litre)	Reference
Asiatic clam (*Corbicula fluminea*)	larva	stat	20			oxide	24	2100[e]	Foster (1981)
Water flea (*Daphnia magna*)	adult	stat[b]	21			chloride	96	5.9 (3.7-9.4)[e]	Meador (1986)
	adult	stat[b]	21			chloride	120	3.4 (1.3-8.8)[e]	Meador (1986)
						acetate	48	3.3 (1.5-6.0)[e,f]	Polster & Halacka (1971)
						oleate	48	8.5 (4.2-10.5)[e,f]	
						benzoate	48	4.3 (1.8-9.5)[e,f]	
						chloride	48	4.5 (1.2-9.3)[e,f]	
						laurate	48	4.7 (1.2-9.3)[e,f]	
						oxide	48	2.3 (1.2-5.2)[e,f]	
	juvenile	stat	20	200	7.5	chloride	24	13[e]	Vighi & Calamari (1985)
	juvenile	stat	20	200	7.5	oxide	24	14[e]	Vighi & Calamari (1985)
	juvenile	stat	19		8.2	oxide	48	4.7	RIVM (1989)
	juvenile	stat	20			oxide	48	70[e]	Foster (1981)
Tubifex worm (*Tubifex tubifex*)						acetate	48	8.0 (2.8-10.3)[e,f]	Polster & Halacka (1971)
						oleate	48	17.0 (10.1-30.0)[e,f]	
						benzoate	48	16.0 (10.1-27.0)[e,f]	
						chloride	48	15.0 (10.1-23.0)[e,f]	
						laurate	48	33.0 (10.6-75.0)[e,f]	
						oxide	48	5.5 (1.6-10.3)[e,f]	

[a] stat = static conditions (water unchanged for the duration of the test unless stated otherwise); flow = flow-through conditions (TBT concentration in water continuously maintained).
[b] Static renewal conditions (water changed periodically).
[c] Hardness expressed as mg/litre $CaCO_3$.
[d] 95% confidence limits are given in brackets; concentrations expressed as the TBT salt used unless otherwise stated.
[e] Nominal concentration.
[f] Concentration expressed as TBT.

completely suppressed. A 30-min exposure to concentrations of 1 µg/litre or less had relatively little effect on motility of cercariae and on subsequent infectivity of mice. The authors also exposed *S. mansoni* miracidia to TBTO and found that 10 µg/litre immobilized the miracidia after a 40-min exposure and completely suppressed the infectivity to snails *(Biomphalaria glabrata)*. However, a concentration of 1 µg/litre had no effect on motility and infectivity after an exposure period of 120 min.

Viyanant et al. (1982) exposed *Schistosoma mansoni* cercariae to TBT fluoride and calculated an LC_{50} of 16.8 µg/litre and an LC_{90} of 21.7 µg/litre for a 1-h exposure. Following a 1-h exposure of *S. mansoni* to TBT fluoride, cercarial infectivity of mice was observed over a period of 30 min. A 100% suppression of infectivity was found at 6 µg/litre; effective doses (99%-100%) were between 2 and 6 µg/litre.

8.2.2 Freshwater molluscs

Summary

The LC_{50} values for target fresh water snail adults in schistosomiasis control range from 30 to 400 µg/litre. This indicates very low selectivity of TBT as a Bilharzia molluscicide, and a high risk to sensitive non-target aquatic species.

The lethal concentrations of TBT to adult Bilharzia snails are also expected to inhibit motility and infectivity of both cercariae and miracidiae in the contaminated water, as the suppressive levels were found to be 10 µg/litre for both cercariae and miracidiae of Schistosoma mansoni *after 5 and 40 min, respectively. The 1-h LC_{50} for cercariae is 16.8 µg per litre.*

Generally, the toxicity of TBT to freshwater snails depends on the species, stage, age, temperature, pH, time of exposure, time of observation, suspended matter, and type of structure and formulation.

Pellets or matrices of natural rubber or synthetic polymers impregnated with TBT produce a slow-release effective level of the molluscicides, which results in low acute toxicity but extended long-term toxicity.

Exposure of adult snails to TBT levels as low as 0.01 to 0.001 µg/litre reduced egg laying, inhibited hatchability of the exposed eggs, and retarded the development of the surviving offspring.

The no-observed-effect level for adult freshwater snails (Limnaea stagnalis) was 0.32 µg/litre in long-term tests.

TBT compounds are strongly adsorbed on to suspended clay and organic particles. These particulates are ingested by the snails and provide one of the inputs for toxicity. Studies of the impact of type and amount of suspended matter on TBT toxicity to snails vary in their conclusions.

Increasing the pH was found to enhance the molluscicidal toxicity of slow-release TBT formulations.

The acute toxicity of TBT to adult freshwater snails is summarized in Table 10. The data are based mainly on species that are intermediate hosts in the life-cycle of the parasite causing Bilharzia (schistosomiasis) in man, TBT being used as a molluscicide to control the disease. The toxic action of TBT is slow, the mortality at the end of a 24-h exposure is often low, and for a more realistic result a post-exposure observation period is required.

Rubber impregnated with TBT to produce a slow-release molluscicide that maintains a low, but toxic, concentration over a long period was developed by Cardarelli and colleagues, and was shown to be very effective against snail pest species such as *Biomphalaria glabrata* and *B. globosus* (Berrios-Duran & Ritchie, 1968).

Molluscicidal activity has been demonstrated against *Bulinus* spp., *Biomphalaria* spp., and certain operculate freshwater molluscs, but organotin compounds have proved to be not as toxic against the amphibious oncomelaniid snails (McCullough et al., 1980).

8.2.2.1 Acute toxicity

Webbe (1963) found that young snails *(Biomphalaria sudanica* and *Bulinus nasutus)* were more sensitive than adults to TBT acetate, the 24-h LC_{50} values being 14 and 15 µg/litre for the two snail species, respectively. When eggs from the same two species were exposed, the 24-h

Table 10. Acute toxicity of tributyltin to freshwater snails

Species	TBT salt	Exposure duration (h)	Post-exposure observation (h)	LC_{50} (µg/litre)	Reference
Biomphalaria glabrata	oxide	6	72	410	Seiffer & Schoof (1967)
	acetate	6	72	290	Seiffer & Schoof (1967)
	oxide	6	24	370	Ritchie et al. (1964)
	oxide	24	24	40	Ritchie et al. (1964)
	acetate	6	24	190	Ritchie et al. (1964)
	acetate	24	24	85	Ritchie et al. (1964)
	acetate	24		100-300	Hopf et al. (1967)
	pentachloro-phenate	24		100-400	Hopf et al. (1967)
	oxide	24		50-100	Hopf et al. (1967)
	oxide	24		30	Deschiens et al. (1966)
	acetate	24	72	170	Paulini (1964)
Biomphalaria contortus	oxide	24		30	Deschiens et al. (1966)
Biomphalaria sudanica	acetate	24	48	34	Webbe (1963)
Bulinus nasutus	acetate	24	48	32	Webbe (1963)
Bulinus tropicus	oxide	17	24	10	de Villiers & MacKenzie (1963)
Limnaea stagnalis	oxide	24	96	60	Temmink & Everts (1987)
	oxide	96	96	24	Temmink & Everts (1987)
	oxide	96		42	RIVM (1989)

LC_{50} values ranged from 100 to 1000 µg/litre. Paulini (1964) found embryos of *Biomphalaria glabrata* to be more susceptible than adults to TBT acetate. The 24-h LC_{50} values for embryos ranged from 26 µg/litre at 5-12 h of age to 46 µg/litre at 77-87 h of age, whereas the value for adults was 170 µg/litre.

2.2.2 Short- and long-term toxicity

Ritchie et al. (1974) found that egg laying in *Biomphalaria glabrata* was completely inhibited by 10 µg TBTO/litre, all the snails being killed within 2 to 5 days. Egg laying was reduced, over a period of 2 to 3 weeks, by more than 90% at 1 µg/litre and by 50% at 0.1 µg/litre. At 0.01 µg/litre, egg laying was unaffected. Newly-laid eggs were exposed to TBTO for 34 days followed by 50 days in clean water. Eggs exposed to 10 µg per litre did not hatch, even after 50 days in clean water. Of those exposed to 1 µg/litre, only 3% hatched during the exposure and 35% of the rest hatched after transfer to clean water (but with a delayed hatching time). When newly-hatched snails were exposed to TBTO, 95% of those exposed to 1 µg/litre from hatching died and those that survived failed to lay eggs for 85 days. At 0.1 µg/litre, 60% of the snails died and egg laying in the survivors was reduced by 80%. Egg laying was also significantly reduced at both 0.01 and 0.001 µg/litre.

Upatham et al. (1980) studied the toxicity to *Bulinus abyssinicus* of various controlled-release organotin molluscicides, i.e. BioMet SRM rubber pellets (6% TBTO), CBL-9B rubber pellets (20% TBT fluoride), and EC-13 floating ethylene propylene co-polymer pellets (30% TBT fluoride). The organotin compounds killed all of the snails within 1 to 2 days at 100 mg/litre (active ingredient) and within 5 to 7 days at 1 mg/litre, there being no significant difference between the compounds. Changing the test water daily had no significant effect. At lower concentrations the molluscicides required 36 to 40 days to kill all the snails at an active ingredient concentration of 0.03 mg/litre, and at 0.3 mg/litre 9 to 10 days was required for BioMet SRM and CBL-9B, and 22 days for EC-13.

In long-term exposure tests, toxic effects on freshwater snails have been found at very low TBT concentrations. Cardarelli (1973) quoted a 120-day LC_{100} of 7 µg TBTO/litre for *Biomphalaria glabrata*. At 0.7 µg per litre, 26% of the snails died within 120 days. RIVM (1989) reported a NOEL for the freshwater snail *Limnaea stagnalis* of 0.32 µg/litre in long-term tests.

8.2.2.3 *Factors affecting toxicity*

Paulini & de Souza (1970) studied the effect of various factors on the molluscicidal activity of TBT to freshly laid eggs of *Biomphalaria glabrata*. A concentration of colloidal clay (the proportion of clay to molluscicide was 1000:1) of 1000 mg/litre reduced the 24-h LC_{50} (with a 7-day recovery period included in the mortality count) by 30% for TBT acetate and by 7% for TBTO. The addition of a yeast *(Saccharomyces* sp.) suspension

(1 g/litre) reduced the 24-h LC_{50} (with a 24-h recovery period) by 95% for TBTO and 72% for TBT acetate. The proportion of yeast to molluscicide was 1000:1 for TBTO and 100:1 for TBT fluoride.

Cardarelli & Evans (1980) studied the effect of various factors on the toxicity to snails of controlled-release organotin molluscicides, i.e. BioMet SRM (6% TBTO in natural rubber) and CBL-9B (20% TBT fluoride in natural rubber). Using 100-mg/kg pellets, they found that increasing the pH from 6 to 8 increased the toxicity (as measured by both LT_{50} and LT_{100}) of BioMet SRM but decreased the toxicity of CBL-9B to both *Biomphalaria glabrata* and *Bulinus globosus*. The authors found no effect of yeast or humic acid (1 to 100 mg/litre) on the toxicity (LT_{100}) of these controlled-release molluscicides, neither did they find an effect of suspended colloidal clays. They concluded that, although the organotin compounds are adsorbed, they are still toxic because the snails ingest the added materials. Therefore, snails are still exposed to TBT even after it is adsorbed to surfaces. In an experiment to compare adsorbed uptake of TBT, soil-browsing snails and isolated snails were compared during exposure to slow-release organotin pellets. The molluscicides were found to be more toxic when the snails were allowed to browse on soil, and, at a distance of 60 cm from the pellets, isolated snails were producing egg masses whereas those browsing on soil were not. The authors also concluded that the organotin molecules that come into contact with soil particles are adsorbed and slowly form ligands of a nontoxic nature, so that soil only remains toxic as long as it is freshly exposed to organotin. Upatham et al. (1980) found that the presence of mud or plant life, compared to exposure in water alone, had no effect on the toxicity (LT_{100}) of either CBL-9B or EC-13 at 1 or 10 mg/litre (active ingredient) to *Bulinus abyssinicus*. When the snails were exposed to BioMet SRM, no effect of mud or plants was found at 10 mg/litre, but at 1 mg/litre a slightly shorter time was required to kill all the snails in water alone. Chu (1976) noted that organic materials such as mud and weeds reduced the molluscicidal activity of TBTO on *Bulinus rohlfsi*, when exposed to a rubber formulation containing 5% TBTO (5 mg/litre TBTO), with a 24-h exposure period every 3 to 5 days for 70 days and twice a month for a further 7 months.

Macklad et al. (1983) found that the toxicity of controlled-release molluscicides containing TBT fluoride was dependent on the pre-exposure soaking time. The 48-h LC_{50} for *Biomphalaria alexandrina* of 10 mg/litre total available toxicant was achieved after 7, 3, and 1 days soaking period for the formulations EC27 (10% TBT fluoride in a plastic polymer), EC1320 (20% TBT fluoride in rubber), and EC1330 (30% TBT fluoride in a polypropylene/polyethylene mixture), respectively. EC1330 produced no mortality following a 3-h soaking period and exposure to concentrations ranging from 1 to 100 mg/litre for 48-h; the authors suggested that the polypropylene/polyethylene mixture (EC1330) needs to be sufficiently wet before it begins to release TBT fluoride. A second experiment to test the aging of slow-release molluscicides was carried out. EC27 gave 89% snail mortality during a 48-h exposure period to 50 mg/litre after a soaking time of 24-h. After being left to age for 1 month the molluscicide was tested again and had lost 80% of its original toxicity.

8.2.3 Marine molluscs

Summary

A large body of data exists on the effects of TBT on marine molluscs and in particular on commercially important bivalves. Sublethal effects occur at very low concentrations. It has been shown experimentally that TBT affects shell deposition of growing oysters, gonad development and gender of adult oysters, settlement, growth, and mortality of larval oysters and of other bivalves, and causes imposex (the development of male characteristics) in female gastropods. The NOEL for shell thickening of the most sensitive oyster species (C. gigas) is about 20 ng/litre. Embryo-larval stages are more susceptible than adults; adverse effects on larval development have been demonstrated at concentrations as low as 50 ng/litre. The NOEL is 20 ng/litre.

The authors of recent work on imposex in Nucella have determined threshold concentrations by extrapolation below the limit of reliable detection. While the circumstantial evidence in support is substantial (see chapter 10), the determination of toxicological thresholds below the limits of chemical detection is not practicable. It is generally agreed that imposex is not a specific index of TBT contamination, in that it can be induced by other factors. The wide distribution of low concentrations of TBT and the incidence of imposex at levels similar to or below the analytical detection limits make long-term controlled experiments difficult. The establishment of NOELs will have to await the development of better analytical techniques.

.2.3.1 *Acute toxicity*

Waldock & Thain (1985) calculated the 24-h EC_{50} (mortality plus moribundity) of two organotin-containing fishnet antifouling preparations for larval oysters to be 12 µg/litre for 'Norimp 200' and 320 µg/litre for 'Flexgard'. These compare with a value for TBTO of 1.7 µg per litre. Thain (1983) pointed out that adult bivalves tend to appear more resistant to pollutants in standard short-term tests since they can close their shell over the test period and thus reduce exposure. Larval stages appear to be much more sensitive in these tests.

.2.3.2 *Short- and long-term toxicity*

Alzieu et al. (1982) kept Pacific oysters *(Crassostrea gigas)* in 150-litre tanks that were successively filled and drained according to the tidal period. To these tanks were added panels coated on one side with TBT fluoride, giving estimated concentrations of 0.2 and 2.0 µg TBT per litre. All oysters died within 30 days in a tank containing the larger panel. In the tank with a panel surface of 50 cm², 30% of oysters died after 110 days of exposure and all oysters within 170 days.

His & Robert (1985) experimentally tested hypotheses regarding the poor performance of Pacific oysters in the Bay of Arcachon, France. Larvae were maintained in the laboratory at TBT acetate concentrations ranging from 0.02 to 100 µg/litre. Growth was affected by all concentrations except 0.02 µg/litre. The next concentration tested (0.05 µg/litre) reduced growth, led to mortality within 10 days, and interrupted normal feeding by day 8. No other effects were noted at 0.02 µg/litre and this was regarded as the NOEL for larvae (see Table 11).

Table 11. Effects of TBT acetate on *Crassostrea gigas* larvae at various water concentrations[a]

Water concentration (µg/litre)	Effect
100	inhibition of fertilization
50	inhibition of segmentation
25	partial inhibition of segmentation (40%)
10	no formation of trochophores
3 to 5	no veligers; malformed trochophores
1	abnormal veligers; total mortality within 6 days
0.5	numbers of abnormal larvae; total mortality within 8 days; perturbation of feeding regime, particularly from 4 to 8 days after exposure; growth greatly reduced
0.2	percentage of D larvae showing abnormalities less elevated; perturbation of feeding regime from day 4; progressive mortality; total by day 12; weak growth
0.1	majority of D larvae normal; marked perturbation of feeding regime from day 6; weak growth until day 6; some survivors after 12 days
0.05	normal D larvae; perturbation of feeding regime, marked on day 8; significant mortality beginning at day 10; reduced growth
0.02	normal D larvae; little mortality; good growth; no effect of TBT

[a] From: His & Robert (1985).

Thain & Waldock (1985) exposed various bivalve spat (common European oyster, *Ostrea edulis;* Pacific oyster, *Crassostrea gigas;* common mussel, *Mytilus edulis;* and carpet shells, *Venerupis decussata* and *Venerupis semidecussata*) to TBT leachate by maintaining them in flowing sea-water tanks containing house slates painted with 'Micron 25R' (containing TBT methacrylate co-polymer). The water concentrations of TBT were 0.24 or 2.6 µg/litre. At 2.6 µg/litre, growth was completely inhibited in all groups and mortality was high (except for *V. semidecussata*) within the 45-day exposure period; all mussels had died within 14 days. At the lower exposure concentration, growth was significantly inhibited in *C. gigas, M. edulis,* and *V. decussata* but not in the other two species. In a second study, the authors reported a severe reduction in growth rate of recently metamorphosed oyster *(Ostrea edulis)* spat after exposure to TBT leachate (0.06 µg per litre) for 10 days under static conditions. Growth rate was reduced between 0 and 10 days of exposure to 0.02 µg per litre, but there was only slight reduction in growth, relative to controls, between days 10 and 20.

Growth curves for oysters *(Ostrea edulis)*, 2-3 mm in size, exposed to different concentrations of TBTO are given in Fig. 3.

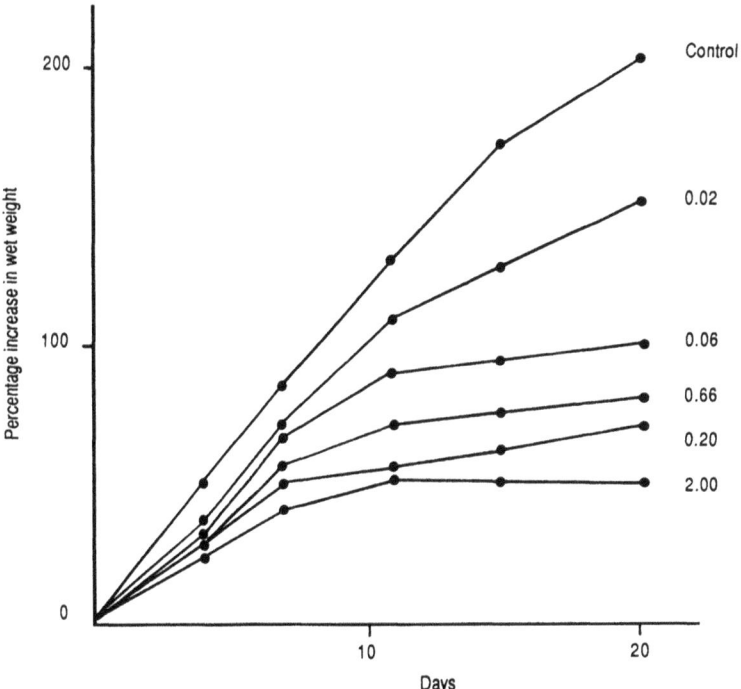

Fig. 3. Growth of oysters *(Ostrea edulis)*, as percentage increase in wet weight, after exposure to various concentrations of TBTO (µg/litre).
From: Thain & Waldock (1985).

Valkirs et al. (1987) calculated the 66-day LC_{50} of TBT chloride for the mussel *Mytilus edulis* to be 0.97 µg per litre under flow-through conditions. Beaumont & Budd (1984) kept larvae of the common mussel, *Mytilus edulis*, in filtered sea water containing TBTO concentrations of 0.1, 1.0, or 10.0 µg/litre. No larvae survived for longer than 5 days at 10 µg/litre, or 10 days at 1.0 µg/litre. Approximately half of the mussel larvae, at 0.1 µg per litre, had died within 15 days. The survivors were moribund, and their growth was significantly slower than that of controls.

Laughlin et al. (1987) exposed the hard-shell clam *Mercenaria mercenaria* to various concentrations of TBTO, under static renewal conditions for larval (veliger) stages and in flowing sea water for juveniles. They found the post-larval settlement stages to be the least sensitive. In a 25-day exposure, only juvenile clams exposed at 10 µg/litre suffered 100% mortality, while those exposed to 7.5 µg/litre or less showed mortality not significantly different from that of controls. When veligers were exposed, none survived TBTO levels of 1 µg per litre or more for longer than 7 days, mortality being 100% within 2 days at 2.5, 5.0, and 7.5 µg/litre. At the end of the 8-day experiment, all controls had become pediveligers. Clams exposed to 0.6 µg/litre showed a survival level of approximately 40% of the control level, but survivors achieved little growth and metamorphosis to pediveligers did not occur. In another set of studies (Laughlin et al., 1987, 1988), clams were exposed, from fertilization to metamorphosis (approximately 14 days), to TBTO concentrations of between 10 and 500 ng/litre. Clams were also exposed for the first 5 days and then kept in clean water for a further 9 days. Survival was found not to be exposure dependent and a recovery period had no effect. Growth was reduced at all concentrations, higher exposure causing greater growth depression. At TBTO concentrations above 100 ng/litre, veligers failed to metamorphose to pediveligers within the 14-day exposure period. Although the 9-day recovery period caused a slight increase in growth, the animals were not significantly larger than clams exposed continuously.

Pickwell & Steinert (1988) exposed adult mussels *(Mytilus edulis)* and oysters *(Crassostrea virginica)* in a flowing sea-water system contaminated with TBT from panels painted with antifouling paint. The TBT concentration was 0.7 µg/litre and exposure lasted for 60 days. Haemolymph was collected from the exposed animals and its protein content measured. Mussel haemolymph protein content at the end of the exposure period was 462 mg/litre, compared with 44 mg/litre in controls. Measurement of haemolymph lysozyme activity and DNA content revealed no difference between controls and treated mussels. This showed that there had been no lysis of the haemocytes and no increase in their numbers. Protein was not, therefore, derived from blood cells. Oysters showed no similar effect of TBT exposure, although haemolymph protein content was much higher than in mussels. Over the course of the experiment, there was approximately 50% mortality in mussels but no deaths among the oysters.

2.3.3 Reproductive effects

Thain & Waldock (1986) reported the results of studies on the reproduction of the European flat oyster *(Ostrea edulis)* exposed to TBT antifouling paints. Three holding tanks were set up each with 50 adult oysters weighing between 50 and 70 g. One tank held controls and the other two were exposed to TBT leaching from painted panels in a mixing tank. A flow rate of 1 litre/min was maintained and the two treatment tanks showed TBT concentrations of 0.24 and 2.6 µg/litre measured at the outflow. Only control oysters released larvae during the course of the 75-day experiment; about five million larvae were released representing probably between four and six spawnings. At the end of the experiment, the gonads of oysters from each treatment were examined histologically. There were no females in either of the treated groups of oysters (20% females in the control group). At 2.6 µg/litre, 18 out of 25 oysters examined were undifferentiated, 7 were male, and none were female. There were 3 undifferentiated gonads out of 27 at the lower exposure level. Gonadal thickness was reduced in a dose-related manner. Mortality was low in all groups (0 in controls and 3 and 5 in the two treatment groups). Shell growth was reduced by TBT exposure; 25 oysters showed growth in the control group, 18 at 0.24 µg/litre, and 4 at 2.62 µg/litre). There were no significant differences between the various groups of oysters using two measures of condition (dry meat weight compared with internal shell volume or compared with wet meat weight). Final body burdens of TBT were 0.19, 0.40, and 1.23 mg/kg wet meat weight for control, low-dose, and high-dose groups, respectively.

Roberts et al. (1987) maintained adult oysters *(Crassostrea virginica)* in TBT solutions containing 0.05, 0.1, 0.5, or 1.0 µg/litre for up to 8 weeks. The oysters were brought into reproductive condition by increasing water temperature. There were no deaths except at the highest exposure concentration, where 20% to 30% mortality occurred between the second and fourth weeks of exposure. Gametes stripped from the exposed oysters were fertilized by gametes from a reference population. There was no evidence that TBT exposure had any effect on the ability of gametes to be fertilized, and there was no statistically significant effect of treatment on the gender of exposed oysters over the 8-week exposure period.

8.2.3.4 *Effects on growth*

Waldock & Thain (1983) maintained spat of the Pacific oyster *(Crassostrea gigas)* in experimental tanks, containing either TBTO, TBT and marine sediment, or just sediment, for 56 days. Weekly growth measurements (measured as wet weight) showed enhanced weight gain in oysters exposed to sediment alone (50 or 100 mg/litre). Low levels of TBTO (0.15 µg/litre) inhibited growth and showed pronounced thickening of the upper valve, and severe inhibition of growth was noted at 1.6 µg/litre. Addition of sediment, along with the TBT, slightly reduced the adverse effect on oyster growth. This experiment was conducted to counter arguments that sediment caused the effects observed in oysters in the field.

Thain (1986) exposed Eastern oyster *(Crassostrea virginica)* spat to TBTO concentrations of 0.02, 0.2, or 2.0 µg/litre under static renewal test conditions for 5 weeks. The percentage increase in growth was substantially reduced at 2.0 µg/litre, whereas at the other two concentrations growth rate was similar to that of controls. No deaths occurred and there was no evidence of shell thickening or deformity in any of the treated animals.

Lawler & Aldrich (1987) exposed Pacific oyster spat to TBTO concentrations of 0.01, 0.02, 0.05, 0.1, or 0.2 µg per litre and monitored the average rate of oxygen consumption before and after exposure. A significant negative correlation was found between TBTO concentration and oxygen consumption. There was also a significant relationship between TBTO concentration in the water and feeding rates. Feeding rates were measured by transmittance, which increases as particulate food matter is removed from the water. Change in transmittance was monitored after 1 h of feeding. As the TBTO concentration in the water increased, feeding rate decreased. Neither oxygen consumption nor feeding was significantly affected below 0.05 µg/litre. Increasing the TBTO level also progressively decreased the ability of the oysters to compensate for hypoxia; this effect was significant down to 0.01 µg/litre. Growth rate (measured as average increase in valve length) was monitored over a 48-day exposure period. There was a significant negative correlation between increasing TBTO concentration and growth. Growth was not significantly affected at the lowest concentration of 0.01 µg TBTO/litre. At levels of 0.05 µg/litre or more, there was an increased incidence of shell thickening. However, reservations must be expressed regarding the experimental design of this work. The authors did not analyse TBT concentrations in the test solutions. In addition, no analyses were carried out on the dilution water, which may have been contaminated by ambient TBT, typically in excess of 10 ng/litre (the lowest threshold determined). Furthermore, the ratio of biomass to water was such that TBT would have been rapidly removed from solution, so that nominal concentrations would have been maintained for only a few hours. Although experimental solutions were replaced daily, the rate of loss invalidates the threshold values cited. Similar criticisms can be made of other work using static or static renewal systems.

Valkirs et al. (1987) exposed adults of both the common mussel *(Mytilus edulis)* and Eastern oyster *(Crassostrea virginica)* to TBT concentrations of 0.04, 0.13, 0.31, 0.73, or 1.89 µg/litre, for a 66-day period, under flowing sea-water conditions. The TBT consisted of leachate from plastic panels painted with antifouling paint. Growth effects were measured by shell length, shell width, and whole body wet weight (soft tissues and shell). Since there was high mussel mortality at a TBT level of

1.89 µg/litre, growth effects were examined in animals exposed to TBT concentrations of up to 0.73 µg/litre. No significant effect on mussel shell width or whole body weight was found, but a significant decrease in shell length was observed at 0.31 and 0.73 µg/litre. More than 90% of all oysters tested within each concentration survived the test period. Statistical analysis of length, width, and weight of oysters could not be carried out since controls were significantly different from exposed groups with respect to initial length of individuals. A condition index (ratio of wet body weight to internal shell volume) was calculated for both mussel and oyster. No significant difference was found at any test concentration for mussels. For oysters, the mean condition indices were significantly lower at concentrations of 0.73 and 1.89 µg/litre, compared both with the indices at lower TBT concentrations and with controls.

Salazar & Salazar (1987) exposed juvenile common mussels *(Mytilus edulis),* in flowing sea water, to TBT concentrations of 70, 80, or 200 ng/litre in a 196-day test and 40, 50, or 160 ng/litre in a 56-day test. Mussel growth (measured as wet weight and length) was not significantly affected up to 56 days in either test. From 63 days to the end of the experiment, there was a significant reduction in growth at all exposure concentrations. No significant mortality was reported in either experiment. A group of controls kept under "field" conditions had growth rates four times that of the laboratory controls over a 56-day period, suggesting that bioassay conditions were stressful for the mussels.

Stromgren & Bongard (1987) exposed juvenile mussels *(Mytilus edulis)* to TBTO concentrations of 0.1 to 10 µg/litre in flowing sea water and measured shell growth (length) at intervals of 24 to 48 h for 7 days. No effect was observed at the lowest exposure concentration, but at 0.4 µg/litre or more there was a significant reduction in shell growth rate. The relationship between TBTO concentration and growth response was approximately hyperbolic. After 7 days of exposure, all groups treated with 0.4 µg/litre or more showed growth rates of approximately 25% (or less) of the control value. The highest exposure concentration reduced growth to approximately 5% of the control value.

.2.3.5 *Shell thickening*

Alzieu et al. (1982) reported that adult oysters *(Crassostrea gigas)* developed gel centres in the shell when they were exposed to TBT fluoride at a concentration of 0.2 µg/litre.

Thain et al. (1987) exposed spat of the Pacific oyster *(Crassostrea gigas)* to TBT concentrations of 2 to 200 ng/litre for 49 days. No effect on shell thickness was observed in controls or at 2 ng TBT/litre. Between 20 and 200 ng/litre, there was a dose-related increase in shell thickness. Severe "balling" occurred at both 100 and 200 ng/litre (where the overall appearance of the oyster shell is spherical rather than having the flattened profile of one valve of a normal oyster) (Fig. 4).

.2.3.6 *Imposex*

The phenomenon of "imposex" was first observed in the field (see section 10.2), the term being used to describe the development of male characteristics by female gastropods. The females develop a penis and ultimately become infertile. Stages in the development of imposex are illustrated in Fig. 5.

Smith (1981a) collected female mud snails *(Nassarius obsoletus)* from three localities designated "dirty", "intermediate", and "clean" on the basis of the degree of imposex noted in the field (see section 10.2). A piece of filter paper with 1.5 to 1.8 g of dried antifouling paint containing TBT and lead arsenate (Alumacide) was placed in 110-litre tanks, and the snails were exposed for 75 days. Halfway through the exposure period, the filter paper was removed because the snails became lethargic. At the end of the exposure period, all snails exposed to the Alumacide had developed significantly more intense imposex. Snails from the "clean" area showed an increase in imposex incidence from 0% to 14.3%, whereas levels of imposex remained constant in snails from "dirty" or "intermediate" areas (> 95% incidence). Penis expression in snails from "dirty" and "intermediate" areas regressed significantly when they were transferred to clean water. However, the extent to which the effects observed in this study can be attributed to TBTO is

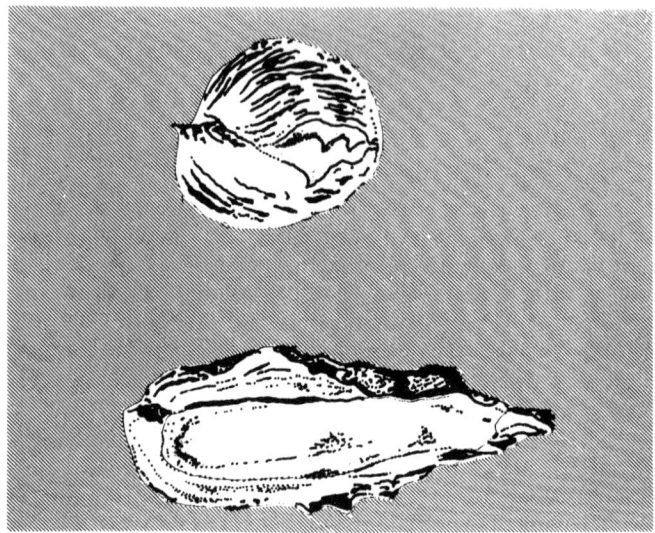

Fig. 4. Diagrammatic cross sections of the oyster *Crassostrea gigas* showing shell-thickening effect ("balling").
Top: thick-shelled oyster from an estuary contaminated with tributyltin
Bottom: normal oyster from an estuary without boating activity
The meat content of the normal oyster is five times more than that of the thickened one.
After: Thain & Waldock (1986).

unclear, since the antifoulant contained two biocides and no analytical measurements were made.

Feral & Le Gall (1983) attempted to identify which part of the neuroendocrine system of a marine gastropod, *Ocenebra erinacea*, was primarily affected in the induction, by TBT, of the development of a penis in female snails. A biological assay was established using isolated female pedal ganglia or complete nervous system (intact complex of pedal ganglia and cerebropleural ganglia) of *Ocenebra erinacea* and isolated presumptive penis-forming areas of a second species *Crepidula fornicata*. When pedal ganglia were cultured with the presumptive penis-forming area in a medium based on either clean or "polluted" sea water (from areas known to have the imposex phenomenon in the field) there was no penis development. Culturing the whole nervous system in a medium based on clean sea water also resulted in no penis growth. However, culturing the complete nervous system with a medium based on "polluted" sea water caused the growth of a penis. Culturing in artificial sea water with added TBT (0.2 µg per litre) also induced penis development. The authors concluded that the primary effect of TBT is on the cerebropleural ganglia of the snails (Fig. 6).

In studies by Bryan et al. (1986), the dogwhelk *Nucella lapillus* was exposed to TBT concentrations of 0.02 µg tin/litre in tidal tanks, the TBT being leached from a co-polymer antifouling paint. Within 4 months, animals of both sexes had accumulated 1 mg tin/kg (as TBT), and females showed a high degree of imposex, which was still increasing. The authors stated that the experiment tended to underestimate the exposure, since the diet of barnacles was initially uncontaminated but would later have contributed TBT to the dogwhelks via an extra route. Gibbs et al. (1987) found that after 12 months of exposure to 18.7 ng tin/litre, penis size in female dogwhelks was increased, and that there was very little difference in size between the sexes. The "control" dogwhelks in this study were actually exposed to TBT at 1.5 ng/litre, which was the background concentration in the sea water used. These control females showed a penis bulk of 10-14% of that of control males. Field observations on populations living in < 0.5 ng/litre showed little penis development (between 2% and 5% of male penis bulk). The NOEL for the development of imposex is, therefore, less than 1.0 ng TBT/litre.

Gibbs et al. (1988) reared dogwhelks in the laboratory for 2 years from hatching in various concentrations of TBT leached from antifouling paints. TBT concentrations in the water were monitored at 1-2, 3-5, 20, and 100 ng tin/litre and tissue concentrations in the whelks were also measured. All exposed females were affected at all concentrations, developing a penis. Penis development (expressed as a relative size index compared to males exposed to the same TBT concentrations) in females was between 50 and 60% of male penis bulk after exposure for 1 and 2 years to TBT

Effects on Organisms in the Environment: Aquatic Organisms

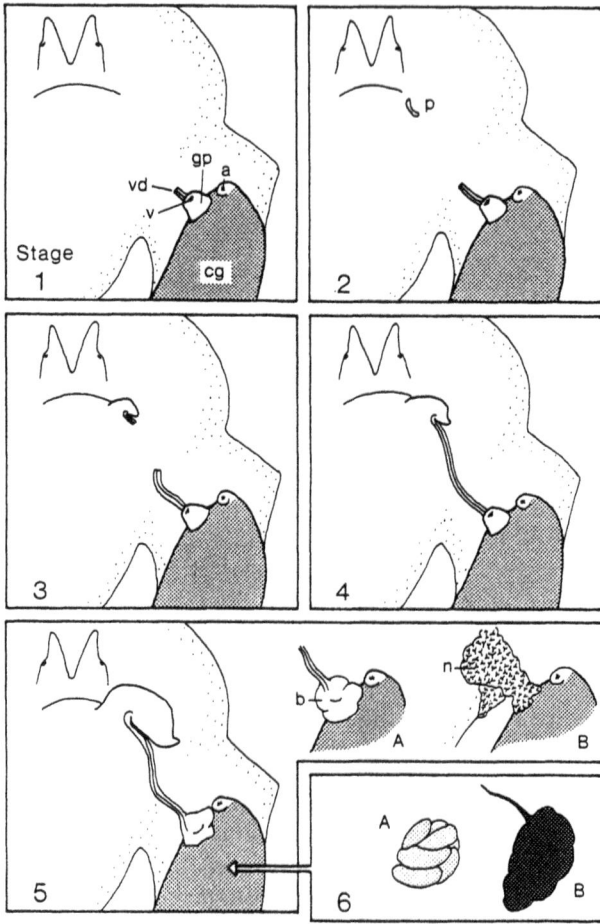

Fig. 5. Stages in the development of imposex in *Nucella lapillus* based on vas deferens sequence.
Stage 0 - the normal female state with no male character being visibly superimposed; pallial oviduct terminates at a clearly defined opening or vulva situated at the apex of a prominent genital papilla which projects into the mantle cavity.
Stage 1 - development of proximal section of vas deferens commencing by infolding of the mantle cavity epithelium in the region ventral to the genital papilla.
Stage 2 - development of penis initiated with the formation of a ridge a short distance behind the right tentacle.
Stage 3 - small penis formed and development of distal section of vas deferens commencing from base of penis.
Stage 4 - proximal and distal sections of vas deferens now fused and penis enlargement to a size approaching that of the male.

Stage 5 - proliferating vas deferens tissue overgrowing genital papilla causing vulva to be displaced, constricted or no longer visible; blister-like protuberances may appear around site of the papilla (5A), and nodules of hyperplastic tissue often develop (5B).
Stage 6 - lumen of capsule gland contains material of aborted capsules; this material may comprise a single capsule or several to many that are compressed together to form a translucent or brown mass (6 A,B).
Abbreviations: a = anus; b = blister; gp = genital papilla; n = nodule; p = penis; v = vulva; vd = vas deferens
From: Gibbs et al. (1987).

at a level of 1-2 ng tin/litre. The female penis reached comparable size to that of the male on exposure to TBT levels of 3-5 ng tin/litre or more. At increasing TBT exposure concentrations, further male characteristics developed and further female characteristics were repressed. At TBT concentrations in the water of 1-2 ng tin/litre, some females retained the capacity to breed although others were sterilized by oviduct blockage. At 3-5 ng/litre, virtually all females were sterilized but oogenesis was apparently normal. At 10 ng/litre, oogenesis was suppressed, oocytes were resorbed, and spermatogenesis was initiated. At 20 ng/litre, there was a functional testis in the "females", with ripe sperm in the most-affected animals.

Bryan et al. (1988) investigated the capacity of various organotin compounds to induce imposex in the dogwhelk. Whelks, already slightly affected by imposex, were taken from the wild and exposed to 200 ng/litre tin, in the form of TBT chloride, tri-n-propyl tin (TPrT), tetrabutyltin (TTBT), dibutyltin (DBT), or triphenyltin (TPhT), for 14 days before being returned to the shore. Penis size, as a percentage of male penis size, increased to 44% in females exposed to TBT chloride, compared with 6% in controls. TPrT increased relative penis size to only 14%, and no other compound had any effect. In an attempt to eliminate differences due to differential uptake of the compounds, the organotin compounds were injected in a second experiment. The females were maintained in the laboratory for up to 105 days. TBT again induced increased penis size but TTBT also showed an effect (19.5% compared to the 34% shown after TBT injection). Other compounds were ineffective. The authors believed the effect of TTBT to be caused by contamination by TBT and conversion to TBT in the tissues. However, the increased imposex after treatment with TPrT could not be explained in this way and the imposex effect is considered to be not totally specific to tributyltin.

8.2.3.7 Genotoxicity

Dixon & Prosser (1986) found that TBTO was not genotoxic, at concentrations of 0.05 to 5.0 µg tin/litre, to the larvae of the mussel *Mytilus edulis*. Results were based on chromosome analysis and sister chromatid exchange (SCE). In 4-day acute toxicity studies, TBTO was found to cause a dose-dependent reduction in both larval survival and development of mussels. Survival ranged from 46% of controls at 0.05 µg/litre to 1.4% at 5 µg/litre. The percentage of animals reaching the D-shell stage of development was 8.7% of controls at the lowest dose, but none reached this stage at either 1 or 5 µg/litre. However, when mussel larvae were exposed to a standard mutagen (mitomycin C) or crude oil, in the presence of TBTO, the SCE frequency increased to approximately twice that found when larvae were exposed to either toxicant in isolation (Dixon & McFadzen, 1987).

8.2.4 Crustaceans

Summary

Most of the available data for freshwater organisms are derived from acute exposure tests with Daphnia. LC_{50} data for similar exposure times are variable (up to 2 orders of magnitude) probably due to age differences in the populations studied. The NOEL for Daphnia has been estimated to be around 0.5 µg/litre, behaviour being the most sensitive parameter.

A range of marine species from copepods to crabs and lobsters has been studied, the lowest NOEL being 0.09 µg per litre for reproductive effects in mysid shrimp.

The presence of sediment in test aquaria greatly reduces the toxic effect of TBTO on estuarine crustaceans.

8.2.4.1 Acute effects

Using TBTO and TBT acetate, Floch et al. (1964) calculated LC_{100} and LC_0 values for various species of freshwater invertebrates. The lethal concentrations of TBTO to

Daphnia magna over 24 and 72 h were 0.12 mg/litre and 0.06 mg/litre, respectively. Another aquatic crustacean, *Cypridopsis hartwigi*, was less sensitive with lethal concentrations of 4 mg/litre for a 24-h exposure, 2 mg/litre for a 48-h exposure, and 0.12 mg/litre for a 96-h exposure. NOELs were 0.03 and 0.06 mg/litre for *Daphnia* and *Cypridopsis*, respectively. For TBT acetate, the LC_{100} was 0.15 mg/litre for a 72-h exposure of *Daphnia* and 0.15 mg/litre for a 96-h exposure of *Cypridopsis*. The LC_0 was 0.075 mg/litre for both species.

However, more recent work has found *Daphnia* to be considerably more sensitive to TBT. Meador (1986) reported a 96-h LC_{50} for *Daphnia magna* of 5.9 µg/litre and noted that TBT is a slow-acting toxicant for *Daphnia* with effects only being shown after 96 h or more of exposure. Polster & Halacka (1971) quoted 48-h LC_{50} values for *Daphnia magna* using various TBT salts, which ranged from 2.2 µg TBTO/litre to 8.5 µg TBT oleate/litre.

RIVM (1989) reported a 48-h EC_{50} for *Daphnia* of 4.7 µg/litre and a NOEL, over the same time period, of 0.56 µg/litre.

Davidson et al. (1986) calculated the 96-h LC_{50} to be 0.42 µg/litre after exposing the mysid shrimp *Acanthomysis sculpta* to a leachate of TBT.

When Walsh (1986) exposed the mole crab *Emerita talpoida* to concentrations of 10 µg TBTO/litre of sea water or 4500 µg/kg of sand, no effect on crab survival was observed after 7 days of exposure. In continuous-flow bioassays, 10 000 µg TBTO/kg of sediment did not kill grass shrimp after a 96-h exposure.

3.2.4.2 *Short- and long-term toxicity*

U'Ren (1983) maintained the marine copepod *Acartia tonsa* in solutions containing TBTO, under static conditions, and calculated a 144-day LC_{50} of 0.55 µg per litre; by combining moribundity and mortality as endpoints, the 144-day EC_{50} was found to be 0.4 µg/litre.

Laughlin et al. (1983) maintained mud crab larvae *(Rhithropanopeus harrisii)*, from hatching, in solutions containing either TBTO at 0.5 to 25 µg/litre or TBT sulfide at 0.5 to 50 µg/litre, under static renewal procedures. The survival of the zoeae, up to 15 days, was unaffected by TBTO at levels up to 10 µg/litre. At 15 µg per litre, 84% successfully moulted to the megalopa stage, but at 5 µg TBTO/litre only 37% survived. Zoeal survival was unaffected by concentrations of TBT sulfide up to 5 µg/litre. Survival at 20, 30, and 50 µg/litre was 78%, 26%, and 4%, respectively. The development rate, over the same time period, decreased with increasing TBT concentration, although this was not statistically significant below 10 µg TBTO/litre or 20 µg TBT sulfide/litre. At the highest exposure concentrations (10 µg TBTO/litre and 20 µg TBT sulfide/litre), metamorphosis was delayed by approximately 2 days in the case of TBTO and 6 days for TBT sulfide. Growth (measured as mean wet weight) was significantly reduced at TBTO concentrations of 15 and 25 µg/litre or TBT sulfide concentrations of 20, 30, and 50 µg/litre, and showed dose dependency. Daily growth was monitored for up to 12 days at concentrations (of both TBTO and TBT sulfide) of 0.5, 1.0, and 5.0 µg per litre. Although the final weights were not significantly different, all TBT treatments caused an initial growth lag during the first three days of exposure. Laughlin et al. (1985) found the LC_{50} for exposure of zoeae of *Rhithropanopeus harrisii* to TBTO during the 12 days of zoeal development to be 55 nmol/litre.

Laughlin & French (1980) exposed shore crabs *(Hemigrapsus nudus)*, 2 to 3 days after hatching, to TBTO (as "Biomet") for up to 14 days under static conditions. At the highest concentrations (500 and 1000 µg/litre), all the zoeae died within 2 days. Survival time increased as the concentration of TBTO decreased from 100 to 25 µg per litre; most larvae died within 8 days even at 25 µg per litre. The estimated values of LT_{50} for 100, 75, 50, and 25 µg/litre were 3.4, 4.8, 5.8, and 6.2 days, respectively. Lobster larvae *(Homarus americanus)* were much more sensitive; 100% being killed within 24 h and 2 days by 20 and 15 µg TBTO/litre, respectively. Concentrations of 10 and 5 µg/litre killed all larvae within 5 to 6 days. In the group exposed to 1 µg/litre, there was a similar mortality pattern to the controls and high mortality at the first ecdysis (3 to 5 days post-hatch). However, in this group only a single larva metamorphosed successfully, compared with 43% in the control group.

Davidson et al. (1986) kept juvenile mysid shrimps *(Acanthomysis sculpta)*, newly-released from the female, in TBT concentrations of between 0.03 and 0.48 µg per litre for a 63-day period under flow-through conditions. The TBT source was leachate from panels coated with antifouling paint. All animals died within 7 days at the higher exposure level. There was no significant difference in shrimp mortality between those exposed at levels up to 0.38 µg/litre and the controls, either at 22 or 41 days. From day 41 to the end of the test (63 days), survival decreased at 0.38 µg/litre and only 22.5% survived to the end of the experiment, compared with 60% in the control group. The authors stated that this indicated a lowering of the NOEL for the entire life cycle of *A. sculpta* from 0.38 µg/litre to 0.25 µg/litre at 41 days. The increase in mortality coincided with the release of juveniles by the females, which indicated a sensitive time in the life cycle. Both mean length and weight of females, at a TBT level of 0.38 µg/litre, were significantly reduced after 63 days of exposure, but no effect of TBT concentrations up to and including 0.38 µg/litre was observed in males. A similar result was found in another study after 28 days at 0.49 µg/litre; again no effect on length or weight was found in males. There was a significant effect on the length of developing juveniles and sub-adults. After 14 days of exposure to either 0.19 or 0.33 µg/litre, mysids were significantly shorter; this was also the case at 0.2 µg/litre after 27 days. At TBT concentrations up to and including 0.33 µg/litre, there was no effect on the number of juveniles released per individual female, the number of individuals in unhatched broods, or the number of days from hatching of a female to the release of its juveniles. However, there was a significant reduction in the number of viable juveniles released at both 0.19 µg per litre and 0.33 µg/litre. The authors suggest a NOEL of 0.09 µg/litre for reproduction, the most sensitive parameter found in the study.

Laughlin et al. (1984) exposed the Baltic amphipod *Gammarus oceanicus* to TBTO or TBT fluoride concentrations of 0.3 or 3.0 µg/litre for 8 weeks, under 48-h static renewal conditions. They also exposed the amphipods to leachates from TBT-containing antifouling paints, by placing a 1 cm^2 plexiglass plate, which was painted with either "Micron 25" or "Interracing", in the tank for

5 weeks. Again the water was changed every 48 h. TBT levels in the experiment with pure compounds, remained constant, but the TBT concentration (measured as TBTO) from the leachates gradually increased over each 48-h exposure period to approximately 5.5 µg/litre for "Interracing" and 0.5 µg/litre for "Micron 25", reflecting the different leaching rates of the two compounds. At the highest concentration of both TBTO and TBT fluoride, 50% of the adults died within 10 to 12 days of the exposure and all had died within 16 days (TBTO) or 33 days (TBT fluoride). The TBT paint "Interracing" caused 100% mortality within 1 week. The lower concentration of the exposures to pure compounds and "Micron 25" resulted in mortality patterns that were not dependent on TBT concentration but on senility. The exposures to 0.3 µg per litre and "Micron 25" had significantly reduced the number of surviving larvae by the end of the experiment. Slight decreases in larval growth were observed after exposure to TBTO and "Micron 25" but, generally, concentrations of less than 1 µg TBT/litre had little effect on growth and no effect on whole animal oxygen consumption rates.

Clark et al. (1987) monitored the survival of the grass shrimp *(Palaemonetes pugio)* in water and water/sediment test aquaria after the addition of TBTO. When added to water and tested in the absence of sediment, TBTO gave 96-h LC_{50} values comparable to other published results at 20 µg/litre. However, when the TBTO was admixed with sediment rather than water, the LC_{50} could not be determined. TBT levels in sediment at 1 mg/kg in static and 10 mg/kg in flow-through tests showed no effects on shrimp survival. Similar tests using *Amphioxus* gave an LC_{50} for sediment containing TBTO of between 1 and 10 mg/kg over 4 and 10 days. The animals were killed by 10 µg TBT per litre in water.

8.2.4.3 Reproductive effects

Hall et al. (1988b) maintained egg-carrying females of the copepod *Eurytemora affinis* in TBT chloride at levels of 0.1 or 0.5 µg/litre for up to 13 days. After 3 days of exposure, the higher concentration had significantly reduced the mean brood size to 0.2, compared with 15.2 in controls. Neonate survival was significantly reduced at 0.1 µg/litre after 6 days (22% of control survival). No offspring survived the higher exposure concentration. In a second experiment, mean brood size, after 2 days of exposure, was not significantly affected at concentrations of between 12.5 and 200 ng/litre. Neonate survival, after 13 days, was unaffected by concentrations up to and including 50 ng/litre; survival at 100 ng/litre was 76% (compared to 22% survival at the same exposure level, in the first experiment, over 6 days) and was further reduced to 24% at 200 ng TBT/litre.

When Johansen & Mohlenberg (1987) exposed fertilized mature female copepods *(Acartia tonsa)* to TBTO, egg production was significantly reduced at the highest exposure level of 0.1 µg/litre after 72 h. After 120 h, all exposure concentrations had significantly reduced egg production by 18%, 19%, and 37% relative to controls, at TBTO concentrations of 0.01, 0.05, and 0.1 µg per litre, respectively.

3.2.4.4 Limb regeneration

Weis et al. (1987a,b) exposed the fiddler crab *(Uca pugilator)* to TBTO concentrations of 0.5, 5.0, or 50 µg per litre under static renewal conditions. Regeneration (autotomy) of 1 chela and 5 walking legs was induced by pinching them off at the merus. Although some growth retardation was observed, the most striking effect was the development in regenerated limbs of deformities, e.g., backward curling or complete absence of the dactyl of the claw, chelae or walking legs, stunted, unjointed, or bent in the wrong direction. The percentage of males exhibiting deformities was 17% at 0.5 µg/litre, 24% at 5 µg per litre, and 67% at 50 µg/litre, the test solution being changed twice weekly. In a second experiment, where the test solution was changed three times weekly, the percentage deformities were as follows: males, 100% at both 5 and 50 µg/litre; females, 29% at 5 µg/litre and 100% at 50 µg/litre. There were no deformities in the control groups during the experiments.

3.2.4.5 Behavioural effects

When Pinkney et al. (1985) gave the grass shrimp *(Palaemonetes pugio)* a choice between TBTO-contaminated water and clean water, it did not avoid total organic tin concentrations of 2.3 to 30 µg/litre. The response data, at both 2.3 and 30 µg/litre, were very similar.

Meador (1986) reported the effects of TBT chloride on the photobehaviour of water fleas *(Daphnia magna)*. The normal response of *Daphnia* to a unidirectional light source is to swim away from the light; this is an adaptive response to avoid predators. The author reported that *Daphnia* exposed to TBT chloride showed a reversal of this behaviour and swam towards the light source (usually with considerably increased swimming intensity). The threshold concentration of TBT chloride causing this behavioural reversal was 0.5 µg/litre (the LC_{50} over the same time period was between 3.5 and 6 µg/litre).

8.2.5 Other aquatic invertebrates

Summary

Few studies have been carried out on other species. The lowest effect level in annelids was observed for Nereis diversicolor; *mortality and behavioural effects were seen after chronic exposure to 2 µg/litre. Limb regeneration was significantly inhibited in a brittle star after exposure to 0.1 µg per litre. Experiments have been carried out on four insect species. The most sensitive was* Notonectes, *the LC_0 being 0.03 mg/litre and the LC_{50} 0.06 mg/litre.*

8.2.5.1 Acute effects

Walsh et al. (1986a) exposed larvae of the lugworm *Arenicola cristata* to either TBTO or TBT acetate, for 96 or 168 h, respectively. The concentrations that killed 100% of the animals were: 4 µg/litre (96 h) for TBTO; 10 µg/litre (96 h) and 5 µg/litre (168 h) for TBT acetate. At 5 µg TBT acetate/litre, all larvae were abnormal after 96 h of exposure. No deaths or abnormalities resulted from exposure to 2 µg TBTO/litre for up to 168 h. When Beaumont et al. (1987) exposed adult polychaetes *(Nereis diversicolor)* to TBT in flowing sea water for up to 22 days, there was 100% mortality by 22 days at 4 µg per litre and 55% mortality at 2 µg/litre (20% control deaths). Eversion of the proboscis was a more sensitive indication of toxicity. No controls showed this effect, whereas 75% of animals exposed to 2 µg/litre showed everted proboscis after 22 days (50% after 20 days of exposure).

Dragonfly larvae *(Aeschna)* sp. showed a 48-h LC_{100} of 0.25 mg TBTO/litre and an LC_0 of 0.12 mg TBTO/litre. Corresponding values for TBT acetate were 0.5 mg/litre (72-h LC_{100}) and 0.025 mg/litre (LC_0). *Notonectes* sp. yielded LC_0 values of 0.03 mg/litre for both TBTO and TBT acetate and 72-h LC_{100} values of 0.06 and 0.15 mg/litre for TBTO and TBT acetate, respectively. Chironomid (midge) larvae revealed a NOEL of 0.075 mg/litre for TBT acetate and a 48-h LC_{100} of 0.15 mg/litre (Floch et al., 1964).

Cardarelli (1978) studied the efficacy of controlled-release organotin compounds as mosquito larvicides. The toxicity (LT_{100}) of BioMet (6% TBTO in natural rubber), CBL-9B (20% TBT fluoride in natural rubber), and ECOPRO-1230 and ECOPRO-1330 (both are ethylene propylene polymers containing 30% TBT fluoride) were tested against larvae of the mosquito *Culex quinquefasciatus*. For BioMet and CBL-9B, LT_{100} values ranged from 4 to 9 days for toxicant concentrations of 0.1 to 10 mg/kg of pellet added to the water, the toxicity increasing with increasing toxicant concentration. A degradation product, TBT carbonate, was found to be less toxic, the LT_{100} being 9 days after exposure to 10 mg/litre. When the polymers were tested at toxicant concentrations ranging from 0.9 to 32.6 mg/kg, toxicity was found to increase with increasing toxicant concentration (LT_{100}s range from 2 days to 16 days). Although initially toxicity tended to decrease as the soaking time of the pellet increased, prior to exposure, between days 100 and 500 of soaking toxicity remained relatively unchanged. The authors observed that the organotin compounds dramatically slowed or even prevented morphogenesis.

3.2.5.2 *Limb regeneration*

In a study on limb regeneration, Walsh et al. (1986b) maintained the brittle star *Ophioderma brevispina* in TBTO concentrations of 0.01, 0.1, or 0.5 µg/litre under flow-through conditions. On the first day of the experiment, autotomy was induced in two arms, at opposite sides of the

Effects on Organisms in the Environment: Aquatic Organisms

disc, by pinching midway between disc and arm tip. The animals were then exposed for four weeks to TBTO. There were no deaths and no effect on disc diameter. Both 0.1 and 0.5 µg/litre significantly inhibited regeneration of arms as measured by length; both groups showed average and median lengths less than those in the lowest-dose group, but variability precluded statistical significance. Average weights of limbs were also reduced in the groups exposed to 0.1 and 0.5 µg/litre, but statistical analysis was not carried out because pooled weights did not provide enough data.

8.3 Fish

Summary

The acute toxicity of tributyltin to marine and freshwater fish is highly variable, LC_{50} values ranging from 1.5 to 240 µg/litre. It is unclear whether this is due to inherent differences in sensitivity or to differences in route of exposure. Many of the acute toxicity studies need to be interpreted with care, since the TBT concentrations cited are often nominal and biologically available concentrations were not measured.

In long-term toxicity tests, the NOEL for general toxicological parameters (growth and behaviour) for trout yolk-sac fry was greater than 0.2 µg/litre, and for medaka it was 3.2 µg/litre. Using histopathological parameters, the NOEL for medaka was found to be 0.32 µg/litre, vacuolation of the retinal epithelium being the most sensitive parameter.

Few embryotoxicity tests have been performed and it has not been possible to establish a NOEL.

8.3.1 Acute effects

The 96-h LC_{50} of TBTO for marine fish ranges between 1.5 and 36 µg/litre (Table 12). Larvae seem to be more sensitive than adults in those few studies examining different life stages in the same test. Fewer LC_{50} values have been published for freshwater fish; they range from 13 to 240 µg/litre.

8.3.2 Short- and long-term toxicity

Matthiessen (1974) measured a lethal threshold concentration of TBTO for *Tilapia mossambica* of between 8 and 16 µg/litre (24-h LC_{50}, 28 µg/litre; LC_5, 24 µg per litre; LC_{90}, 33 µg/litre) as a preliminary to studies at sublethal concentrations. A temporary opacity of the surface of the eyes developed at concentrations below this threshold (> 8 µg/litre) but disappeared after a few days. Other symptoms included sluggishness and difficulties with balance. Melanophores in the skin were found to be constricted, giving treated fish a paler appearance than controls. The fish did not produce behaviourally related display patterns, an activity important in the species. As with the eye opacity, these other symptoms disappeared after a few days or weeks, suggesting that the fish develop some tolerance to the TBTO. The growth of *Tilapia* exposed to 0, 5, or 8 µg TBTO/litre was monitored over a 5-week period. These concentrations of TBTO were estimated, on the basis of release rates, in water after the TBTO had been used to control mollusc vectors for schistosomiasis. There was no difference in growth between fish exposed to 5 µg/litre and controls. *Tilapia* exposed to 8 µg/litre showed negative growth and lost about 6% of body weight over the experimental period. Eye opacity was only found in the fish exposed to 8 µg per litre, but this effect did not seem to affect feeding behaviour. The only other change in the high-dose group was an increase in aggressive encounters between males. There was an increased reluctance amongst attacked males to avoid conflict, which led to the death of several individuals. Fatal engagements between males are normally very rare in this species.

When Seinen et al. (1981) exposed rainbow trout *(Salmo gairdneri)* yolk-sac fry to TBT chloride concentrations of 0.2, 1, or 5 µg/litre for up to 110 days, all fry died within 10 to 12 days (at the transition from yolk-sac fry to the swimming fry stage) at 5 µg/litre, but there were no deaths at lower doses. The major histopathological change in fish that died after exposure to 5 µg per litre was hydropic degeneration of tubule segments of the pronephros. At 0.2 and 1 µg/litre, there was a dose-related

Table 12. Toxicity of tributyltin to fish

Organism	Size/age	Stat/flow[a]	Temperature (°C)	Salinity (°/oo)	pH	TBT salt	Duration (h)	LC_{50}[c] (µg/litre)	Reference
Marine and estuarine species									
Sheepshead minnow (*Cyprinodon variegatus*)	sub-adult	flow	19.4-21.3	9.8-12.1	8.15-8.31	chloride	48 72 96	> 31[d,f] 28.1 (24-36.5)[d,f] 25.9 (22.8-30.1)[d,f]	Bushong et al. (1988)
Bleak (*Alburnus alburnus*)	8 cm	stat	10	7	7.8	fluoride oxide	96 96	6-8[e] 15 (13-17)[e]	Linden et al. (1979)
Inland silverside (*Menidia beryllina*)	larva	flow	20	10		chloride	48 72	7.7 (5.5-10.9)[d,f] 4.6 (3.3-6.2)[d,f]	Bushong et al. (1987)
Atlantic silverside (*Menidia menidia*)	sub-adult	flow	20	10		chloride	48 72 96	12.7 (7.8-15.2)[d,f] 9.3 (7.1-12.4)[d,f] 8.9 (6.7-11.6)[d,f]	Bushong et al. (1987)
Atlantic menhaden (*Brevoortia tyrannus*)	juvenile	flow	20	10		chloride	48 72 96	6.8 (4.1-∞)[d,f] 5.2 (3.7-6.5)[d,f] 4.5 (3.6-6.4)[d,f]	Bushong et al. (1987)
Sole (*Solea solea*)	larva larva adult adult	stat[b]				oxide	48 96 48 96	8.5 2.1 88 36	Thain (1983)

Table 12 (contd).

Species	Stage	Test	Weight/Size	Temp (°C)	Salinity	pH	Compound	Duration (h)	Value	Reference
Armed bullhead (*Agonus cataphractus*)	adult	stat[b]					oxide	48 96	26 16	Thain (1983)
Girella (*Girella punctata*)	2.4 g	stat[b]		19.9-20.5		7.8-8.1	oxide	48 96	5.2[d] 3.2[d]	Kakuno & Kimura (1987)
Saltwater goby (*Chasmichthys dolichognathus*)		stat[b]		20.2-21.0	32.5-32.8	8.1-8.3	oxide	24 48 96	12[d] 9[d] 4[d]	Shimizu & Kimura (1987)
Chinook salmon (*Oncorhynchus tshawytscha*)	juvenile	stat		3-5	28		oxide	6 12 96	54[d] 20[d] 1.5[d]	Short & Thrower (1987)
Mummichog (*Fundulus heteroclitus*)	larvae larvae larvae sub-adult sub-adult sub-adult	flow		19.4-21.3	9.8-12.1	8.15-8.31	chloride	48 72 96 48 72 96	> 32.2[d,f] 28.2 (15.1-∞)[d,f] 23.4 (15.2-30.9)[d,f] > 32.2[d,f] 28.3 (23.4-43.2)[d,f] 23.8 (20.8-28)[d,f]	Bushong et al. (1988)

Table 12 (contd).

Organism	Size/age	Stat/flow[a]	Temperature (°C)	Hardness[g] (mg/litre)	pH	TBT salt	Duration (h)	LC$_{50}$[c] (µg/litre)	Reference
Freshwater species									
Rainbow trout (Salmo gairdneri)	yearling	stat	18	250		oxide	24	28[e]	Alabaster (1969)
	yearling	stat[b]	18	250		oxide	48	21[e]	
Guppy (Lebistes reticulatus)	3-4 weeks	stat[b]	23			oxide	96	21	RIVM (1989)
						chloride	168	21 (16-29)[e,f]	Polster & Halacka (1971)
						oleate	168	33 (19-60)[e,f]	
						benzoate	168	25 (19-32)[e,f]	
						laurate	168	30 (18-50)[e,f]	
						acetate	168	28 (21-33)[e,f]	
						oxide	168	39 (28-50)[e,f]	
Medaka (Oryzias latipes)	4-5 weeks	stat[b]	23			oxide	96	17	RIVM (1989)

Table 12 (contd).

Stickleback (Gasterosteus aculeatus)	4-5 weeks	stat[b]	19	oxide	96	13	RIVM (1989)
Carp (Cyprinus carpio)				oxide	24	75	Temmink & Everts (1987)
				oxide	96	32	
Golden orfe (Leuciscus idus melanotus)				oxide	48	50[e]	Plum (1981)
				naphthenate	48	70[e]	
Bluegill sunfish (Lepomis macrochirus)		stat	20	oxide	96	240[e]	Foster (1981)

[a] stat = static conditions (water unchanged for the duration of the test unless stated otherwise); flow = flow-through conditions (TBT concentration in water continuously maintained).
[b] Static renewal conditions (water changed periodically).
[c] 95% confidence limits are given in brackets.
[d] Measured concentration.
[e] Nominal concentration.
[f] Concentration expressed as TBT.
[g] Hardness expressed as mg $CaCO_3$/litre.

retardation of growth, resulting in a 44% decrease in body weight (relative to controls) in the 1 μg/litre group after 110 days. At the end of the experiment, both remaining groups showed significant reductions in the haemoglobin titre in the blood and in body weight. Only at the higher concentration was there a significant decrease in blood cell number. Relative liver weight was significantly increased at both concentrations but relative numbers of thymus cells were unaffected. The authors also measured the relative area distribution of the various hepatic compartments in liver sections. The area occupied by nuclei significantly increased at both concentrations, whereas glycogen storage area decreased, but this was significant only at the highest exposure level. Cytoplasmic area was unaffected, as were all non-parenchymal compartments.

Pinkney et al. (1988) exposed 13- and 16-day-old larvae of striped bass *(Morone saxatilis)* to varying concentrations of TBT from methacrylate-painted panels for 6 to 7 days. They found significant reductions in survival at measured concentrations of 0.766 μg TBT/litre or more. At lower exposure concentrations (0.067 μg/litre), growth parameters changed in the 13-day-old larvae only. No changes occurred in the growth parameters of 16-day-old larvae exposed to 0.444 μg/litre or less. The authors did not know whether this apparent difference in sensitivity between larvae of different ages was a true effect or simply the result of differences between the various batches of larvae.

Wester et al. (1988) reported NOELs for the medaka *(Oryzias latipes)* of 3.2 μg TBTO/litre for general toxicological parameters (mortality, growth, general appearance, abnormal behaviour) and 0.32 μg/litre for histopathological effects during 1 month of exposure. The most sensitive histopathological effect was the development of vacuolation in the retinal epithelium of the eye. There was a dose-related increase in hepatocellular vacuolation, with swelling in pronounced cases. The vacuoles appeared to be glycogen deposits, although, at higher doses, lipid vacuoles were also noted. The NOEL for liver effects was 1 μg TBTO/litre. Kidney effects mostly involved the tubule and included dilation, epithelial atrophy, degeneration and regeneration, and proteinaceous casts including cellular debris (tubulonephrosis). Severe cases also showed glomerular effects. Similar lesions were reported after 3 months of exposure, with, in addition, effects on the swim bladder, skin, oral cavity, and thyroid gland at the highest concentration tested (10 µg/litre). Thymus atrophy, reported by the same authors in the guppy, was not found in the medaka, indicating some species specificity regarding the effects of TBT. Increased glycogen in liver and muscle after TBTO treatment was demonstrated analytically in the medaka, confirming histochemical suggestions of increased glycogen in the guppy.

Shimizu & Kimura (1987) exposed the marine goby *Chasmichthys dolichognathus* to TBTO in short (4 day) and long (12 week) experiments, and reported a 96-h LC_{50} of 4 µg/litre. Long-term exposure to 2.1 µg/litre during the season of gonadal recrudescence led to a significant depression of the gonadosomatic index in male fish. There was no effect on female fish in terms of gonadosomatic index or ovarian histology.

8.3.3 Embryotoxicity

Newton et al. (1985) exposed eggs, embryos, and larvae of the California grunion *(Leuresthes tenuis)* to plates painted with 9.4% TBT methacrylate (0.5% TBTO; 44.7% cuprous oxide; 45.5% inert ingredient) and aged for 30 days in flowing sea water. The authors claimed that the exposure to concentrations of between 0.14 and 1.72 µg TBT per litre had no adverse effect on hatching, growth, or development. In fact the presence of TBT at such concentrations enhanced both hatching success and stimulated growth. A concentration of 10 µg TBT/litre had no effect on hatchability, but at 74 µg/litre hatching success was reduced by approximately 50%. The authors observed no effect on the survival of larvae, hatched from eggs exposed to concentrations of 0.14 to 1.72 µg/litre, up to 7 days post-hatch. The presence of copper, however, should be taken into consideration in the interpretation of these results.

Weis et al. (1987a) reported considerable variation in the response of embryos of the killifish *(Fundulus heteroclitus)* to concentrations of TBTO ranging between 3 and 30 µg/litre. Two batches of embryos developed abnormalities at the highest concentration of TBTO tested

(30 µg/litre) and showed some mortality. Other batches of embryos showed embryotoxicity for all tested concentrations (down to 3 µg/litre) but no abnormalities in the embryos. Owing to this difference in sensitivity of different batches of eggs and the separation of embryotoxic and teratogenic effects, it is difficult to establish a NOEL for this species.

Fent (1989b) exposed fertilized eggs of the freshwater minnow *Phoxinus phoxinus* to two TBT concentrations in petri dishes in an environment chamber. The eggs were exposed from the blastula stage (20 to 24 h after spawning), and the water was renewed daily. Analytical determination of TBT showed that the actual concentration had reduced over the 24-h exposure period from 1.5 to 0.5 µg/litre in the low-dose group and from 8.4 to 7.9 µg/litre in the high-dose group. There were no differences in survival between the control and low-dose groups. Hatching was normal but some fish showed vertebral malformations. At the high dose, hatching was delayed or reduced and all hatched larvae had severe vertebral malformations; many were unable to uncurl. These larvae remained motionless at the bottom of the dish. Some had oedema in the region of the heart. Within 3 to 4 days of hatching, all of the larvae in the high-dose group had died. A further series of experiments similarly showed malformation at an exposure level of 4.5 µg TBT/litre.

8.3.4 Behavioural effects

The avoidance response of the mummichog *(Fundulus heteroclitus)* to TBTO has been studied by Pinkney et al. (1985). When given a choice between TBTO-contaminated and clean water, 4 out of 6 groups of fish avoided a total organic tin level of 1 µg/litre. There were significant avoidance responses for all test groups at total organic tin levels of 3.7, 8, and 13.8 µg/litre. However, the higher concentrations of tin did not result in an increase in avoidance response. The authors found that, under the same conditions, no avoidance response was shown by the grass shrimp (see section 8.2.4.5). This shrimp is a major food item of the mummichog in tidal marshes. Hall et al. (1984) studied the avoidance response of two species of juvenile estuarine fish, the striped bass *(Morone saxatilis)* and Atlantic menhaden *(Brevoortia tyrannus)*. An avoidance response to TBTO was exhibited by bass at a total organic tin concentration of 24.9 µg per litre. Atlantic menhaden were more sensitive, showing a "mild" avoidance at 5.5 µg/litre and a "strong" avoidance at 9.1 µg/litre.

Chliamovitch & Kuhn (1977) measured an EC_{50} for the loss of positive rheotaxis of 30.8 µg/litre for the rainbow trout *(Salmo gairdneri)* and 53.2 µg/litre for a tilapia *(Tilapia rendalli)*.

8.4 Amphibians

Summary

There are few data on the effects of tributyltin on amphibians. Survival of frog larvae was at least 80% of control levels after exposure to 3 µg TBT/litre.

Floch et al. (1964) reported a NOEL for mortality of tadpoles of two species of amphibians *(Rana* and *Alytes* sp.) of 30 µg/litre. For both species, the 24-h LC_{100} for TBTO was 75 µg/litre, the 48-h LC_{100} 50 µg/litre, and the 48-h LC_{100} for TBT acetate was 75 µg/litre.

Laughlin & Linden (1982) exposed eggs of the frog *Rana temporaria* to concentrations of either TBTO or TBT fluoride of 0.3, 3, or 30 µg/litre, for 5 days from the postgastrula stage of development, under static renewal conditions. All surviving larvae hatched on either day 4 or 5 of exposure. Survival was at least 80% of control levels after exposure to 0.3 or 3 µg/litre. Only at the highest concentration (30 µg/litre) did TBT affect survival (40% mortality with TBT fluoride and 50% mortality with TBTO). The authors collected all surviving tadpoles and measured wet and dry weight. Wet weights were significantly lower in tadpoles exposed to 30 µg/litre but unaffected at lower exposure concentrations. Tadpoles exposed to TBT always showed higher mean dry weight than controls, although increases were not consistently dose dependent. The percentage of body water declined from 86-88.5% for controls to 73.8% after exposure at the highest concentration of TBT. The changes resulting from TBT treatment were significant, but not the differences produced by the different TBT compounds.

8.5 Multispecies studies

Summary

The few available microcosm studies indicate that the most sensitive organism(s) within the microcosm are affected by TBT at concentrations greater than 0.05 µg/litre. Recovery of these organisms occurred a few months after exposure. Simultaneous exposure of snails and fish yields conflicting results, snails appearing somewhat more sensitive than fish.

Beaumont et al. (1987) exposed sandy-substrate microcosms of flowing sea water to TBT derived from slate panels painted with "Micron 25" antifouling paint. Three replicate microcosms were exposed for 4 months at high (1-3 µg/litre) and at low (0.06-0.17 µg/litre) TBT concentrations in water, together with three control microcosms. Flow rates were maintained by gravity from a header tank at approximately 1 litre/min; the painted panels were located in the header tank where water was passed over them using a circulating pump. The substrate sediment was sieved after collection (to 2 mm) to remove larger organisms and allowed to settle in the microcosms for 3 weeks before the addition of animals. The sediment was 10 cm deep and the overlying water 15 cm deep in each microcosm. At the beginning of the trial, 50 specimens of a bivalve *(Cerastoderma edule)*, a crustacean *(Corophium volutator)*, and two polychaetes *(Nereis diversicolor* and *Cirratulus cirratus)* were introduced. After 4 weeks, 12 specimens of the gastropod *Littorina littorea* were added and, after 6 weeks, 26 specimens of a second bivalve *(Scrobicularia plana)* were added. Other species were found at the end of the trial derived from small (< 2 mm) juveniles in the sediment and inflowing sea water. Each day, 10 litres of a suspension of the microalga *Pavlova lutheri* (5×10^6 cells/ml) were added to the header tank as additional food supply. The most sensitive of the introduced species was the cockle *(C. edule)*; 100% died within 2 weeks at the high concentration of TBT and there was cumulative mortality at the low TBT concentration over 17 weeks (14% of controls died). Two-way analysis of variance indicated significant differences between all three groups (i.e. control, and low and high concentrations of TBT; $p < 0.05$). The other bivalve *(S. plana)* showed high mortality at the highest exposure level (100% after 10 weeks). At the low TBT concentration there were no time-related deaths in this species and no significant difference from controls. Among the polychaetes, high death rates were recorded for *N. diversicolor* in all microcosms, including the control, possibly because adults introduced were ripe and died after spawning during the experiment. The other polychaete *(C. cirratus)* survived well even after exposure to the high concentration of TBT. Only one gastropod *(L. littorea)* died in any of the microcosms. Juvenile bivalves were the most common species found; their numbers and diversity were lower in the low-dose microcosms (66 to 109) than in control microcosms (137 to 179), and they were virtually absent from the high-dose microcosms (0, 1, and 1 for the 3 replicates). The size of juvenile mussels *(Mytilus edulis)* was also significantly reduced at the low TBT concentration, relative to controls; other self-introduced bivalve species were not affected by the low TBT exposure. Measurements of chlorophyll *a* in sediment cores, as a measure of algal biomass, indicated a significant rise after exposure to high TBT levels. This is explained by the relative insensitivity of algae to the toxic effects of TBT and by reduced (or non-existent) animal life available to consume the algae. The authors emphasize the sensitivity of some species, for which TBT is toxic at levels of 1 to 2 μg/litre under conditions approximating natural exposure. They further emphasize the great variation in sensitivity between species; for example, while *Mytilus edulis* and *Cerastoderma edule* were clearly affected at very low levels of TBT, other related bivalves were largely unchecked. Differences in feeding behaviour, leading to different effective exposure levels, is offered as one possible explanation for differences in response. Differential absorption or subsequent loss, observed in laboratory studies with other molluscs, is also proposed as a possible mechanism.

Henderson (1986) conducted long-term flow-through microcosm studies on communities of marine organisms from Pearl Harbour, Hawaii, where the organisms had been exposed to leaching TBT from naval ships for some time. Panels (20 x 25 cm) of roughened plexiglass were suspended in the harbour for 14 weeks prior to the experiment to allow settlement and growth of organisms, and 30 different species were found on the panels. Prior to exposure, the panels were kept for a further 5 weeks in the experimental tanks. These tanks had a capacity of 155 litre and were supplied with sea water pumped directly from the harbour and through the tanks at a rate of 4 litres/min. The sea water was passed through a 1 cm mesh with no further filtration; organisms could, therefore, enter the tanks easily and settle on the panels. The water was rich in plankton consisting largely of diatoms, copepods, and chaetognaths. Exposure to TBT derived from painted panels treated with antifouling paint containing 9.4% TBT methacrylate, 0.5% TBTO, 44.7% cuprous oxide, and 45.4% inert ingredients. Nominal concentrations of TBT were 0, 0.05, 0.13, 0.31, 0.78, and 1.95 µg/litre, but actual mean concentrations were 0.01, 0.04, 0.10, 0.54, 1.77, and 2.52 µg/litre, respectively. The measured copper levels in the same samples were 1.0, 1.2, 1.2, 3.1, 4.4, and 5 µg/litre, respectively. Changes in coverage of the panels was assessed using photographs taken with an underwater camera at weekly or biweekly intervals throughout the experimental period of approximately 60 days of exposure and a further 60 days of recovery. One week after the start of exposure, a further plastic panel was introduced to monitor new colonization. There was a clear decline in both total number of species and in species diversity (reductions of 55%, 60%, and 80% at the three highest exposure levels, respectively) on pre-fouled panels exposed to TBT at 0.5, 1.8, and 2.5 µg/litre but no effect at lower concentrations. The mortality of individual species, in relation to TBT exposure, showed considerable variation. The most sensitive of the six most common species on the panels was *Botrylloides* spp, an orange-coloured colonial tunicate, which showed 100% mortality at TBT concentrations of 0.1 µg/litre or more. An encrusting bryozoan, *Schizoporella errata,* showed 49% mortality at 0.1 µg/litre and 80 to 100% mortality at higher concentrations. Specimens of a second colonial tunicate, *Didemnus candidum,* and the saddle oyster *(Anomis nobilis)* were all killed at concentrations of 0.5 µg/litre or more. A tube worm *(Hydroides elegans)* and a solitary tunicate *(Ascidia* spp.) survived even the highest exposure level, though with considerable mortality at 1.8 and 2.5 µg/litre. Recovery of populations was complete 60 days after cessation of treatment. Settlement on the panels not previously exposed was reduced by TBT concentrations of 0.1 µg/litre or more, but not by 0.04 µg per litre. Algal settlement and growth on the walls of the tanks was not affected by exposure to TBT at any concentration; coralline algae increased their coverage of prefouled panels. A total of 18 oysters *(Crassostrea virginica)* placed in each tank prior to treatment was monitored after 60 days. There was 50% mortality after TBT exposure at 1.8 µg/litre but no significant reduction in survival at lower concentrations. However, the condition index of the oysters was affected by exposure to 0.1 µg/litre or more, but had returned to near normal after 2 months recovery in clean water. The author regarded 0.05 µg/litre as a reliable NOEL for the most sensitive organisms exposed.

When Salazar & Salazar (1985) exposed copepods *(Acartia tonsa)*, mysids *(Acanthomysis sculpta)*, and fish *(Citharichthys stigmaeus)* to suspended sediment at a TBTO concentration of 0.49 µg/litre water for 96 h, no significant mortality was found. In a second experiment, mysids *(A. sculpta)*, worms *(Neanthes arenaceodentata)*, and clams *(Macoma nasuta)* were exposed to TBTO-contaminated sediment with overlying water for 10 days in the case of mysids and 20 days in the case of clams and worms. Levels of TBTO in the sediment varied from 155 to 610 µg per kg, falling during the exposure period, while measured levels in the overlying water were about 0.2 µg/litre. No mortality was observed during the exposure period.

Cardarelli (1973) exposed snails *(Biomphalaria glabrata)* and fish *(Lebistes reticulatus)* to slow-releasing molluscicides containing either TBTO or TBT fluoride. At a daily release rate of 35 µg TBTO/litre, 100% mortality was achieved in snails within 60 days but all of the fish also died within this period. At a TBTO release rate of 7 µg/litre per day, snail mortality was 100% after 120 days exposure and fish mortality only 2%. However, a second experiment gave a much higher fish mortality of 46% after 120 days exposure to only 3.5 µg TBTO per litre per day. Exposure to TBT fluoride at 7 µg per litre per day killed all snails and fish within 60 days, and 52% of fish and 100% of snails were killed after 90 days of exposure to 3.5 µg/litre per day.

In order to simulate the effect of molluscicides containing 6% TBTO on biota, Jordan (1985) set up a model ecosystem as follows: filtered river water was allowed to flow into a tray containing washed mud (to simulate a marsh), and overflow from this upper tank was allowed to flow into a lower tank containing washed coarse sand (to simulate a river). Snails *(Biomphalaria glabrata* and *Potamopyrgus coronatus)* and guppies *(Lebistes reticulatus)* were added to the "marsh", while snails *(B. glabrata* and *Pomacea glauca),* shrimps *(Macrobrachium faustinum),* and *L. reticulatus* were added to the "river". The molluscicide was added to the "marsh" as pellets at levels of 2, 5, 10, or 20 g/m² of marsh surface. The percentage of both *B. glabrata* and *L. reticulatus* surviving 14 days of exposure was recorded (see Table 13). The authors concluded that, in this model ecosystem, there was higher mortality of *B. glabrata* than of *L. reticulatus* at low doses of slow-release TBTO, i.e. 2 and 5 g of pellet per m² of "marsh".

Table 13. Percentage of *B. glabrata* and *L. reticulatus* surviving 14 days exposure to slow-release pellets containing 6% TBTO added to the "marsh" in a "marsh" or "river" model ecosystem[a]

Dose of molluscicide	B. glabrata		L. reticulatus	
	"marsh"	"river"	"marsh"	"river"
20 g/m²	00.0* (0/240)	00.0* (0/240)	00.0* (0/240)	00.0* (0/240)
10 g/m²	00.0* (0/240)	00.0* (0/240)	00.0* (0/240)	2.5* (6/240)
5 g/m²	00.0* (0/240)	16.3** (39/240)	23.3** (56/240)	60.0+ (144/240)
2 g/m²	52.9+ (127/240)	75.4++ (181/240)	75.8++ (182/240)	78.8 (189/240)

[a] From: Jordan (1985).
The percentages represent percent survival at various doses for all weeks of exposure in replicate experiments. The values marked with the same symbol are not statistically different from each other at the 0.05 probability level. The numbers in parentheses represent the number of survivors compared to the number of animals exposed.

9. EFFECTS ON ORGANISMS IN THE ENVIRONMENT: TERRESTRIAL ORGANISMS

Summary

Exposure of terrestrial organisms to TBT derives primarily from its use as a wood preservative. However, little information is available. TBTO has proved toxic to honey-bees coming into close contact with TBTO-treated wood. TBT compounds are toxic to insects exposed either topically or via feeding on treated wood. The acute toxicity to wild small mammals is moderate (between 37 and 240 mg/kg per day). The toxicity of TBTO to bats is probable but not proven. There is no information on other species.

9.1 Microcosm studies

Gile et al. (1982) introduced TBTO into a terrestrial microcosm on pine posts, each microcosm containing four posts (3.3 x 2.6 x 14 cm) treated with ^{14}C-labelled TBTO (167 mg/cm^3). The microcosms consisted of soil and endogenous soil organisms, ryegrass, earthworms, pillbugs (woodlice), mealworms, crickets, garden snails, and a gravid female gray-tailed vole. There were no effects on any of the organisms over a period of 77 days. About 95% of the TBTO remained in the posts for the whole of the exposure period. A similar system set up to investigate cricket mortality, with and without predation, showed no effect of TBTO (Gillett et al., 1983).

9.2 Terrestrial insects

When Gardiner & Poller (1964) exposed larvae of the common clothes moth *(Tineola bisselliella)* to wool treated with a TBTO concentration of 1% by weight, all of the exposed larvae were killed within the exposure period of 14 days. The action appeared to be that of a contact insecticide because none of the cloth was eaten. Phenyltin compounds were not as toxic as TBTO. Baker & Taylor (1967) found that the action of TBTO more closely resembled the slow toxicity of a stomach insecticide after exposing wood-boring beetles *(Lyctus brunneus)* to impregnated wood.

Contact insecticides such as lindane (γ-hexachlorocyclohexane) and dieldrin were 100 times more toxic than TBTO. The LD_{50} of TBTO for another wood-boring species, *Anobium punctatum*, was 0.254 kg/m^3 (application rate to wood).

Saxena & Crowe (1988) applied TBTO, TBT chloride, and TBT linoleate topically to the thorax of newly-emerged insects of three species. The LD_{50} values ranged from 0.48% to 0.72% (dilutions with acetone) for the house fly *Musca domestica*, 0.29% to 0.69% for the mosquito *Anophelese stephensi*, and 0.52% to 0.87% for the cotton stainer *Dysdercus cingulatus*. TBT compounds were more toxic than the other organotin compounds tested (triphenyltin, tricyclohexyltin, dimethyltin, phenyltin, and diethyltin). The authors pointed out that TBT compounds are considerably less toxic than trimethyltin compounds to *Musca* sp.

In studies by Kalnins & Detroy (1984), wood was treated with TBTO (1.9 kg/m^3) after sawing and before use in the construction of beehives. Five hives made from the treated wood were stocked with bees. Tin residues of 3.24 mg/kg were found in bees during the first summer, and residues of 8.67 mg/kg were found in the wax of the combs. However, there were no detectable tin residues in honey. There was high mortality in the bee colonies over winter, only one colony surviving. No control colonies died over winter. Residues in bees and wax in the second year (1.3 and 4.6 mg/kg, respectively) were lower than in the first year in the one surviving colony.

9.3 Terrestrial mammals

Racey & Swift (1986) housed pipistrelle bats *(Pipistrellus pipistrellus)* in roosting cages treated with TBTO. The bats were pregnant females collected from nursery roosts, and they were trained to feed on mealworms before transfer to the experimental cages. The cages were made of metal, lined with plywood, and were painted with TBTO as a 1% solution in white spirit (the manufacturers recommended rate for use of TBTO as a fungicide). The wood was treated 2 months before the bats were introduced into the cages. During the course of the 142-day experiment, seven of the ten bats died. Median survival time was 100 days, with a range between 49 and 142 days. Two deaths in the white spirit control group and three in the untreated control group meant that results for TBTO were not statistically significant.

Schafer & Bowles (1985) conducted toxicity and repellency tests on deer mice *(Peromyscus maniculatus)* and house mice *(Mus musculus)* using various TBT salts. Treatment of feed seeds with 2% (by mass) produced clear repellent effects of TBT in both species. The approximate lethal dose (estimated by increasing the TBT dose until the test animals died) for TBT acetate and fluoride was 320 mg/kg. The estimated dietary LC_{50}, based on consumption of treated seed used in the repellency tests, varied between 37.5 mg/kg per day for TBT acetate and 238 mg/kg per day for fluoride and sulfate. The LC_{50} for TBTO was 200 mg/kg per day.

10. EFFECTS ON ORGANISMS IN THE ENVIRONMENT: FIELD OBSERVATIONS

Summary

Tributyltin compounds have had a wide range of uses. Most concern has focussed on their use in the marine environment, where TBT has been associated with mortality and failure of settlement of bivalve larvae, reduced growth, shell thickening, and other malformations in oysters, imposex (the development of male reproductive appendages in female animals) in mud snails, and imposex concurrent with population decline in dogwhelks. Controls on the use of TBT in antifouling paints has led to recovery of economically important shellfish growth and reproduction. Water concentrations of TBT are still high enough in some areas to affect marine gastropods.

Field and laboratory results for marine molluscs are in good agreement. Both imposex in dogwhelks and shell growth and chambering in Pacific oysters are effective biological indicators of TBT contamination.

There have been few studies into the effects on organisms of TBT in sediment. There are indications that TBT is bioavailable to burrowing organisms and can cause mortality in the field.

Gross toxic effects and histopathological changes have been reported in farmed marine fish exposed to TBT through the use of antifouling paints on retaining nets.

Although TBT has been detected in fresh water at high concentrations in some areas, there have been few studies on its effects. Spills of large amounts of TBT from timber treatment plants have caused ecological damage, but recovery occurred within 9 months.

Field testing of tributyltin derivatives, mainly slow-release formulations of TBTO, has shown that it is difficult to apply TBT without damaging non-target organisms. Recovery occurs through recolonization.

10.1 Effects on bivalves

In the 1970s, the French oyster industry was undergoing a crisis. During the 1977, 1978, and 1979 seasons, very poor spatfalls were reported, together with increasing reports of poor shell growth and shell malformations. An extensive survey of the occurrence and intensity of malformations related to metal residues in oysters suggested, for the first time, a connection with organotin compounds (Alzieu, 1981). The shell thickening was found to be due to the appearance of chambers in the oyster shell and interlamellar gel formation in these cavities (Alzieu, 1981; Alzieu et al., 1982). The authors of these reports described in detail the shell abnormalities and the process of calcification of the oyster shell, and suggested mechanisms of TBT action. TBT is known to inhibit oxidative phosphorylation and it has been suggested that this forms the basis of its action on the shell. It is also known to complex amino acids. The effect on calcification derives from inadequate calcium addition to the organic matrix (a process dependent on ATP) and incorrect deposition of this matrix. Alzieu et al. (1982) found good correlation between the occurrence of shell thickening and the proximity of ports where large numbers of boats were usually moored. These field observations were corroborated by the finding of similar shell abnormalities in the laboratory when oysters were exposed to TBT fluoride, an organotin compound present in antifouling paint used on the boats. Oysters placed in flowing sea-water tanks containing plates coated with TBT antifouling paints died after a 30-day exposure to an estimated water concentration of 2 μg/litre (organotin leachate) and shell thickening was found to occur at water concentrations of 0.2 μg/litre.

Alzieu et al. (1982) assessed the shell quality of 18-month-old Pacific oysters *(Crassostrea gigas;* also known as the Japanese oyster) sampled along the eastern coast of Oleron Island and in the vicinity of La Rochelle, France. They concluded that the proximity of pleasure craft ports or a commercial harbour could badly affect the quality and growth of oyster shells. However, the presence of other chemicals, along with TBT in the sea water made direct assessment difficult. The authors, therefore, carried out a set of experiments to confirm their conclusions. Groups of oysters from areas with no shell abnormalities were distributed to other locations, i.e. a marina, a river, and the laboratory (three groups: a control group; a group exposed to 50-cm² panels coated with TBT fluoride; and a group exposed to coated panels 500 cm² in area). All oysters died within 30 days after exposure to the larger panel in the laboratory and within 170 days after transfer to the marina. Oysters exposed to the smaller panels showed a mortality rate of 30% after 110 days of exposure. Oysters transferred to the marina site and those exposed to 50-cm² TBT-coated panels developed gel-filled shell cavities after 100 and 110 days, respectively, during the period of shell growth. Analysis of the oysters for total tin content revealed levels of < 1 mg/kg (dry weight) in "unpolluted" groups, 110 mg/kg after 80 days at the marina site, and up to 25 mg/kg after exposure to 50-cm² panels in the laboratory.

Maurer et al. (1985) found TBT levels to be related to inhibition of settlement of Pacific oyster in the Bay of Arcachon and the Gironde estuary, France. The authors used arrays of settling tubes mounted around a central tube which was painted with "International TBT Antifouling" at a rate of 6.4 g of paint on a surface of 8 dm². The settling tubes were mounted at varying distances (between 4.5 and 13 cm) from the central painted tube. In control arrays, the central tube was unpainted. The arrays of tubes were placed out in the two study areas in July 1982 and observations on settlement and growth were made in September and November 1982. In the Gironde region, a second method was also used; slates were painted with TBT paint (21 g of "International TBT Antifouling" on a surface of 26 dm²) and mounted 10 cm apart, alternating unpainted with painted slates on a rod. The spacing of tubes in the arrays was up to 25 cm from the central painted tube. In the Gironde estuary, settlement was comparable with controls except on the painted tube; tubes 5 cm or more away from the TBT paint had similar numbers of settling larvae as the control. However, deaths among the settled larvae were high; 100% on tubes 15 cm away (or less), 99.3% on the tube at 20 cm distant, and 78.3% on the tube 25 cm distant from the paint. Slates showed high settlement rates and a mortality of 82.5% at 10 cm away from the paint. In the Bay of Arcachon, there was a much lower settlement of larvae; in the Villa Algerienne area there were 178 settlements/dm² on the treated tubes compared with 440 on controls, and in the Comprian area

81 or 83 settlements/dm^2 on treated tubes compared with 323 on controls. Barnacles, which were less sensitive to the paint, were also found to settle on the tubes. The settlement period in this area was longer than that in the Gironde estuary; some larvae settling later in the season showed reduced growth compared with controls.

Thain & Waldock (1986) reported that the Pacific oyster was introduced into the United Kingdom during the mid-1970s. At this time, growth trials were performed at several coastal locations. The oysters grew well at most sites, but at some east coast sites, such as the estuary of the River Crouch, they exhibited poor growth, reduced meat yield, and shell thickening. At other sites, such as the north Norfolk coast, there were good growth results with none of the deformities found at the Crouch. The cause of the poor growth results in some areas was investigated, and Key et al. (1976) found good correlation between poor growth and high levels of fine suspended particles. Areas of poor performance in the trials were not used for the cultivation of the newly-introduced oyster species. The types of shell abnormality exhibited by oysters in France were very similar to those observed in oysters from the east coast of England, which had been attributed to sediment. The sediment in the marinas used by Key et al. (1976) for resettlement studies was probably contaminated with TBTO (Personal communication by M.J. Waldock to IPCS). In 1982 it was decided to reassess the causes of poor oyster shell growth in Britain. Levels of TBT were measured in the estuaries of the Rivers Crouch and Blackwater, on the east coast of England, and were found regularly to exceed 0.2 µg/litre, a level shown by the French studies to be harmful to the oyster (Thain & Waldock, 1986). In a laboratory study, Waldock & Thain (1983) investigated the effect of both suspended sediment and TBT on growth and shell thickening in spat of the Pacific oyster. They found that TBT levels of 0.16 µg per litre inhibited and 1.6 µg/litre stopped growth. Shell thickening was observed in the oysters exposed to TBT. Exposure to sediment in "clean" water (i.e. containing no TBT) actually enhanced growth. Thain & Waldock (1986) reported that, during 1983, the laboratory finding that TBT and not suspended sediment was affecting growth and causing shell abnormalities in oyster was corroborated in the field by studying oysters from different sites.

Alzieu & Portmann (1984) reported that although the findings clearly implicated TBT as a major cause of growth problems and abnormalities, they did not completely exclude the possibility that other chemicals present might have caused similar effects. They reviewed the effects of a 1982 ban by French authorities on use of TBT paints on boats shorter than 25 m. In the Bay of Arcachon area (where, in 1980 and 1981, 95% to 100% of oysters had shown deformities), the 1982 figures for deformities were 70% to 80% and by 1983 deformities had declined to 45% to 50%. The number of oysters from the same area showing deformities in *both* upper and lower shells was between 70% and 90%, in 1980 and 1981, and zero by 1983. The spatfall, which in both 1980 and 1981 failed completely, subsequently recovered; it was described as good in 1982 and excellent by 1983. The authors also reported, however, that these results were not reflected in another area (La Rochelle Bay). This was attributed both to its close proximity to a major commercial harbour and the fact that the ban on the use of TBT antifouling paints on pleasure craft in this area had not been as strictly observed as in the Bay of Arcachon.

His et al. (1986) reported bioassays conducted on oysters *(Crassostrea gigas)* using sea water collected from the Bay of Arcachon both before and after the imposition of a ban on the use of TBT paints on small boats. The sea water collected in 1981 caused abnormalities in 40% of larval oysters over 12 days of observation (compared with 4% in controls), whereas the sea water from 1982 produced only 12% abnormalities over the same period. Growth of the oyster larvae was also improved relative to the period when TBT paints were still being used. In 1981, mean growth of larval shells over 12 days was 133 μm, in Bay of Arcachon sea water, compared with 142 μm in controls. In 1982, mean growth was 162 μm, as opposed to 168 μm in controls. Alzieu et al. (1986) stated that between 1980 and 1982 about 90% of oysters displayed anomalies in shell calcification. Each year anomalies became apparent in April and reached maximum intensity during June and July. During the period 1983 to 1985, the percentage of oysters displaying shell anomalies fell steadily. By 1985 none of the oysters examined had malformations in both valves and less than 40% had shell anomalies in one of the valves (usually the upper valve). Alzieu et al. (1989) monitored oysters in 1986 and 1987 and found that, although oysters with deformities in both valves had stabilized at < 10%, those with deformities in at least one valve had risen again to a peak of 70% for both years.

Effects on oysters have also been reported near to fish farms containing nets treated with TBT antifoulants. Davies et al. (1987a) maintained caged Pacific oysters (obtained from a nursery unit distant from any significant sources of TBT) at varying distances from fish farms at Loch Sween, Scotland. They found that significant accumulation of tin was restricted to within 200 m of the fish farms and that effects on oyster shell structure were observed at a distance of 1000 m but not at 5000 m. A comparison of shell thickness index and tin accumulation showed significant tin accumulation in those oysters with the most severe shell thickening.

Studies in the USA and Japan have revealed similar effects. Stephenson et al. (1986) transplanted culched and culchless Pacific oysters *(Crassostrea gigas)* and two species of mussel *(Mytilus edulis* and *Mytilus californianus)* to areas of San Diego Bay, California, USA, along a gradient of known sea-water TBT concentrations (0.01-0.93 µg/litre). Reduced shell growth was observed in all three species in areas where TBT levels were highest. Oyster and Californian mussel samples (but not *M. edulis)* showed marked trends of reduced growth with increasing TBT levels. Shell thickening in the oysters also correlated with increasing TBT levels. Wolniakowski et al. (1987) found Pacific oysters in Coos bay, Oregon, USA, to have thickened and ball-shaped shells. When these oysters were analysed, they were found to contain high levels of TBT (49.7 to 189 µg/kg). The most marked deformities occurred in animals collected in a marina and near to where boats were painted. Okoshi et al. (1987) transplanted spat of two different strains of Pacific oysters *(Crassostrea gigas)* to two different experimental field sites in northern Japan for 41 weeks. The number of chambers in the oyster shells increased gradually in the Miyagi strain at one site. In contrast, few chambers were observed in the Hiroshima strain at either site. The authors concluded that both genetic and environmental factors were involved in the formation of shell chambers.

Crassostrea gigas is a non-indigenous species in the United Kingdom and France. Stocks for breeding were introduced into both countries in the late 1960s and originated from the Miyagi region of Japan (Walne & Helm, 1979).

When Paul & Davies (1986) maintained scallops *(Pecten maximus)* and Pacific oysters *(Crassostrea gigas)* in nets coated with a TBTO-based paint, the mortality of scallop spat was 24%, compared with a control mortality of less than 6%, over the 31-week exposure period. Adult scallop mor- tality was less than that of controls in the treated group, and no effect was observed on growth. No oysters died. Scallop spat in TBT-treated nets grew significantly less rapidly than the control spat. Oyster growth, as measured by mean shell length, was significantly reduced and had largely ceased after 10 weeks of exposure. A significant thickening of the oyster shell was observed within 10 weeks of exposure and continued throughout the 31-week exposure. It was maintained even after transfer to untreated nets for 10 weeks.

Minchin et al. (1987) monitored bivalve settlement in Mulroy Bay, Ireland, between 1979 and 1986 using settling panels placed in the sea. They found that, during this period, settlement either failed or was reduced. Scallop numbers fell from an average of > 1000 per panel in 1979 to zero in 1983. In 1984, no settlement of any bivalve species was recorded on the panels. This reduced settlement corresponded to the introduction of organotin fishnet dips in local salmonid farms. The first use of TBT paints appears to have been in 1981. This use of organotin compounds ceased after 1985. In 1986, in all bivalves monitored (except flame shells), there was again good settlement. Scallops *(Pecten maximus)* and flame shells *(Lima hians* and *Chlamys varia)* (all members of the Pectinacea) were found to be particularly sensitive to organotin compounds. It is not known whether the effect of the TBT was on the reproduction of the bivalves or a toxic effect on the larvae.

10.2 Effects on gastropods: imposex

Between the years 1972 and 1976, Smith (1981c) sampled mud snails *(Nassarius obsoletus)* from four locations bordering Long Island Sound in Westport and Fairfield,

Connecticut, USA. The snails were examined for imposex (see section 8.2.3.6), and the results were quantified by measuring the percentage of snails in a sample showing any imposex and estimating the degree of imposex within individual snails. In two of the areas, adjacent to a yacht yard in Southport Harbour and at the mouth of the harbour, 95% to 100% of snails had some degree of imposex. Both showed significantly more imposex than the other two sites, an area used to moor a few old boats and an area protected from human interference. The mud snails in this last area showed no imposex. The area with a few old boats showed imposex levels of 30% to 50%, much less than in the first two areas. Smith (1981a) collected mud snails from three of the locations, the yacht yard in the harbour (where all female snails were abnormal and degree of imposex greatest), the mouth of the harbour (where almost all snails were abnormal but the degree of imposex changes was intermediate), and the area protected from human impact (at least 3.5 km from the nearest marina, where all female snails were normal). The author labelled these areas as "dirty", "intermediate", and "clean". Snails transferred from the "clean" area to the "dirty" area developed imposex. In those transferred from the "dirty" area to the "clean" area the degree of imposex was reduced. An analysis of chemicals present in water from the "dirty" area was then carried out and snails were exposed to some of the contaminants individually, i.e. marina disinfectants, detergents, copper antifouling paints, leaded gasoline, combustion emissions, and two types of TBT-based antifouling paints. Only the tin-containing antifouling paints increased the level of penis expression in female snails.

In a survey of the dogwhelk *Nucella lapillus* around the south-west of England, Bryan et al. (1986) found imposex to be widespread. The south coast of England was the most severely affected. Populations showing the highest incidence and highest intensity of imposex were close to areas of boating or shipping activity. The degree of imposex had increased markedly between 1969 and 1985 in Plymouth Sound (an area on the south coast with large numbers of small boats and ships), coinciding with the introduction and increasing use of TBT-containing antifouling paints in the area. Imposex correlated with concentrations of sea-water tin (TBT fraction) and residues of tin in the dogwhelks (Fig. 6). Transferring whelks from an area with little boating activity to Plymouth marina resulted in a marked increase in the degree of imposex. Bailey & Davies (1988b) found an increase in the degree of imposex and also a higher incidence of penis development in female dogwhelks collected in 1987 in the Firth of Forth, Scotland, compared with those caught in 1975.

One of the effects of imposex on the female dogwhelk is the blocking of the pallial oviduct, preventing the release of egg capsules and rendering the female sterile. A high incidence of females carrying aborted capsules was found in declining populations close to sources of TBT. The build-up of aborted capsules seemed, eventually, to be lethal to the female; there were fewer females than expected in affected areas (Gibbs & Bryan, 1986). The same authors reported that the gross morphological changes occurring in late imposex in the dogwhelk seem to be irreversible, since animals transferred from a moderately-contaminated site to a "clean" site showed no resorption of the penis. Gibbs & Bryan (1987) stated that imposex in the dogwhelk was seen in sea water with TBT concentrations of less than 1 ng tin/litre. They reported that the reproductive failure, along with a lack of recruitment, had led to population declines, almost to the point of extinction, in areas of heavy TBT contamination. Gibbs et al. (1988) experimentally transferred dogwhelks from an uncontaminated area to one showing water concentrations of 9-19 ng tin/litre (TBT fraction) and demonstrated the development of imposex within 18 months at the new location. These transferred adults were able to spawn for much of this period. The authors compared these results with results for juveniles, which developed imposex earlier and were sterile before reaching maturity. They discussed the implications for the recolonization of areas where reproduction in the dogwhelk has been eliminated. Adults are irreversibly affected by imposex. Recolonization is unlikely until the TBT levels in sea water fall to around 2 ng tin/litre, a concentration at which the juveniles are not sterilized before they reach sexual maturity. The extent of recovery of populations would, therefore, depend on the success of control measures and the water

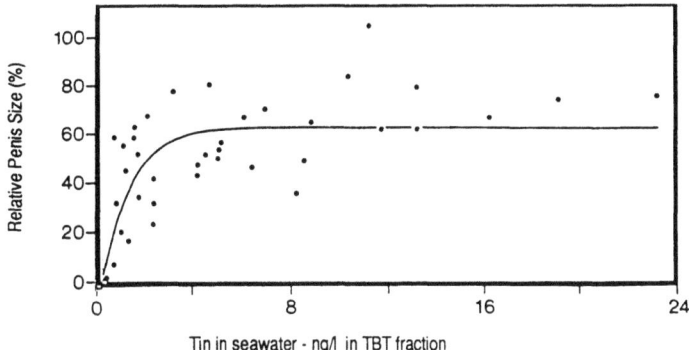

Relationship between relative penis size and concentration of TBT tin in ambient seawater for samples of animals and water taken at the same time around south-west England; 1984 to 1986.

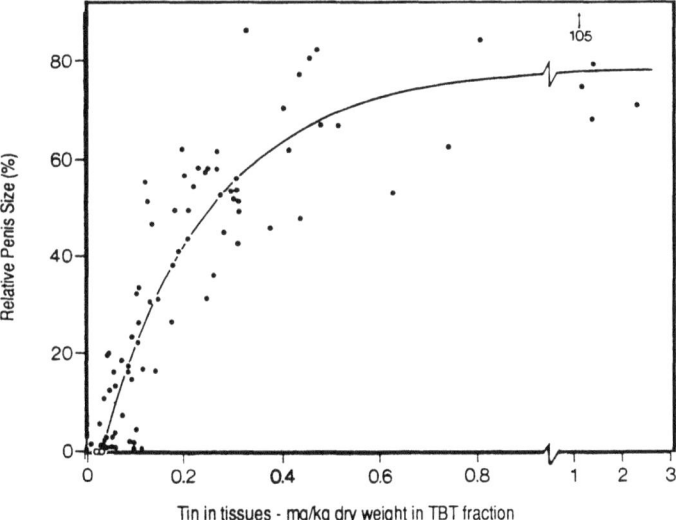

Relationship between relative penis size and concentration of TBT tin in tissue (whole body) samples of animals taken around south-west England; 1984 to 1986.

Fig. 6. Relationship between tin (TBT fraction) in sea water and tissues of the dogwhelk and degree of imposex in females from south-west England. From: Gibbs et al. (1987).

concentrations resulting from bigger ships exempt from the ban on TBT-containing antifouling paints.

Bryan et al. (1987) stated that while the evidence did not show conclusively that TBT is solely responsible for imposex in the dogwhelk, circumstantial evidence was considerable. Imposex is related to the level of boating activity. There is a significant relationship between imposex and the body residue of organotin. Populations that are in decline show the highest levels of TBT. Female populations are declining faster than males and also have the higher levels of TBT. The rise in the degree of imposex coincided with the introduction and use of antifouling paints containing TBT. Imposex has been shown to be caused by TBT in other species of stenoglossan snails, i.e. mud snails (Smith, 1981b). A significant decline in imposex in monitored juvenile *Nucella* (Personal communication by P.E. Gibbs & G.W. Bryan to IPCS) followed the introduction of TBT legislation in the United Kingdom.

10.3 Effects on farmed fish

Wooten et al. (1986) reported the effects of exposure to TBT antifouling paints applied to retaining nets for farmed salmon. Fish exposed to newly-treated cage nets were reported to be blind. The authors examined diseased post-smolt salmon from cages treated with TBT at the time of smolt transfer. Elevated tin levels were found in all salmon exposed to the TBT paint; liver residues ranged between 1.01 and 1.62 mg tin/kg wet weight. Residues in the liver of blind fish ranged between 1.01 and 1.07 mg tin/kg wet weight. Blindness had been caused by rupturing of the eye; the eye lens was missing. Eye tissues appeared normal histologically apart from the rupture; there were no histological lesions. The kidney, liver, stomach, heart and muscle of the blind fish appeared normal histologically. The intestine showed mucosal sloughing, vasodilation, and pyknotic nuclei. The spleen had an "open structure" with increased numbers of erythrocytes. There was thickening of secondary gill filaments and some necrosis and capillary separation in the epithelium. Other fish in the affected population were reported to have swellings along the lateral line. These were shown histologically to be thick folds of epidermis under which there was cellular infiltration of necrotic collagen forming an abscess. Pancreas disease was also reported in affected fish. In the liver there was a breakdown of lobular structure with lack of cohesion between cells. The effects were thought to be consistent with poisoning by organotin.

10.4 Effects of TBT-contaminated sediment

Matthiessen & Thain (1989) studied the recolonization by marine organisms in the field of sediment contaminated with TBT-containing paint. Sediment was collected from mudflats, and macroorganisms present were killed by repeated freezing and thawing. TBT was added to the sediment in the form of abraded paint. The paint was abraded with scourers used on yachts to produce material of the kind likely to contaminate sediments normally. Sediment samples containing 0.1, 1, 10, and 100 mg TBT/kg were prepared. The contaminated sediment was returned to the mudflats and placed in excavated trenches (3 m x 30 cm wide x 20 cm deep) lined with polyethylene mesh (5-mm apertures). Recolonization of the sediment could, therefore, take place both by settlement of organisms from above and by lateral transfer of organisms from adjoining mud. The sites were revisited five times during the next 160 days when samples were taken both to count recolonizing organisms and to measure TBT levels at various depths. Surface sediment decontaminated rapidly; water movement would have removed sediment and deposited new. The subsurface TBT levels remained reasonably stable throughout the experiment. Burrowing activity (estimated by counting casts on the surface) of the polychaete *Arenicola marina* was reduced at all concentrations of TBT, though the effect of 0.1 mg TBT/kg disappeared after 3 months. A dose-related reduction in populations of the burrowing polychaete *Scoloplos armiger* and burrowing amphipod *Urothoe poseidonis* was observed over the whole concentration range. There were no clear effects on other species, including molluscs. The authors pointed out that some unaffected groups were associated with the surface sediment, where TBT was lost rapidly. Feeding behaviour of these surface dwellers, such as the cockle *(Cardium edule)*, would lead to little TBT exposure, since they filter overlying sea water and ingest little or no sediment. Species associated with deeper layers of sediment and feeding on fine particles, such as *Urothoe poseidonis*, showed greater effects of TBT, resulting, presumably, from greater exposure rather than greater inherent sensitivity. The authors also noted the wide range of sensitivity of different species in laboratory tests without sediment. The bioavailability of TBT associated with sediment would probably be different from that dissolved in water.

10.5 Effects of freshwater molluscicides

Following earlier laboratory trials on the use of TBT as a molluscicide for schistosomiasis control (Deschiens & Floch, 1962), Deschiens et al. (1966) applied TBTO to a pond used for fish culture, in Cameroon, of approximately 1 metre in depth and with an area of 50 m^2 (approximately 50 tonnes of water) and a water temperature of 23 °C. Caged pond snails *(Biomphalaria [Australorbis] glabratus* and *Bulinus contortus)*, 10 to a cage supplied with food, were placed in the pond in different areas and at different depths. Renewal of cages was performed to study the persistence of the compound. The pond was treated with TBTO, as "Biomet" (50% TBTO and 50% toxicologically inert dispersant), at rates giving TBTO concentrations in water of 0.015, 0.03, or 0.045 mg/litre, and the side effects on fish and plankton were investigated. At 0.045 mg/litre, TBTO killed 100% of the snails and 70% of the fish within 24 to 48 h. At 0.03 mg/litre, TBTO killed 100% of snails within 2 to 3 days, but no effect on the fish was observed within 15 days. At 0.015 mg/litre, the TBTO killed all of the snails within 4 to 7 days and again had no observable effect on the fish. The authors considered this to be a practical concentration to achieve full effect on snails without killing non-target organisms. Various planktonic organisms (desmids, daphnids, and aquatic insect larvae) were killed by TBTO at 0.5 mg/litre experimentally. However, no effect was found on any of these species in the pond treated at 0.015 mg/litre, although there was some inhibition (but no deaths) of these organisms at 0.03 and 0.045 mg/litre.

Gilbert et al. (1973) applied slow-release TBTO in underseal (quick-drying asphalt-rubber-asbestos-clay paste) to four sites, in Brazil, at concentrations of 15, 15, 50, or 300 g TBTO/m^2, to control *Biomphalaria tenagophila* and *B. straminea*. Dead fish were observed at the sites treated with 50 or 300 g/m^2 and also at one of the two sites treated with 15 g/m^2, a static man-made pit. At the other site, with a flow rate of 100 to 200 litre/min, there was a 100% reduction in the snail population *(B. tenagophila)* maintained for up to 12 months, while both fish and aquatic insect life were apparently normal one month after treatment. At this site abundant natural vegetation flourished in the immediate vicinity of the molluscicide. Toledo et al. (1976) found that 15 g TBTO/m^2 eliminated snails from 76% of treated sites for 1 year. Guppies, which are often present in highly polluted sites, normally suffered some mortality at the beginning of molluscicidal treatment but in general they tolerated it well. The authors found no lasting effect on plant or insect life, and concluded that, because of the ability of an unidentified fungus to grow profusely, microbiological life continued in treated areas.

Shiff et al. (1975) applied BioMet SRM pellets (containing TBTO) at concentrations of 20 and 30 g/m^2 to a night-storage dam in Zimbabwe. At the lower application rate, pellets remained active against the snails (various *Biomphalaria* spp.) for up to one year. At 30 g/m^2, 100% mortality of snails was achieved within 2 weeks of application and was maintained up until the last sampling time 2 months after application. Prior to treatment, 80 specimens of *Tilapia* fish sp. and 1 of *Clarias gariepinus* were caught. Four weeks after treatment 26 *Tilapia* were caught and one dead *Clarias* was found. Eight weeks after treatment 400 *Tilapia* were caught, of which 80 were examined and all appeared normal.

Ayala et al. (1980) applied slow-release molluscicide (rubber impregnated with 11% TBTO) at a rate of between 5 and 15 g/m^2 to a site in Brazil and studied the effect on non-target organisms. The TBTO molluscicide was initially herbicidal towards floating vegetation but did not affect either plants rooted in the mud or marginal plants. The chemical was initially repellent to aquatic animals, some of which were killed by the molluscicide. Within 3 months, populations of non-target snails such as *Pomacea* sp., *Drepanotrema* sp., and a *Physa* sp. had returned to normal. Although no fish had returned within 3 months, after 5 months numbers had returned to normal. In fact, 5 months after application all but *Spirogyra* sp. were normal, and the molluscicidal activity of the TBTO was retained for more than one year. The authors concluded that after 3 to 5 months the action of the TBTO molluscicide is confined to the bottom mud where *Biomphalaria glabrata* snails spend much of their time.

10.6 Effects from spills

According to Waldock et al. (1987a), major inputs of TBT into the environment may have arisen from spills of timber-treatment products, often containing dieldrin and pentachlorophenol as well as the organotin. They reported that a detailed study was carried out after a spill contaminated a section of the Newmill Channel, Kent, United Kingdom. There was a major kill of fish and all macroinvertebrates (except oligochaetes, chironomid larvae, and elmid beetles) were also killed. Concentrations of TBT in the water shortly after the spill were 540 µg per litre, falling to 10 µg/litre after 3 weeks and 0.75 µg per litre after 6 weeks. Nine months after the incident, macroinvertebrate populations were reported to have recovered. The authors stated that five such major spills from timber treatment plants had been reported in the United Kingdom within 2 years.

10.7 The use of indicator species for monitoring the environment

Both shell growth and shell chambering in Pacific oysters and imposex in dogwhelks have been used as biological indicators of TBT contamination. Smith et al. (1987) transferred juvenile Pacific oysters to major bays and harbours of California, USA, known to contain elevated levels of TBT. They observed a graded increase of stunted growth and/or shell deformation, which was associated with poor flushing and the proximity of large numbers of boats. Gibbs et al. (1987) used the dogwhelk to monitor water around the south-west peninsula of England. They found the species to be a very sensitive indicator, especially if the individuals were about 1 year old and in the early stages of ovarian development. Davies et al. (1987a) found imposex in dogwhelks to be a far more sensitive indicator than either shell thickening in oysters or tin accumulation. The dogwhelk has been used to identify areas of contamination associated with seasonal small boat activity and salmon farm cages in Scottish sea lochs (Davies et al., 1987b), in areas of pleasure craft activity, fishing harbours and a boat yard in the Firth of Forth (Scotland) (Bailey & Davies, 1988b), and to investigate contamination from an oil terminal in Sullom Voe, Shetland (Bailey & Davies, 1988a).

11. EFFECTS ON EXPERIMENTAL ANIMALS AND *IN VITRO* TEST SYSTEMS

11.1 Single exposure

Summary

The acute toxic effects of the various TBT compounds that have been studied are comparable and are characteristically delayed for several days. Oral LD_{50} values in laboratory animals range from approximately 40 to 250 mg/kg body weight. These compounds exhibit greater lethal potential when administered parenterally, relative to the oral route, probably because they are only partially absorbed from the gut. Acute toxicity via the dermal route is low.

TBT compounds are potent skin irritants and extreme eye irritants. Dermal exposure to TBTO appears to have little sensitization potential.

Aerosols of TBT compounds are highly toxic. However, TBT vapour/air mixtures at room temperature produce no effect, even at saturation.

Other effects of acute exposure may include alterations in blood lipid levels, the endocrine system, liver, and spleen, and transient deficits in brain development. The toxicological significance of these effects, reported after high single doses of the compounds, is questionable and the cause of death remains unknown.

11.1.1 *Oral and parenteral administration*

The acute toxicity of tributyltin to laboratory mammals by various routes of administration is summarized in Table 14. The acute oral LD_{50} for the rat ranges between 94 and 234 mg/kg body weight and for the mouse between 44 and 230 mg/kg body weight. Truhaut et al. (1976) pointed to the delayed toxicity of tributyltin and, therefore, the necessity to continue the observation of animals, after a single acute dose, for several days. The period of post-dosing observation is therefore indicated in Table 14.

LD_{50} values for ip and iv administrations of TBT are very much lower than in the case of the oral route (10 mg/kg for rat ip and 6 mg/kg for mouse iv).

Table 14. Acute toxicity of tributyltin to laboratory mammals

Species	TBT	Route	Observation period[a] (days)	LD_{50} (mg/kg body weight)	Reference
Rat	oxide	oral	7	194 (165-227)[b]	Elsea & Paynter (1958)
	oxide	oral	7	148 (113-195)[c]	Elsea & Paynter (1958)
	oxide	oral	7	180 (132-228)	Truhaut et al. (1976)
	oxide	oral	21	197 (137-273)	Funahashi et al. (1980)
	oxide	oral		127	Schweinfurth (1985)
	oxide	ip	14	20 (18-21)	Poitou et al. (1978)
	oxide	oral		234	Sheldon (1975)
	fluoride	oral		200	Sheldon (1975)
	fluoride	oral	14	94	Schweinfurth (1985)
	chloride	oral	14	122	Schweinfurth (1985)
	acetate	oral		113.5	Klimmer (1969)
	benzoate	oral		141	Klimmer (1969)
	benzoate	oral	14	99/203	Schweinfurth (1985)
	oleate	oral		225	Klimmer (1969)
	linoleate	oral	14	190	Schweinfurth (1985)
	abietate	oral	14	158	Schweinfurth (1985)
	naphthenate	oral	14	224	Schweinfurth (1985)
Mouse	oxide	oral	7	85 (52-130)	Polster & Halacka (1971)
	acetate	oral	7	46 (25-85)	Pelikan & Cerny (1968)
	oleate	oral	7	230 (175-301)	Pelikan & Cerny (1968)
	benzoate	oral	7	108 (74-156)	Pelikan & Cerny (1968)
	chloride	oral	7	117 (80-170)	Pelikan & Cerny (1968)
	laurate	oral	7	180 (136-237)	Pelikan & Cerny (1968)
	oxide	sc	7	200 (140-270)	Polster & Halacka (1971)
	oxide	iv	7	6 (5.5-6.5)	Truhaut et al. (1976)
	oxide	ip	14	16 (15-17)	Poitou et al. (1978)
Rabbit	fluoride	dermal		680	Sheldon (1975)

[a] Following a single application of TBT, the observation period was as indicated.
[b] Application as aqueous suspension.
[c] Application in corn oil.

Pelikan & Cerny (1968) administered TBT (as the acetate, benzoate, chloride, laurate, or oleate) to white mice (body weight 25 g) in a single oral gavage dose of 500 mg/kg body weight, dissolved in sunflower oil. Ten animals were used for each TBT compound. The mice were observed for 8 h before being killed, and the viscera were examined histologically. Four hours after treatment, all animals showed signs of intoxication with the exception of those given the laurate; after 8 h all showed toxic symptoms. Gross damage was seen in the digestive tract, liver, and spleen. Histological findings included a steatosis of the liver cells in all animals (but to varying degrees), traces of lipid in renal tubule cells (in those animals receiving oleate or laurate) and many haemorrhages in the digestive tract and kidneys. Effects on the liver and spleen were also noted after dermal absorption of TBTO (Pelikan & Cerny, 1969). However, no real conclusions can be drawn from these studies as there was no clear reported evidence that steatosis was caused either by the TBT or by the fatty acids.

In studies by Funahashi et al. (1980), Sprague-Dawley rats were given a single dose, in olive oil, of 100 mg TBTO/kg body weight by intubation and were examined over the following 21 days. Adrenal weight was slightly increased 12 h after treatment and reached a maximum on the second day. Histological changes in the adrenal had returned to normal by day 14. The thyroid follicles showed signs similar to those produced by hypophysectomy, i.e. distension with colloid, flat epithelial cells. These changes were severe after 72 h, but had returned to normal within 14 days. Absolute pituitary weight was increased slightly (and not significantly) 1 and 2 days after dosing, while relative weight increased significantly. There was atrophy of pituitary adrenocorticotrophin (ACTH) cells 6 h after dosing. After 72 h, the staining of ACTH cells became more intense. There were marked reductions in the circulating levels of both thyroid stimulating hormone (TSH) and thyroxine (T_4) during the 72 h following dosing, serum titres falling to one half and one sixth of control values for the two hormones, respectively. The authors concluded that TBTO had both a direct and an indirect effect on the thyroid, since initially there was a simultaneous rise in T_4 and fall in TSH. Serum cortisol levels increased to twice the control level 96 h after treatment with TBTO at a level of 100 mg/kg body weight. Intramuscular ACTH administration, 8 h after dosing, led to increased cortisol in the blood of both treated and control rats. After 16 h, controls showed release of cortisol after ACTH stimulation, but treated rats showed a decrease in circulating levels of cortisol after similar stimulation.

Matsui et al. (1982) reported the effects of a single dose of TBT fluoride (100 mg/kg body weight) given by gastric intubation to Japanese white rabbits. A reversible but pronounced hyperlipidaemia was observed, particularly involving triglycerides and total cholesterol. Ultracentrifugation showed a marked increase in the chylomicron plus VLDL (very low density lipoprotein) fraction. The activity of lipoprotein lipase (LPL) in plasma was reduced to about 50% of control levels. Fasting levels of blood glucose were elevated, and the response to iv infusion of glucose (given 3 days after the TBT fluoride) was inhibited (insulin release reduced). The authors suggested that the hyperlipidaemia was the result of reduced LPL activity, which in turn was brought about by inhibition of insulin release.

Calley et al. (1967) investigated the effects of TBT acetate on liver function in rabbits. Following a single oral dose of TBT acetate at 50 mg/kg body weight (half of the measured LD_{50} in rabbits), only the serum glutamic-pyruvate transaminase (SGPT) activity was affected. This activity was not elevated after 48 h but was increased within 144 h of dosing. Prothrombin time, alkaline phosphatase, and thymol turbidity showed no significant changes from control values. SGPT is a highly specific indicator of liver damage, directly reflecting liver cell injury. Tributyltin acetate also significantly increased the hexabarbitol-induced sleeping times of mice; a 50 mg/kg body weight oral dose increased the sleeping time from 29 to 43 min following a standard dose of the narcotic.

When Aldridge et al. (1977) administered TBTO (and its gamma-keto, gamma-hydroxy, and delta-hydroxy metabolites) intraperitoneally to mice on two consecutive days (at dose levels of 12.5, 25, and 50 μmol/kg body weight), they found no evidence of cerebral oedema after any of the treatments.

Crofton et al. (1989) gave rat pups a single dose of TBTO on day 5 following birth by gastric intubation with 0, 40, 50, or 60 mg/kg body weight. The monitoring of behavioural parameters up to 62 days post-dosing showed no persistent effect on motor activity or acoustic startle response.

When Barnes & Stoner (1958) fed rats with tributyltin acetate during the first 3 months after birth, they found increased brain and spinal cord water content at the highest dose tested (100 mg/kg diet). This increase was not sufficiently great to be seen in histological sections. Bouldin et al. (1981) found no light or electron microscopic evidence of neuronal damage in the hippocampus or the pyriform cortex of neonate or adult rats exposed daily to tributyltin acetate at 10 mg/kg body weight by gavage for up to 30 days.

O'Callaghan & Miller (1988) reported the effects of a single ip injection of TBTO on neonatal rat brain. The rats were injected when 5 days old with 2, 3, or 4 mg/kg. They were sacrificed at 13, 22, or 60 days of age, and various proteins in homogenates of brain tissue were measured by radioimmunoassay. Brain weight was reduced in a dose-dependent manner, the cerebellum being most affected. There was no evidence of altered brain histology under the light microscope. Dose-dependent and region-dependent decreases were found in P-38 (a synaptic-vesicle-associated protein) and myelin basic protein (a protein associated with oligodendroganglia and the myelin sheath); there were decreases in both total (per tissue) and concentration (per mg) levels of these proteins in the cerebellum and forebrain but not the hippocampus. These effects were seen at a dose level that did not affect body weight. However, in contrast to the neurotoxic effects of trimethyltin compounds, which are irreversible and persist into adulthood, these neurotoxic effects of TBTO were transitory at dose levels that did not affect body weight.

Robinson (1969) monitored tissue levels of catecholamines after ip administration of TBTO, in corn oil, to rats at a level of 10 mg/kg body weight. This dose exceeded the 6-day LD_{50}, determined by the same authors to be 7.21 mg/kg. Brain noradrenalin levels were significantly reduced at 2, 24, and 48 h after dosing, whereas 5-hydroxytryptamine levels were only reduced (though markedly) after 48 h. Noradrenalin levels in heart tissue were also significantly reduced after 2, 24, and 48 h. Adrenal adrenalin and noradrenalin levels were reduced after 24 and 48 h, but only adrenalin was affected after 2 h.

11.1.2 Dermal administration

The acute LD_{50} of TBTO administered to rabbits via the dermal route is very high, i.e. approximately 9000 mg/kg body weight (Table 14). Although there is dermal absorption of TBT (see later), the degree of absorption is not great enough to lead to acute toxic effects systemically, except at very high exposure levels.

11.1.3 Administration by inhalation

In a "nose only" inhalation exposure (to minimize dermal exposure and exposure through ingestion) lasting 4 h, the acute LC_{50} of TBTO for the rat was estimated to be 77 mg/m^3 by measurement of airborne droplets. This value decreased to 65 mg/m^3 when "inhalable" particles, 10 μm or less in diameter, were considered. There was evidence of lung irritation and oedema in this study (Schweinfurth, 1985). When groups of 10 male and 10 female rats were each exposed to atmospheres containing almost saturated vapours of TBTO, TBT benzoate, or TBT naphthenate once for 7 h, no deaths occurred during exposure or in a 14-day observation period following exposure. Only minor clinical signs were noted occasionally during the experiment, such as slight nasal discharge (Schweinfurth, 1985).

Truhaut et al. (1979) exposed mice to an aerosol of TBTO in olive oil, for either a single 1-h period or seven 1-h periods on successive days, using TBTO concentrations in air ranging between 0.05 and 0.4 mg/litre (50 to 400 mg/m^3). Exploratory behaviour was scored over 5-min periods 2 h after the single exposure was complete or 24 h after the last of the seven exposure periods. The lower two exposure doses caused significant increases in exploratory behaviour (17% and 5% for 42 and 84 mg/kg, respectively) while the higher exposure doses reduced exploratory behaviour (-18% and -38% for 170 and 340 mg/kg, respectively). Truhaut et al. (1981) found a median survival time for mice of 22 min and for guinea-pigs of 9 min after exposure to an aerosol of tributyltin (concentration not stated). They reported that only tissues in the respiratory system showed significant lesions. There was diffuse congestion of the pulmonary blood vessels extending to the septal capillary beds. There were also inflammatory responses in the trachea and bronchii, secretion of mucus in the bronchii and bronchioles, and distension and rupture of the alveoli.

Anger et al. (1976) exposed guinea-pigs to aerosols of TBTO ranging between 0.1 and 1 mg/litre air for 1 h. All males exposed to 0.2 mg/litre died, and 12 out of 15 females exposed to 1 mg/litre died. No particular lesions were observed in those animals that died, with the exception of a general congestion of the lungs. Exposure of either males or females to 0.17 mg/litre caused no deaths, though nasal irritation was observed; all these animals survived a further 7 days of observation.

11.1.4 Irritation and sensitization

11.1.4.1 Skin irritation

In a study by Elsea & Paynter (1958), undiluted TBTO was applied to the closely-clipped skin of the abdominal area of rabbits, which was then covered with rubber dental damming, gauze, and adhesive tape. After an exposure period of 24 h, the covering was removed, and the TBTO was washed off, as far as possible, by sponging with warm water. This single application of doses up to 11.7 g/kg body weight caused some of the rabbits to die from the effects of TBTO absorbed into the body. There was, however, only moderate dermal irritation, characterized by reddening, oedema, atonia, blanched areas, and areas of brown discolouration. Examination of the skin at autopsy showed some subcutaneous oedema. Repeated dermal application of TBTO, impregnated into paper at 8 mg/kg, daily for 5 days, only affected one animal out of four. This rabbit showed slight erythema and oedema following the first and second applications. Later in the experiment, the skin appeared normal. No detailed histological examination of the skin was carried out.

Pelikan & Cerny (1969) applied to the shaved skin of rats two preparations of TBTO, i.e. "Lastanax T" (containing 20% TBTO plus a medium of water, alcohols of short chain length, and n-alkyl-polyethylene oxide) and "Lastanax P" (containing 15% TBTO plus a medium also containing bis-(5-chloro-2-hydroxyphenyl)-methane). Actual doses applied, corresponding to water dilutions of 100%, 33%, 10%, and 1% of the preparations, were 185, 61.5, 18.5, and 1.85 mg TBTO/kg body weight for Lastanax T and 145, 47, 14, and 1.4 mg TBTO for Lastanax P. Controls received either water or the medium without TBTO. The experiment was carried out in duplicate. In the first series, clinical observations were made twice daily for

60 days, whereas in the second series rats were killed on day 10 and the skin was examined histologically. Control rats showed no clinical or histological effects on the skin. However, clinical and histological changes were found in all treated rats, even with the 1% dilution, though severity increased with exposure dose. On the first and second days after application, there was reddening of the skin and oedema developed. From day 3, haemorrhagic eschars developed with well defined borders; there was no inflammation of the surrounding areas of skin. Between these foci, numerous papules and pustules developed, some with bleeding; the apices of some papules were necrosed. Later the eschars joined to create larger areas of ulceration. Healing of the areas began between the 9th and 12th days; necroses disappeared by day 20, pustules 3 to 4 days before, and papules by the 30th to 33rd day. All signs had disappeared after 35-38 days (exposure to 1% and 10% solutions) or after 45-50 days (exposure to 33% or 100% solutions). Changes with Lastanax P were similar, but less severe, than with Lastanax T. In the histological study, numerous large bullae, filled with leucocytes and coagulated exudate (proteins), were found under the stratum corneum of the epidermis after 10 days. Akanthosis and vacuolation of epidermal cells occurred following exposure to the 10% and 33% solutions and, to a lesser extent, the 1% solution. Small haemorrhages were found. Epidermal changes were dispersed and alternated with areas of skin appearing normal. The authors suggested that the TBTO NOEL for human skin should be set at 0.005% to 0.01%.

In a study by Middleton & Pratt (1977), TBT chloride was applied to a shaved area of dorsal skin of male Alderley Park (Wistar-derived) rats, four-weeks old (body weight 50-80 g), in absolute ethanol as a solution of 10 mmol/litre. This dose was equivalent to 67 nmol/cm^2. The TBT had produced microscopic changes in the skin within 2 h of application. Polymorphonuclear leucocytes accumulated in capillaries and in dermal tissues. Epidermal cells showed progressive degenerative changes between 2 and 8 h after application until, by 8 h after application, separation of the epidermis and dermis had occurred and fluid collected in this separation. Many inflammatory cells were present in both dermis and epidermis. There was widespread epidermal necrosis within 12 to

24 h, and separation of necrotic epidermis from the dermis was almost complete by this time. The vesicles formed by this separation were frequently packed with inflammatory cells as well as exudative fluid. Regeneration of the epidermal layer was observed after 18 to 24 h and dermal inflammatory infiltration was regressing by this time. Erythema, visually assessed and scored, reached a maximum within 5 h of application and remained at this level for 48 h. The erythema had subsided by 72 h after application. Vascular permeability of the skin was assessed by injecting rats with a dye, tryphan blue, 45 min before sacrifice. There was a biphasic response. At 2 h after application of TBT chloride, there was an initial increase in permeability of the skin to 135% of control levels. A second peak began at 12 h and persisted for more than 25 h after application. The effect was still evident after 48 h and had occurred in both the treated and untreated flanks of the animal, indicating absorption of the compound and a systemic effect. The water content of the skin was increased by TBT chloride, reaching a peak within 2 h of application; by 10 h this effect had disappeared. Middleton & Pratt (1978) reported that TBT produced focal epidermal necroses and dermal inflammation at levels as low as 33 nmol/cm^2, fairly extensive epidermal necroses and dermal inflammation at 67 nmol/cm^2, and almost total epidermal necrosis at 167 nmol/cm^2.

11.1.4.2 Eye irritation

Pelikan (1969) applied TBTO, as "Lastanax T or P", in a single dose of 0.03 ml to the left eye of rabbits. Lastanax T is 20% TBTO in alcohols of short chain length, non-ionic surface active substances (n-alkyl-polyethylene oxide) and water. Lastanax P is 15% TBTO in the same vehicle with the addition of bis-(5-chloro-2-hydroxyphenyl) methane. A 10% and a 1% solution in water were used. The 10% solution represented an actual TBTO dose of 6.1 and 4.6 mg/kg body weight for the two formulations, respectively. With the 10% solution, both rabbits died, 11 and 12 days after application. Severe ulceration of the eye preceded death. Histopathological examination of internal organs after death revealed hyperaemia of the brain and medulla oblongata and hyperplasia of reticuloendothelial cells of the spleen. Necrotic changes were seen on the cornea of eyes treated with the 1% solutions within 3 h of application, and symptoms worsened over the next 2 to 5 days. Recovery was incomplete 100 days later.

1.4.3 Skin sensitization

Poitou et al. (1978) investigated the skin-sensitizing potential of TBTO in guinea-pigs using the Magnussen-Kligman method. The concentrations used for sensitization were 1% (intradermal phase) and 5% (topical phase). Using challenge concentrations of 0.25% and 0.1%, no sensitizing action was demonstrated in the 20 test animals.

11.1.5 In vitro studies

Johnson & Knowles (1983) demonstrated that incubation of rat blood platelets with TBT chloride or TBTO, *in vitro*, inhibited their ability to take up ^{14}C-labelled 5-hydroxytryptamine (5-HT). The organotin also caused release of ^{14}C-labelled 5-HT, taken up before exposure, along with endogenous 5-HT. Treating rats ip with TBT chloride at 5.0 mg/kg body weight also led to reduced uptake of 5-HT (37% inhibition) 30 min after treatment. The level of 5-HT in platelets, however, was unaffected by the *in vivo* treatment with TBT chloride. Knowles & Johnson (1986) reported that exposure of rat platelets to TBT chloride inhibited aggregation induced with ADP or collagen. The inhibition of ADP-induced aggregation was dependent on the dose of TBT and on the exposure time prior to ADP addition. Exposure of the platelets to 5 μmol TBT per litre for 5 min or 10 μmol/litre for 0.1 min produced inhibition. However, exposure to 1 μmol/litre for 5 min was ineffective. With an incubation time of 1 min, TBTO was effective in lengthening the time taken for aggregation after collagen induction at 0.625 μmol/litre, but not at 0.5 μmol/litre.

The trialkyltins, including tributyltin, have been shown to inhibit oxidative phosphorylation in rat mitochondria (Aldridge & Street, 1964). TBT stimulated adenosinetriphosphatase (ATPase) activity and caused limited swelling of rat liver mitochondria. These last two effects occurred at similar concentrations of TBT in the medium. The authors postulated that the two effects were linked; the ATPase activity increased over a concentration range of TBT and was always mirrored by a decrease in the mitochondrial swelling. This relationship persisted despite a complex response to TBT over the concentration range; at higher concentrations there was a sudden, much smaller mitochondrial swelling and a concomitant rise in ATPase activity. TBT also inhibited the hydrolysis of ATP by rat brain microsomes, although the concentrations required were much higher than those affecting phosphorylation. The authors postulated that a combination of trialkyltin compounds with negatively charged lipids is involved in their biological activity.

Elferink et al. (1986) treated polymorphonuclear leucocytes (PMNs), obtained from the peritoneal cavity of rabbits, with an unspecified tributyltin (1 μmol/litre). Uptake of opsonized zymosan was used as a measure of phagocytosis, and enzyme (lysozyme) release to the supernatant during incubation was also monitored. There was almost complete inhibition of both parameters at 10^{-6} mol TBT/litre but no effect at 10^{-7} mol/litre. Inhibition of phagocytosis was exactly paralleled by inhibition of enzyme release. At concentrations of between 10^{-6} and 10^{-5} mol/litre, tributyltin caused lysis of the cells with release of LDH, suggesting damage to the plasma membrane. Exocytosis, induced by FMLP in the presence of "cytocolasin B", was also inhibited by the TBT at concentrations of 10^{-6} mol/litre or more. There was little effect of the compound on ATP levels in PMNs, and the authors suggested that interference with ATP production was not the basis for the effect of the TBT. Activation of PMNs is accompanied by an increase in plasma membrane permeability to Ca^{2+}; this was strongly inhibited by the TBT. The authors proposed two alternative explanations. Either the Ca^{2+} permeability change is directly affected or an earlier step is inhibited which, in turn, affects calcium permeability. The observation that the exocytosis effect could be counteracted by the addition of sulfydryl compounds led the authors to conclude that the earliest stages of activation of the PMNs were affected. Arakawa & Wada (1984) reported a suppression of the chemotactic response of rabbit leucocytes (neutrophils) towards formyl-methionyl-leucyl-phenylalanine by tributyltin chloride at concentration between 0.1 and 10 μmol/litre *in vitro*.

Reinhardt et al. (1982) used cell detachment and cloning efficiency of baby hamster kidney cells (BHK-21 C13) to quantify the cytotoxicity of organotin compounds. The two parameters are independent, but each covers a range of cellular damage. Cell detachment indicates irreversible damage to the cytoskeleton over a 4-h period, while cloning efficiency covers influence on growth of single cells over a 6-day period and includes cell reattachment followed by clone formation. The IC_{50} (concentration at which there was a 50% reduction in cloning efficiency) for TBTO was 5×10^{-7} mol/litre (0.3 mg/litre medium) and for TBT chloride was 1.4×10^{-6} mol per litre (0.5 mg/litre). The CD_{50} (50% effect on cell detachment) was less sensitive to TBT, i.e. 3×10^{-5} mol/litre for TBTO (18 mg/litre) and 4.3×10^{-5} mol/litre for TBT chloride (14 mg/litre).

When Snoeij et al. (1986a) incubated isolated rat thymocytes with TBT chloride, there was membrane damage and disintegration of the cells at concentrations higher than 1 μmol/litre. Various parameters of cell function were investigated. The TBT chloride increased the consumption of glucose in a dose-related manner at concentrations in the culture medium higher than 0.1 μmol/litre; production of lactate was also increased in parallel. The effect peaked at 1 μmol TBT/litre and thereafter declined; damage to cell integrity occurred at these concentrations. Over the same effective range of concentrations (0.1 to 1 μmol/litre), TBT decreased ATP levels. The ATP diminished very rapidly, within 2.5 min, and remained low for at least 3 h. The incorporation of radiolabelled nucleotide precursors into DNA and RNA and of amino acids into protein was also affected. Thymidine incorporation into DNA was reduced, relative to TBT dose, to a minimum of 20% of control incorporation at 1 μmol TBT/litre. Uridine incorporation was similarly reduced, but less effectively. Inhibition of amino acid incorporation was substantial at 0.25 μmol TBT chloride/litre and protein synthesis was virtually totally inhibited at 1 μmol/litre. The median inhibitory concentrations (IC_{50}) for thymidine, uridine, proline, and leucine were 0.32 ± 0.04, 0.95 ± 0.06, 0.38 ± 0.04, and 0.36 ± 0.03 μmol/litre, respectively. TBT chloride concentrations of 0.1 μmol/litre or more markedly reduced the production of cyclic AMP by the thymocytes under stimulation from prostaglandin E_1. TBT chloride, therefore, has marked effects on the energy metabolism of isolated thymocytes at concentrations well below those affecting membrane integrity, and, as a result, the authors stated that TBT chloride is best characterized as an energy poison.

Snoeij et al. (1988a) similarly isolated rat thymocytes, but separated them into fractions based on size. The same parameters of cell function were investigated in each of three fractions. Fraction 1 consisted of small, non-proliferating thymocytes. Fractions 2 and 3 showed some overlap in size, but fraction 2 was enriched in cells actively synthesizing macromolecules, while fraction 3 was enriched in dividing cells and showed the greatest proliferative capacity. Resting ATP levels were highest in the bigger cells, steady state levels increasing with fraction number. TBT chloride reduced ATP levels in each subfraction proportionally to between 62 and 64% of control values. Thus, TBT reduces intracellular ATP concentrations irrespective of cell volume or number of mitochondria. As with unfractionated thymocytes, TBT chloride at both 0.25 and 1.0 μmol/litre inhibited thymidine incorporation (to around 40% of control values at 0.25 μmol/litre and between 21 and 37% of control values at 1 μmol/litre) and leucine incorporation (to between 13 and 29% of controls at 0.25 μmol/litre and 1 to 3% of controls at 1 μmol/litre) in all fractions. In the case of uridine incorporation, although there was inhibition in most cases, 0.25 μmol TBT chloride/litre caused a stimulation to 184% of control levels in fraction 1, the non-proliferating cells.

11.2 Short-term toxicity

Summary

TBT compounds have been studied most extensively in the rat (all the data in this section refer to the rat unless otherwise indicated).

At dietary doses of 320 mg/kg (approximately 25 mg/kg body weight), high mortality rates were observed when the exposure time exceeded 4 weeks. No deaths were noted at 100 mg/kg diet (10 mg/kg body weight) or after daily administration of 12 mg per kg body weight by gavage. In rats dosed during early postnatal life, 3 mg/kg body weight resulted in increased deaths. The main symptoms at lethal doses were loss of appetite, weakness, and emaciation.

Borderline effects on rat growth were observed at 50 mg/kg diet (6 mg/kg body weight) and 6 mg/kg body weight (gavage studies). Mice are less sensitive, effects being observed at 150 to 200 mg/kg diet (22 to 29 mg/kg body weight).

Structural effects on endocrine organs, mainly the pituitary and thyroid, have been noted in both short- and long-term studies. Changes in circulating hormone concentrations and altered response to physiological stimuli (pituitary trophic hormones) were observed in short-term tests, but after long-term exposure most of these changes appeared to be absent. The mechanism of action is not known.

Exposure to TBTO aerosol at 2.8 mg/m^3 produced high mortality, respiratory distress, inflammatory reaction within the respiratory tract and histopathological changes of lymphatic organs. However, exposure to the highest attainable vapour concentration (0.16 mg/m^3) at room temperature produced no effects.

Toxic effects on the liver and bile ducts have been reported in three mammalian species. Hepatocellular necrosis and inflammatory changes in the bile duct were observed in rats fed TBTO at a dietary level of 320 mg/kg (approximately 25 mg/kg body weight) for 4 weeks and in mice fed 80 mg/kg diet (approximately 12 mg/kg body weight) for 90 days. Vacuolization of periportal hepatocytes was noted in dogs fed a dose of 10 mg/kg body weight for 8 to 9 weeks. These changes were occasionally accompanied by increased liver weight and increased serum activities of liver enzymes.

Decreases in haemoglobin concentration and erythrocyte volume in rats, resulting from dosing with 80 mg/kg diet (8 mg/kg body weight), indicate an effect on haemoglobin synthesis, leading to microcytic hypochromic anaemia. The decrease in splenic haemosiderin levels suggests alterations in iron status. Anaemia has also been observed in mice.

The formation of erythrocyte rosettes in mesenteric lymph nodes has been observed in certain short-term investigations but not in long-term studies. The biological significance of this finding (possibly transient) is unclear.

The characteristic toxic effect of TBTO is on the immune system; due to effects on the thymus, the cell-mediated function is impaired. The mechanism of action is unknown, but may involve the metabolic conversion to dibutyltin compounds. Nonspecific resistance is also affected.

General effects on the immune system (e.g., on the weight and morphology of lymphoid tissues, peripheral lymphocyte counts, and total serum immunoglobulin concentrations) have been reported in several different studies with TBTO using rats and dogs, but not mice, at overtly toxic dose levels (effects in mice have been seen with tributyltin chloride at 150 mg/kg). Only the rat exhibits general effects on the immune system without other overt signs of toxicity and is clearly the most sensitive species. The NOEL in short-term rat studies was 5 mg/kg diet (0.6 mg/kg body weight). In studies with tributyltin chloride, analogous effects on the thymus were seen. These were readily reversible when dosing ceased. TBTO has been shown to compromise specific immune function in rat in vivo host resistance studies. Decreased clearance of Listeria monocytogenes was seen after exposure to a dietary level of 50 mg/kg (the NOEL being 5 mg/kg per day), and decreased resistance to Trichinella spiralis was seen at 50 and 5 mg/kg diet, but not at 0.5 mg/kg diet (2.5, 0.25, and 0.025 mg/kg per day body weight, respectively). Similar effects were seen in aged animals, but these were less pronounced.

With present knowledge, the effects on host resistance are probably of most relevance in assessing the potential hazard to man, but there is insufficient experience in these test systems to fully assess their significance. However, some data on the significance of the T. spiralis model are provided by findings in athymic nude rats after the standard challenge. In these studies, the complete absence of thymus-dependent immunity resulted in a 10- to 20-fold increase in muscle larvae counts; by contrast, exposure to TBTO concentrations of 5 and 50 mg/kg diet resulted in a 2-fold and a 4-fold increase, respectively.

Although some data are now available from studies on the effects of tributyltin compounds on the developing immune system, there is no information on host resistance.

It would be prudent to base assessment of the potential hazard to humans on data from the most sensitive species. Effects on host resistance to T. spiralis have been seen at dietary levels as low as 5 mg/kg (equivalent to 0.25 mg/kg per day body weight), the NOEL being 0.5 mg/kg (equivalent to 0.025 mg/kg per day). However, the interpretation of the significance of these data for human risk assessment is controversial. In all other studies a concentration of 5 mg/kg per day in the diet (equivalent to 0.5 mg/kg body weight, based on the short-term studies) was the NOEL with respect to general, as well as specific, effects on the immune system.

11.2.1 Oral dosing: general body effects

Iwasaki et al. (1976) reported some oedema and destruction of nerve axons following the administration of 0.01 ml TBTO/kg directly to the stomach of rats every day for 28 days. No details of procedures or results were presented in this report.

Schweinfurth (1985) found no evidence of brain oedema after dosing rats with TBTO orally in arachis oil. Even doses producing marked toxic effects on other organs (25 mg/kg body weight) failed to produce noticeable brain oedema. However, triethyltin chloride produces brain oedema at a dose of 1.5 mg/kg body weight.

Krajnc et al. (1984) investigated the short-term effects of bis-tributyltin oxide in the rat. In experiments lasting 4 weeks, Wistar rats were fed technical TBTO at levels of 0, 5, 20, 80, or 320 mg/kg diet. All animals survived the dosing period. Various symptoms of poisoning were seen within 1 week of dosing in the group fed 320 mg/kg diet, i.e. weakness, emaciation, roughened fur, and blood-tinged discharge around the eyes and nose. Some of these signs were seen at the lower doses after 4 weeks. Body weight gain was not affected by doses up to 20 mg/kg diet in males and 80 mg/kg in females. Males showed reduced weight gain (96 g compared to control weight gain of 117 g) over 4 weeks at 80 mg TBTO/kg. At 320 mg/kg diet, TBTO caused a reduction in body weight of 13 g in males and 21 g in females. Almost all of this weight loss occurred in the first week of dosing, body weight remaining constant after that. A 50% reduction in food consumption was seen at this dose rate, compared to control animals. Urine analysis, during the fourth week of dosing, revealed no differences in urine volume, protein concentration, or creatinine clearance related to treatment.

Funahashi et al. (1980) conducted histopathological and biochemical studies on Sprague-Dawley rats given bis-tributyltin oxide (TBTO) dissolved in olive oil. The rats were dosed by intubation 5 times weekly for 13 or 26 weeks. Body weight was reduced after 13 weeks dosing at 6 mg/kg body weight, but not significantly so. After 26 weeks, body weight was significantly reduced relative to controls (382 g compared to the control value of 439 g). Dosing at 12 mg/kg reduced body weight significantly at both 13 and 26 weeks (to 311 and 356 g, respectively). There was a slight decrease, but unrelated to either dose or time, in spleen weight. This decrease was just significant at 6 mg/kg over 13 weeks and 12 mg/kg over 26 weeks, but at no other time or dose.

When Mushak et al. (1982) dosed neonatal rats with TBT acetate at levels of 1, 3, or 10 mg/kg per day from day 2 to day 29 of age, all rats given 1 mg/kg per day survived with no apparent gross or histopathological effect. Totals of 9 out of 24 and 17 out of 24 rats survived at dose levels of 10 and 3 mg/kg per day, respectively, but all showed reduced body weight. There were liver effects in survivors.

11.2.2 Inhalation studies

A "nose only" inhalation study (lasting 4-5 weeks) by Schweinfurth (1985) with rats exposed for 4 h/day (on weekdays only; 21 to 24 exposure periods) to an aerosol of TBTO (2.8 mg/m^3) produced mortality (50% of males and 60% of females), apathy, and respiratory distress. Food consumption and body weight gain were reduced. There were inflammatory reactions within the respiratory tract and lymphotoxic effects (depletion of lymphocytes in the thymic cortex, atrophy of the thymus, and lymph nodes). Inhalation of TBTO vapour/air mixtures produced no observable effect. A concentration of 0.16 mg/m^3 in the inhalation chamber, which corresponds to the equilibrium vapour pressure of TBTO at room temperature, was considered to be the NOEL for rats.

When Gohlke et al. (1969) exposed rats to TBT chloride in a 4-month inhalation study at nominal concentrations of

4 to 6 mg/m^3, all animals survived the exposure. Towards the end of the exposure, in the final month, the rats showed minor irritation of the eye and nose. There was an initial increase in relative liver weight but a significant reduction over the whole experimental period. Fat droplets were seen in the livers at autopsy, together with a diffuse oedema of the brain. However, controls also showed oedema. The oedema disappeared slowly as recovery time after exposure increased. There were also inflammatory changes in the respiratory tract of exposed animals.

Crofton et al. (1989) exposed pregnant female rats to TBTO by intubation at 0 to 10 mg/kg per day on days 6 to 20 of gestation. There was no effect on the age at which the testes of male offspring descended. However, females showed a delay of approximately 2 days in vaginal opening, compared to controls, after their mothers were exposed to 10 mg/kg per day.

11.2.3 Histopathological effects

Snoeij et al. (1985) reported that weanling rats fed tributyltin chloride at a level of 150 mg/kg diet showed marked reductions in body weight (treated rats, 87 g; control rats, 119 g) and brain weight (treated rats, 1.54 g; control rats, 1.67 g) associated with a reduced food intake of 25%. Thymus weight was reduced to 39% of the control value over the 2-week feeding period.

Krajnc et al. (1984) found histopathological changes in male and female Wistar rats exposed to 5, 20, 80, or 320 mg TBTO/kg diet for 4 weeks. No treatment-related changes were found in the brain, heart, kidney, pancreas, adrenals, popliteal lymph nodes, intestinal tract, or bone marrow. Slight atrophy of hepatocytes (reduction in size) in the centrilobular region was noted in some livers at 80 mg/kg and marked atrophy in 16 out of 20 livers at 320 mg/kg. The authors reported dystrophic calcification in the liver at the highest dose level. Three animals showed multiple-focus inflammation with necrosis of hepatic parenchyma, which was associated with mononuclear and polymorphonuclear infiltration, fibrosis, and hyperplasia of the intrahepatic bile duct. In one animal there was inflammation of the common bile duct. No bacteria or viruses were found in the lesions. Similar necrotic lesions were observed, in two animals, in a repeat study at 320 mg TBTO/kg diet.

Mori et al. (1984) painted the shaved dorsal skin of guinea-pigs daily for 50 days with an ethanolic solution of TBTO at 10 or 40 mg/kg body weight. Monitoring of urine and blood electrolyte levels during the course of the treatment showed increased loss of sodium, chloride, phosphate, glucose, and amino acids in the urine. There was a concomitant loss of electrolytes from serum. The effect was most marked between 40 and 50 days of treatment. Histological lesions of the kidney tubules were observed when the animals were killed after the 50th day.

11.2.4 Haematological and biochemical effects

Measurements of blood biochemical parameters of rats fed TBTO for 4 weeks indicated few significant effects at dietary dose levels below 320 mg/kg diet. Alanine amino transferase (ALAT) activity was significantly increased, in a dose-related manner, at 20 mg/kg or more, in both males and females. The highest dose significantly decreased blood glucose in males, aspartate amino transferase (ASAT) in both males and females, and liver glycogen in both sexes. Serum triglycerides, alkaline phosphatase, and creatinine kinase activities were unaffected at any dose level, as were blood lactate and pyruvate. At 80 mg/kg diet, TBTO significantly reduced blood haemoglobin in both sexes and haematocrit in females. Mean erythrocytes volume was reduced in both sexes, as was mean corpuscular haemoglobin content (mass), but mean corpuscular haemoglobin concentration and erythrocyte numbers were not affected (Krajnc et al., 1984). A 6-week study at dietary doses of 5, 20, and 80 mg/kg showed significant reductions in haematocrit at 20 and 80 mg/kg and in blood haemoglobin levels at 80 mg/kg. Iron concentration was reduced at 80 mg/kg, as was the isocitrate dehydrogenase (ICDH) activity of erythrocytes. Numbers of erythrocytes, thrombocytes, and reticulocytes were not significantly affected at any dose level of TBTO, though there was a trend towards increased numbers of reticulocytes. The authors suggested an effect on haemoglobin synthesis and other indicators, implying either reduced iron uptake or increased iron loss. The enhanced ICDH activity and increasing reticulocyte numbers indicated the presence of immature erythrocytes, and the authors could not exclude the possibility of an *in vivo* haemolytic action of TBTO comparable to the reported *in vitro* haemolysis (Krajnc et al., 1984).

Rosenberg et al. (1984) measured the activity of haem oxygenase in mucosal cell fractions from control mice and mice dosed by intubation with TBTO at 60 mg/kg body weight. The activity of the enzyme, monitored by the bilirubin absorbance spectrum, was substantially elevated, compared to controls, 16 h after administration of the TBTO. The activity of the same enzyme in liver and kidney microsomes was not affected by this dose of TBTO given by gavage, but was elevated when TBTO was given parenterally. The activities of cytochrome P-450 and benzo(a)pyrene hydroxylase were substantially reduced in the intestine of TBTO-treated mice, this reduced activity being statistically significant for the latter but not for the former. Similar results were obtained in liver fractions when TBTO was applied parenterally.

11.2.5 Effects on lymphoid organs and immune function

Funahashi et al. (1980) reported the effects of feeding TBTO in olive oil (0, 3, 6, or 12 mg/kg body weight per day) for 13 or 26 weeks by gavage to groups of ten male Sprague-Dawley rats, aged 5 weeks at the beginning of the study. No analyses of haematology, immunoglobulin levels, or specific aspects of immune function were performed. A marked dose-related reduction in absolute and relative thymus weight was seen following dosing for both periods. Relative thymus weights were 682, 629, 340, and 313 mg/kg body weight after 13 weeks of dosing and 449, 313, 278, and 248 mg/kg body weight after 26 weeks of dosing in the rats given 0, 3, 6, and 12 mg/kg per day, respectively. All results, with the exception of those for the group given 3 mg/kg body weight per day for 13 weeks, were statistically significant ($p < 0.003$). Despite the considerable reductions in thymus weight, the only histological observation was a slight reduction in the width of the thymic cortex. A dose-related reduction in relative spleen weight was seen after 26 weeks, which was statistically significant ($p < 0.05$) at the dose level of 12 mg/kg body weight per day. Reduced body weight and increases in relative pituitary and relative adrenal weights were statistically significant ($p < 0.01$) at 12 mg/kg body weight per day for 13 and 26 weeks and at 6 mg/kg body weight per day for 26 weeks, and there was a significant ($p < 0.05$) increase in relative adrenal weight at 6 mg/kg body weight per day for 13 weeks. The relative pituitary weight was also increased following 26 weeks of dosing at 3 mg/kg body weight per day ($p < 0.01$). Based on thymus weight, the NOEL was the most sensitive end-point in this study, 3 mg/kg body weight per day for 13 weeks. However, an effect was seen at this dose when it was given for 26 weeks.

Funahashi et al. (1980) also reported that the reduction in relative thymus weight, present 3 days after a single dose of TBTO in olive oil of 100 mg/kg body weight to 5-week-old male Sprague-Dawley rats, showed signs of reversal at day 8. The reversibility of TBT-induced thymus atrophy was also demonstrated by Snoeij et al. (1988b). Groups of 4 or 5 young (4-5 weeks old) male Wistar rats received a single gavage dose of TBT chloride (0 or 16 mg/kg body weight) in corn oil. A 30% reduction in relative thymus weight was evident in animals killed on days 2, 3, or 4, but there was complete recovery by day 7. A similar effect and recovery was seen in the thymus cell counts. An equimolar dose of dibutyltin chloride produced more pronounced effects, the recovery period being prolonged until day 9.

Krajnc et al. (1984) reported the effects of feeding TBTO-containing diets (0, 5, 20, 80, or 320 mg/kg diet) to groups (10 males and 10 females per group) of young SPF Wistar rats for 4 weeks. These dose levels are equivalent to approximately 0, 0.5, 2, 8, or 32 mg/kg body weight per day, respectively, based on actual food consumption measurements. Total leucocyte and circulating lymphocyte counts were significantly reduced in males receiving 80 mg/kg diet ($p < 0.01$) and in both sexes receiving 320 mg/kg diet ($p < 0.001$). Eosinophil counts were significantly reduced ($p < 0.05$) in males receiving 5, 80, or 320 mg/kg diet and in females given the highest dose. Monocyte counts were increased significantly ($p < 0.05$) in males receiving 20, 80, or 320 mg/kg diet but not in females. Total immunoglobulin levels were significantly affected at 80 and 320 mg/kg diet. At 80 mg/kg diet, TBTO significantly increased serum IgM to 132% ($p < 0.01$) and 145% ($p < 0.001$) of control levels for males and females, respectively. At the same dose, IgG in males was reduced significantly ($p < 0.05$), but in females IgG was unaffected. A significant reduction ($p < 0.001$) in serum IgG was found in both sexes fed TBTO at 320 mg/kg diet. Thymus and relative thymus weights were significantly reduced in both sexes ($p < 0.001$) at 80 and 320 mg/kg diet and in females given 20 mg/kg diet ($p < 0.05$). Relative spleen weight was significantly increased in males receiving 320 mg/kg diet but this was probably related to the decreased body weight of these animals. Histological examination showed that all the animals given the highest dose exhibited lymphocyte depletion from the thymic cortex, resulting in an indistinct cortico-medullary junction and an increase in ceroid/lipofuschin-loaded macrophages. Slight atrophy of the thymic cortex was seen in two males fed 80 mg/kg diet. Diffuse atrophy of the white pulp of the spleen was seen in all animals at 320 mg/kg, the periarteriolar lymphocyte sheaths (PALS) being particularly affected. At 80 mg/kg diet, one male and two females showed slight splenic atrophy. Depletion of T lymphocytes, determined by pan-T immuno-staining, was seen in the PALS at 320 mg/kg diet. There was an increase in the incidence of mesenteric lymph nodes atrophy, observable in some animals fed 20 mg/kg and increasing with dose to affect all animals given 320 mg/kg diet. Both the paracortex and medulla of lymph nodes were reduced in size and cellularity, and the numbers and size of follicles were reduced by the highest TBTO dose level. Again, the total number of T lymphocytes was strikingly reduced in the paracortex by TBTO at 320 mg/kg diet, as determined by immuno-staining. Although thymic involvement was marked, it was not only thymus-dependent areas that were affected. In rats exposed to the highest dose level, which was overtly toxic, B lymphocyte areas also showed low level activity, as indicated by fewer follicles and inconspicuous germinal centres in lymph nodes and spleen. An increase in the number of animals with rosettes in sinuses in the mesenteric lymph nodes, composed of erythrocytes surrounding mononuclear cells, was seen. This was dose related: half of the animals dosed at 5 mg/kg and all the animals treated with 80 or 320 mg/kg showed erythrocyte rosettes. The biological significance of these rosettes is unclear. Specific aspects of immune function were not tested. In further studies (personal communication by E.I. Krajnc to IPCS, 1989; Wester, in press), no increase in rosette formation was observed at 5 mg/kg diet or 50 mg/kg diet. Signs of general toxicity were observed in animals treated with 320 mg/kg diet, i.e. reduced body weight ($p < 0.001$) and increased serum ALAT activity. At 80 mg/kg, there was reduced body weight gain in males ($p < 0.05$) and increased ALAT, and at 20 mg/kg increased ALAT in males only. The liver was the only non-lymphoid organ displaying histological changes: centrilobular hepatocyte atrophy, reduced glycogen retention, parenchymal necrosis, and hyperplasia of the intrahepatic bile duct were seen in some animals treated at 320 mg/kg diet. Three animals from the group given 80 mg/kg showed slight hepatocyte atrophy. This study indicated a NOEL of 5 mg/kg diet (approximately 0.5 mg/kg body weight per day).

Vos et al. (1984) investigated functional aspects of the immunological effects reported by Krajnc et al. (1984) in *in vivo* and *ex vivo* experiments using weanling (3 to 4 weeks old) male SPF Wistar rats fed diets containing TBTO. Haematological parameters were not studied. Levels of total circulating immunoglobulins (IgG and IgM) were determined in animals fed diets containing 80 or 320 mg TBTO/kg. At 320 mg/kg diet, IgM was significantly increased ($p < 0.05$) and IgG was significantly decreased ($p < 0.001$) on day 28 (no assays were performed on day 42 for this group). At 80 mg/kg diet, IgM was elevated by 30% on day 42 ($p < 0.01$), while IgG was decreased by 30% on days 28 and 42.

The effects of TBTO on lymphocyte counts and cell viability in lymphoid organs was investigated, and several specific tests of immune system function were also performed. Numbers of B and T lymphocytes were significantly reduced in the spleens (by 15% and 48%, respectively) of animals fed diets containing 80 mg/kg diet. The ratio of total T:B lymphocytes was decreased in a dose-related manner following 9 weeks of exposure.

A significant reduction occurred in the numbers of viable cells (trypan blue exclusion) obtained from the thymus, spleen, and bone marrow of rats treated with TBTO at 80 or 320 mg/kg diet. At 320 mg/kg diet, viability and cell numbers were significantly ($p < 0.05$) reduced for both thymus and spleen following 3, 8, and 20 days of exposure, and bone marrow counts were significantly reduced on days 8 and 20. Doses of 80 mg/kg diet produced significant reductions in thymus cell count and viability on day 8 and thymus, spleen, and bone marrow counts on day 20.

The antibody response to sheep erythrocytes (ip), tetanus toxoid (iv), ovalbumin (sc into the foot pad, included H37Ra adjuvant), and the worm *Trichinella spiralis* (oral) was assessed in animals receiving 20 or 80 mg TBTO per kg diet for 6 weeks. The primary response to sheep erythrocytes (0.5 ml of a 20% suspension, ip) was determined 10 days post inoculation (pi) and the secondary response was determined on day 20 pi following an iv booster inoculation on day 15 pi. The primary response was unaffected, but there was a dose-related decrease in the secondary response seen both in untreated and 2-mercaptoethanol-treated (IgM-inactivated) sera, reaching statistical significance ($p < 0.05$) in treated sera from the highest-dose group. The response (IgG and IgM titres) to tetanus toxoid inoculation measured only on day 21 pi was equivocal, and that to ovalbumin measured on days 15, 21, and 28 pi was unaffected by TBTO. IgG response to oral *T. spiralis* infection was significantly ($p < 0.05$) increased on day 21 pi at 20 mg/kg diet, but not on day 42 or at 80 mg/kg diet at either time. IgM response was unaffected. IgE response, possibly the most relevant to resistance to parasitic infection, was decreased in a dose-related manner on days 21 and 42 following *T. spiralis* infection; log titres were 3.8, 2.5 ($p < 0.05$), and 1.8 ($p < 0.001$) on day 21 and 4.4, 3.6, and 3.4 ($p < 0.05$) on day 42 in the control, 20-, and 80-mg/kg groups, respectively. Delayed-type hypersensitivity was determined as change in skin thickness following a challenge of ovalbumin to the skin of the ear or tuberculin challenge to the skin of the flank, made 3 and 4 weeks, respectively, following initial immunization (sc into a footpad) 6 weeks after starting dietary dosing of TBTO at 20 or 80 mg/kg. Compared to controls similarly injected intradermally with medium, significant reductions in response to ovalbumin challenge were found 24, 48, and 72 h after dosing at 20 mg/kg (all $p < 0.05$), and 24 h ($p < 0.01$) and 48 h ($p < 0.05$) after dosing at 80 mg/kg. With tuberculin challenge, significant effects were found in the group given 80 mg/kg diet after

24 h ($p < 0.01$), 48 h ($p < 0.001$), and 72 h ($p < 0.001$), but only after 72 h ($p < 0.05$) at the lower dose level. Reduced responses were seen at all three times after both doses.

Thymus or spleen cells, obtained from rats fed TBTO at 20 or 80 mg/kg diet, were cultured with and without mitogens (PHA = phytohaemagglutinin; Con A = concanavalin A; PWM = pokeweed mitogen) for 24 h before the addition of ^{3}H-thymidine to monitor DNA synthesis. PHA and Con A are both T cell mitogens and PWM is a mitogen for both T and B cells. Due to a reduction in the number of viable cells in thymic cultures from the high-dose group, responsiveness to mitogens was expressed per culture and per thymus. Significant reductions in ^{3}H-thymidine uptake (expressed per thymus) were found in unstimulated (48% reduction), PHA-treated (64%), Con A-treated (62%), and PWM-treated (50%) cultures derived from the high-dose group; PHA (48%) and PWM (28%) were the only responses reduced at 20 mg/kg diet. Similar effects were seen on splenic cultures, with a reduced number of viable cells per spleen and significant reductions in response (expressed per spleen) to PHA (50% reduction) and Con A (45%) in cultures from the high-dose group; responses to PWM and *E. coli* lipopolysaccharide (a B cell mitogen) were significantly increased on a per culture basis but not a per spleen basis. Cultures from the low-dose group showed reduced response to PHA (25% reduction) and Con A (20%), but these were not statistically significant.

TBTO, at both 20 and 80 mg/kg diet, reduced the resistance of rats to infection by *T. spiralis*. The number of worm larvae in muscle significantly increased in a dose-dependent manner (74 000 in controls; 106 000 in rats fed 20 mg TBTO/kg, $p < 0.01$; 198 000 in rats fed 80 mg/kg $p < 0.001$) after standard infection with 1000 larvae by mouth. The number of adult worms in the small intestine also increased significantly after 10 ($p < 0.05$), 12 ($p < 0.001$), and 14 ($p < 0.01$) days in the high-dose group, and after 12 ($p < 0.05$) and 14 ($p < 0.001$) days in the low-dose groups. In a study of the inflammatory reaction around larva-containing muscle cells in the tongues of animals killed 14 days after infection, the response (mononuclear cells and eosinophilic granulocytes) after treatment with TBTO at 20 mg/kg diet was described as "slightly reduced". However, there was a marked reduction after treatment at 80 mg/kg diet.

The clearance of *Listeria monocytogenes* from the spleen (a measure of host resistance) was monitored in rats fed 20, 80, or 320 mg TBTO/kg diet for 6 or 7 weeks. Statistically significant increases in the number of viable bacteria were seen 2 days after an iv injection into animals treated with 320 mg/kg diet for 6 ($p < 0.01$) or 7 ($p < 0.001$) weeks and with 80 mg/kg diet for 6 weeks ($p < 0.001$). A dose-related reduction, statistically significant ($p < 0.05$) at 80 mg/kg diet, in viable bacteria was seen 1 day post injection in the group receiving TBTO for 7 weeks, but this was not seen in the 6-week study. The *ex vivo* phagocytosis of *L. monocytogenes* by spleen- and peritoneal-derived macrophages from TBTO treated (20 or 80 mg/kg diet) animals was not significantly affected, although a dose-related reduction in the phagocytic activity of splenic macrophages was seen.

Cells derived from the spleen and peritoneal cavity were tested for spontaneous cell-mediated cytotoxicity against murine YAC lymphoma target cells labelled with ^{51}Cr. "Specific release" of the chromium label (release in experimental minus spontaneous release in the controls) was used as the end-point of the assay. Statistically significant reductions in specific release were found with spleen cells from rats fed TBTO at 80 mg/kg diet ($p < 0.05$), but not in spleen cells from those fed 20 mg/kg diet. Statistically significant effects ($p < 0.05$) were found in peritoneal macrophages derived from rats receiving 20 and 80 mg/kg diet, but there were no significant effects on non-adherent cells ("natural killer cells").

These studies were designed to investigate immune function rather than to determine a no-observed-effect-level, and the lowest dose used (20 mg/kg diet) produced statistically significant effects (in particular, depression of host resistance to *T. spiralis* and *L. monocytogenes*). No evidence of general toxicity was seen at this dose level. The only sign of general toxicity recorded was a significant reduction in body weight gain seen after exposure to 320 mg/kg diet for 3, 8, and 20 days and to 80 mg/kg diet for 20 days.

A study of TBTO (0, 0.5, and 50 mg/kg diet) administered to groups of weanling Wistar rats (five animals of each sex per group) for 2 years was briefly reported by Vos et al. (1985) and Wester (in press). It should be noted that the intakes in this study were lower, on a body weight basis, than in the shorter-term studies, being equivalent to 0, 0.025, 0.25, and 2.5 mg/kg body weight per day for the controls, and low, medium, and high doses, respectively (based on actual intake measurements). A significant decrease in peripheral lymphocyte count and a statistically significant increase in platelets were seen in the females fed 50 mg/kg diet for 1 year. Circulating levels of total IgM and IgA were significantly increased at 4-6 and 16-18 months, in rats given 50 mg/kg diet, while significant reductions in IgG levels were recorded, particularly in females.

General effects on the lymphoid organs were not recorded, though several specific tests of immune function were performed using the methods of Vos et al. (1984). A dose-related decrease in resistance to *T. spiralis* infection was seen at 5 and 16 months, achieving statistical significance ($p < 0.05$) at 5 and 50 mg/kg diet. IgE titres were reduced, but IgA levels increased approximately 50-fold at the highest dose level. No effects on delayed-type hypersensitivity were seen, in contrast to results in the short-term study by Vos et al. (1984). Host resistance to *L. monocytogenes* (as measured by the number of viable organisms in the spleen) was significantly reduced at 5 and 17 months in the 50-mg/kg group, but a significant increase was seen at 17 months in the 5-mg/kg group. Natural killer cell activity against YAC lymphoma cells was reduced significantly at the highest dose level after 15-17 months. It will not be possible to fully assess this study until the final report is published, although it would appear that 0.5 mg/kg diet (0.025 mg/kg body weight per day) was the NOEL.

A preliminary report on a study where diets containing TBTO (0, 0.5, 5, or 50 mg/kg diet) were fed to Wistar rats (12 months old) for 6 months, has been issued (personal communication by E.I. Krajnc to IPCS, 1989). Specific tests of immune function were measured after 5 months of dosing. Significant ($p < 0.05$) reductions in host resistance to *T. spiralis* and *L. monocytogenes* were seen at

50 mg/kg only. These results suggest that aged rats are less sensitive to TBTO in the diet than weanlings animals, although this may be due to a lower intake on a per kg body weight basis. Full assessment of this study will need to await the completion of the statistical analyses and final report.

A series of studies have been performed to investigate certain aspects of immune function (Schering, 1989a,b,c,d). When groups (10 animals of each sex) of young (4 to 5 weeks old) Sprague-Dawley rats were fed diets containing TBTO (0, 0.5, 2, 5, or 50 mg/kg diet) for 4 weeks, no significant effects were seen on total or differential white blood cell counts. Serum immunoglobulin levels were not measured. A statistically significant decrease in absolute and relative thymus weight ($p < 0.01$) was seen in males fed 50 mg/kg. A decrease in absolute and relative spleen weight was also seen in this group, though it was not significant statistically. The viability of cultured spleen cells (monitored with trypan blue exclusion) obtained from females fed 5 mg/kg was reduced ($p < 0.05$), but other groups were unaffected. A significant decrease in total thymus cell count was seen in preparations from males fed 50 mg/kg only ($p < 0.05$). A slight but significant ($p < 0.05$) reduction in the thickness of the thymic cortex was also seen in these males, this being the only significant histological finding. Specific measures of immune function were not performed in this study but in parallel studies. The NOEL in this study was 5 mg/kg diet (approximately 0.6 mg/kg body weight per day, based on measured intake) (Schering 1989a).

An assay of plaque-forming cells, a measure of humoral immunity, revealed no effects due to TBTO (at levels of 0.5, 2, 5, or 50 mg/kg diet) fed to groups (10 animals of each sex) of young (4 to 5 weeks old) Sprague-Dawley rats for 5 weeks. The response was measured on day 36, following an iv inoculation of sheep erythrocytes. The only sign of toxicity was a reduction in body weight in males fed 50 mg/kg, but this was not statistically significant. No investigation of general toxicity was performed. The NOEL was 50 mg/kg diet (approximately 5.6 mg/kg body weight per day) in this study (Schering, 1989b).

To assess the effects of TBTO on host resistance to infection, the number of viable *Listeria monocytogenes* cells in the spleen, 4 days after inoculation with 1.4×10^6 cells, was counted. No effects were produced in groups (10 animals of each sex) of young Sprague-Dawley rats fed diets containing TBTO at 0.5, 2, or 5 mg/kg diet for 34 days. However, statistically significant increases in numbers of viable bacteria were seen in the spleen of males ($p = 0.055$) and females ($p < 0.01$) fed 50 mg/kg diet. No investigations of general toxicity were performed. The NOEL was 5 mg/kg diet (approximately 0.6 mg/kg body weight per day) (Schering, 1989c).

The effects of TBTO on delayed-type hypersensitivity reactions, a measure of cell-mediated immunity, were assessed in groups (10 animals of each sex) of 4- to 5-week-old Sprague-Dawley rats fed diets containing 0, 0.5, 2, 5, or 50 mg/kg diet for 37 days. A sensitizing dose of 100 µg bovine serum ablumin (BSA) mixed with Freund's complete adjuvant was given on day 29, followed by a challenge dose of heat-inactivated BSA injected into a hindfoot pad on day 37. No difference in response (increased footpad thickness) was seen between test and control groups. Body weight gain was unaffected, but no other investigations of general toxicity were performed. The NOEL in this study was 50 mg/kg diet (approximately 5.8 mg/kg body weight per day) (Schering 1989d).

The effects of inhaled TBTO were studied in groups (10 animals of each sex) of young (initial weights 86-131 g) SPF Wistar rats exposed to 0, 0.03, 0.16, or 2.8 mg/m^3 for 4 h/day, 5 days per week, for 21 to 24 exposures. The two lower doses were provided by filtered vapour, and the highest dose was provided by an aerosol with over 90% of the particles < 5 µm in diameter (Schering 1983). Lymphocyte and total leucocyte counts, measured at 2 or 4 weeks, were unaffected by TBTO. Some inconsistent changes in reticulocyte counts were found, but these appeared to be primarily related to use of the respiration chamber and not to TBTO exposure. Immunoglobulins were not measured. Thymolysis and lymphocyte depletion of the thymus-dependent areas of the spleen and lymph nodes were reported in the 11 animals (five males, six females) from the highest-dose group that died during the study. No such lesions were detected in the survivors, although in three survivors from the highest-dose group an increase in the number of macrophages containing nuclear debris was seen in the thymic cortex. No significant (p > 0.05) changes were seen in absolute or relative weights of the thymus, spleen, or iliac lymph node in animals surviving the study, but no organ weights were recorded for those animals dying or sacrificed during the study. No specific aspects of immune function were studied. Histological signs of general toxicity were limited to those consistent with inflammatory reactions within the respiratory tract and, with one exception, were confined to animals exposed to the aerosol. Food intake and body weight gain were reduced in both sexes, the reduction being statistically significant (p < 0.01) in male rats exposed to 2.8 mg/m^3. The cause of death in the 11 animals from the highest-dose group was not ascertained (Schering, 1983).

When TBTO (0, 4, 20, 80, or 200 mg/kg diet) was fed to groups (10 animals of each sex) of CD-1 mice, aged 6 to 7 weeks at commencement of the study, for 3 months, leucocyte counts were increased at 80 and 200 mg/kg in both sexes, although this increase did not reach statistical significance (p > 0.05). Immunoglobulins were not measured. Thymus weight was reduced in both sexes at 200 mg/kg, but this was not statistically significant (p > 0.05). Spleen weights were increased in both sexes at 80 and 200 mg/kg (reaching statistical significance (p < 0.05) at 200 mg/kg), possibly secondary to effects on erythrocytes. No specific immune function tests were performed. Histological changes were seen in the livers of both sexes at 80 and 200 mg/kg. Dose-related, statistically significant (p < 0.01) increases in absolute liver weights were seen at 80 and 200 mg/kg, and adrenal weights were significantly (p < 0.01) increased in the male rats fed 200 mg/kg. The NOEL in this study was 20 mg/kg diet (approximately 4 mg/kg body weight per day) (Biodynamics, 1989a).

In studies by Schering (1989e), groups (two animals of each sex) of beagle dogs received variable doses of TBTO in arachis oil by oral gavage:

Group 1: controls;
Group 2: 0.1 mg/kg body weight per day for 5 weeks, 0.2 mg/kg body weight per day for 4 to 5 weeks, then 10 mg/kg body weight per day for 8 to 9 weeks;
Group 3: 0.5 mg/kg body weight per day for 5 weeks

then 1 mg/kg body weight per day for 13 to 14 weeks; Group 4: 2.5 mg/kg body weight per day for 5 weeks then 5 mg/kg body weight per day for 13 to 14 weeks.

All males in groups 2 and 4 died as a result of mis-dosing to the lungs. Increased leucocyte and neutrophil counts were seen in group 4 at weeks 9 and 18 ($p < 0.05$), and there was a statistically significant increase in leucocyte count recorded at 13 weeks in group 2 ($p < 0.05$). Non-statistically significant reductions in leucocyte, neutrophil, and lymphocyte counts were found in group 2 at 18 weeks. Specific immunoglobulins were not measured. Thymus weights were reduced in the two survivors of group 2 (0.9 ± 0.1 g compared with 4.0 ± 0.6 g in controls), and slight increases in thymus weights were seen in groups 3 and 4. Iliac and mesenteric lymph node weights were reduced, though spleen weights were increased, in the two survivors from group 2. Histological changes in lymphoid organs were confined to group 2 where a reduction of lymphocyte numbers in the thymus, spleen (particularly PALS), and lymph nodes was seen. A dose-related increase in relative liver weight (33.1, 41.7, 49.9, and 57.6 g/kg body weight in groups 1, 3, 4, and 2, respectively) was accompanied by cytoplasmic vacuolation of hepatocytes in group 2 (Schering, 1989e).

11.2.6 Mechanism of immunotoxicity

The precise mechanism of the immunotoxic effects of TBTO is not yet clear. However, a hypothesis has been put forward, based on the work of Snoeij (1987) and Pieters et al. (1989).

a) Absorbed TBTO is present as the TBT^+ cation or a salt (chloride or carbonate). Studies using TBT chloride are, therefore, relevant to TBTO immunotoxicity.

b) As dibutyltin chloride (DBT chloride), a metabolite of TBT chloride, is, mole for mole, more potent that TBT chloride at producing effects in the thymus and thymic cells, it is probable that DBT chloride or another DBT salt is the active species in TBTO toxicity.

c) The primary action of DBT is to suspend the maturation of immature thymocytes by inhibiting their interaction/binding with thymic epithelial cells. The turnover period of thymocytes is 3 to 4 days. Therefore, as cell proliferation/maturation is inhibited, rapid depletion of thymocyte numbers without cytotoxicity is expected, followed by a rapid proliferation (observed by Snoeij et al. (1988b) and Funahashi et al. (1980)) on removal of DBT.

Other evidence indicating that TBT compounds have a particular effect on the thymus is provided by the *in vitro* studies of Snoeij (1987), which show TBT chloride to be cytotoxic to thymocytes.

The demonstration of reduced thymus weights in certain fish species (e.g., the freshwater guppy) indicates that TBT may have immunotoxic effects on a wide range of species.

11.2.7 Effects on the endocrine system

The weights of both the adrenal and pituitary glands of Sprague-Dawley rats were significantly increased after exposure to 6 mg TBTO/kg body weight daily, by intubation, for 26 weeks. Pituitary weight was also significantly increased by 3 mg TBTO/kg body weight given daily for 26 weeks (Funahashi et al., 1980).

After 4 weeks, the serum insulin concentration of rats was not significantly affected by dosing with TBTO at up to 80 mg/kg diet, but was undetectable (< 2 milliIU/litre) in rats fed 320 mg/kg (control levels of insulin in serum were 111 and 74 milliIU/litre for males and females, respectively) (Krajnc et al., 1984). In a further study, the same authors monitored endocrine changes in male Wistar rats exposed to TBTO in the diet (0, 20, or 80 mg/kg) for 6 weeks. Serum thyroxine, thyroid stimulating hormone (TSH), and insulin levels were reduced significantly at the higher dose level, but serum follicle stimulating hormone (FSH) and corticosterone levels were unaffected. Only insulin was significantly affected at 20 mg TBTO/kg. The luteinizing hormone (LH) concentration in serum was significantly increased by TBTO at 80 mg/kg, but was unaffected by 20 mg/kg. The authors further examined endocrine function by monitoring hormone release following physiological stimulus. Insulin release, following iv administration of glucose, was unaffected by a 6-week exposure to TBTO at either 20 or 80 mg/kg diet. The effect of TBTO on insulin was attributed by the authors to a decreased food intake. The release of TSH, after iv administration of thyrotrophin releasing hormone (TRH), showed a tendency ($p < 0.1$) to be inhibited in rats fed at 80 mg/kg. The titre of circulating TSH, 20 min after TRH administration, was significantly reduced compared with controls. Release of both LH and FSH, in response to luteinizing hormone releasing factor stimulation, was enhanced in rats fed TBTO at both 20 and 80 mg/kg diet, but only significantly so at the higher dose rate. Histological examination of endocrine organs after a 6-week exposure to TBTO revealed some changes. No differences were observed in either insulin- or glucagon-producing cells in the pancreas. Some flattening of the epithelial lining of the thyroid follicles was observed after exposure of rats to 80 mg/kg but not to 20 mg/kg. Immunocytochemical staining of the pituitary gland identified each cell type producing the different pituitary hormones. There was a dose-related decrease in both the intensity of staining of TSH cells and the number of cells stained. Conversely, there was a dose-related increase in the staining intensity of LH cells. No effects were found on FSH, growth hormone, or adrenocorticotrophin cells in the pituitary (Krajnc et al., 1984).

11.3 Long-term toxicity

Wester (in press) carried out a 106-week toxicity and carcinogenicity study with groups of 50 weanling Wistar rats of each sex. An additional group of 10 rats was used for an interim sacrifice after 1 year. TBTO was fed at 0, 0.5, 5, or 50 mg/kg diet (equivalent to 0, 0.025, 0.25, or 2.5 mg/kg body weight). Increased food consumption occurred in all treated males (not clearly dose-related), and there was increased water consumption in males at 5 and 50 mg/kg. During the second year, the body weight of the highest-dose group was significantly lower than that of controls. Excess mortality, compared with that of controls, was confined to the 50 mg/kg group towards the end of the experiment (see section 11.6). Haematological changes (anaemia, lymphopenia, and thrombocytosis) and increases in plasma enzyme activities (ALAT,

ASAT, and AP) were noted mainly at the high-dose level. Serum IgM and IgA levels increased, while the IgG level decreased (females). No effect was observed on circulating concentrations of T_4, free T_4, TSH, LH, FSH, or insulin; only the free $T_4:T_4$ ratio was decreased. Organ weight changes consisted of increased liver, kidney, adrenal, and pituitary weights and decreased thyroid weight. Non-neoplastic histological alterations consisted of a decrease in cell height of the thyroid follicles (at 50 mg/kg diet after 1 and 2 years), decrease in splenic iron content (at 5 and 50 mg/kg after 1 year only), slight bile duct proliferation (at 50 mg/kg after 1 year only), and vacuolation of kidney proximal tubular epithelium and nephrosis (at 50 mg/kg after 2 years only).

11.4 Genotoxicity

Summary

The genotoxicity of TBTO has been the subject of extensive investigation. Negative results were obtained in the vast majority of studies, and there is no convincing evidence that TBTO has any mutagenic potential.

Davis et al. (1987) conducted a comprehensive study of the genetic effects of TBTO using a wide range of techniques in order to assess possible hazards in the use of the compound as a molluscicide for the control of schistosomiasis. TBTO did not produce gene (point) mutations in Salmonella typhimurium strains TA1530, TA1535, TA1538, TA97, TA98, or TA100, either in the presence or absence of an exogenous metabolic activation system (rat liver S9). The compound did give some evidence of gene mutation in Salmonella typhimurium TA100 using the fluctuation method in the presence of S9, but no dose-response relationship was seen; negative results were seen in the absence of S9. TBTO did not induce point mutations in the yeast *Schizosaccharomyces pombe*. Negative results were obtained when TBTO was tested in the sex-linked recessive lethal assay using *Drosophila melanogaster*, the compound being given in food and by injection, indicating that TBTO did not produce gene mutations in *Drosophila*. Negative results were also obtained when the ability of TBTO to produce DNA damage in *Bacillus subtilis* (recombination assay) or the yeast *Saccharomyces cerevisiae* (mitotic gene conversion) was tested.

The ability of TBTO to produce gene mutations in Salmonella has also been studied by Reimann & Lang (1987). Negative results were obtained using Salmonella typhimurium strains TA1535, TA1537, TA1538, TA98, and TA100, both in the presence and absence of rat S9. Similarly, negative results were obtained with six TBT esters (abietate, borate, linoleate, naphthenate, phosphate, and tallate). Further negative results were obtained when the ability of TBTO to produce mitotic gene conversion in *Saccharomyces cerevisiae* was tested.

The ability of TBTO to produce gene mutations in mammalian cells *in vitro* was extensively investigated by Davis et al. (1987), and negative results were consistently obtained. TBTO did not induce gene mutations in V79 Chinese hamster cells (using resistance to 8-azaguanine, ovabain, or 6-thioguanine as markers) in the presence of rat liver S9. Negative results were also obtained in the V79 cell assays when epidermal cells of mice and humans (primary cultures) were used as the source of metabolic activation in cell-mediated assays.

The *in vitro* clastogenic potential of TBTO has been investigated in mammalian cells in two sets of studies. When Davis et al. (1987) used Chinese hamster ovary (CHO) cells, harvested at 8, 15, and 24 h, an increase in structural aberrations (mainly deletions), together with endoreduplication, was seen, but only at the highest concentration tested (5 μg/ml in the presence of S9 and 1.5 μg/ml in its absence). The increase in the presence of S9 was seen only after 15 h, "toxicity" precluding any analysis of results at this concentration after 8 h. The increase in the absence of S9 was seen only at 8 h, there being no increase at either 15 or 24 h. The results of these studies are difficult to interpret, since the effect was limited to concentrations associated with high toxicity and no data on mitotic index was reported. No increase in sister chromatid exchange was seen at any concentration.

Reimann & Lang (1987) used human lymphocytes to test the clastogenic potential of TBTO and obtained negative results both in the presence and absence of S9. In the latter case, TBTO was added 22 h after stimulation of the cultures with phytohaemagglutinin, and cells were harvested 31 h later. In the former case, TBTO was added with S9 after 26 h; 3 h later the S9 was removed, and the cells were harvested 22 h later. Parallel studies on blood cultures that were differentially stained with BUdR indicated that almost all cells analysed for chromosome aberrations were in the first mitotic stage. The highest TBTO concentrations used (0.1 µg/ml in the absence of S9 and 1 µg/ml in its presence) were associated with a marked reduction in mitotic index (57% and 58%, respectively). No increase in aberrations was seen at any dose level. This study, therefore, failed to confirm the suggestion of some clastogenic potential in the studies using CHO cells.

The ability of TBTO to produce chromosomal damage *in vivo* has been investigated in two separate studies using the micronucleus test. In one study, four doses of TBTO (31.25, 62.5, 125, or 250 mg/kg body weight) were given by gavage, in arachis oil, to NMRI mice, and bone marrow cells were analysed for micronuclei in polychromatic erythrocytes 24, 48, and 72 h after treatment (Reimann & Lang, 1987). The highest dose level resulted in marked lethality (16 out of 36 animals died), precluding any analysis of the results. The 126-mg/kg dose level was also associated with some deaths (4 mice died), but 5000 polychromatic erythrocytes were analysed from five male and five female mice at each harvest interval. Similar analyses were carried out at the two lower dose levels. There was no increase in micronuclei at any dose level or harvest time. This study provided no evidence to indicate that TBTO produces chromosomal damage in bone marrow *in vivo*. A second micronucleus study (Davis et al., 1987) used Balb/c mice. Groups of 10 male and 10 female animals were given 30 or 60 mg TBTO/kg as a solution in olive oil. Bone marrow cells were harvested from five males and five females after 30 h and 48 h, and 1000 polychromatic erythrocytes were analysed from each for micronuclei. An increase in micronuclei was seen only in the male mice after 48 h and at the highest dose level. These results conflict with those of Reinmann & Lang (1987). Furthermore, there was an unusually high spontaneous incidence of micronuclei (up to 5.8 per 1000 polychromatic erythrocytes) in the study of Davis et al. (1987). These factors prompted a re-analysis of the slides from this study by the Institute of Occupational Health, Helsinki, Finland (Schering 1986). This re-analysis, again using 1000 polychromatic erythrocytes per animal, failed to confirm the increase in micronuclei seen after 48 h in the male animals given 60 mg TBTO/kg. A slight, but statistically significant, increase in micronuclei was seen in the female mice on re-analysis, but this was thought to be biologically non-significant due to the high variability in the control data. The re-analysis highlighted the problem of interpreting studies in which only relatively few polychromatic erythrocytes are analysed (1000) and there is marked variability in the control data (with an incidence outside the normal range at some time points). Thus, no conclusions can be drawn from the micronucleus study of Davis et al. (1987).

The ability of TBTO to inhibit metabolic cooperation between V79 Chinese hamster 6-thioguanine-resistant and sensitive cells has been investigated by Davis et al. (1987). This assay has been suggested as a model for tumour promoter activity. Negative results were obtained. The significance of the assay is, however, unclear.

In summary, the genotoxicity of TBTO has been the subject of extensive investigation. Negative results were obtained in the vast majority of studies, and there is no convincing evidence that TBTO has any mutagenic potential.

11.5 Reproductive toxicity

Summary

The potential embryotoxicity of TBTO has been evaluated in three mammalian species (mouse, rat, and rabbit) after oral dosing of the mother. The main malformation noted in rat and mouse fetuses was cleft palate, but this occurred at dosages overtly toxic to the mothers. These results are not considered to be indicative of teratogenic effects of TBTO at doses below those producing maternal toxicity. The lowest NOEL, with regards to embryotoxicity and fetotoxicity for all three species, was 1 mg/kg body weight.

11.5.1 In vivo

Reproductive toxicity has been studied in NMRI mice. The highest dose used (35 mg/kg body weight) was chosen to give minimal maternal mortality based on acute toxicity tests. An increase in cleft palate was seen in the fetuses of mice treated orally with 11.7 mg TBTO/kg body weight (7% cleft palate), 23.4 mg/kg (24%), and 35 mg/kg (48%), compared to the incidence in controls (0.7%). However, 11 out of a total of 15 affected mice were clustered in one of the 18 litters and 15 litters contained none. The two highest doses of TBTO also increased the frequency of irregular ossification centres of sternabrae and of minor abnormalities, such as fusion of the bases of os occipitalis. The strain of mice used in the study has a tendency to produce these particular abnormalities as a result of non-specific stress on the mother. The authors considered that TBTO has a very low teratogenic potential; electron microscopy 26 and 48 h after treatment showed no evidence of damage to the embryos but considerable damage to the maternal liver. At a level of 6 mg/kg body weight, TBTO produced no increase in fetal abnormalities (Davis et al., 1987).

Nemec (1987) investigated the maternal, embryotoxic, and teratogenic effects of TBTO in New Zealand white rabbits. The TBTO was administered in corn oil by gavage, once a day from day 6 of gestation to day 18 inclusive, at doses of 0.2, 1, and 2.5 mg/kg per day body weight in a volume of 0.5 ml. Twenty female rabbits were dosed with corn oil as controls and 20 rabbits were used at each dose level. The rabbits were artificially inseminated and injected iv with human chorionic gonadotrophin immediately afterwards to ensure ovulation. With the exception of a single female dosed at 1 mg/kg, all treated rabbits survived to day 29 of gestation when the experiment was terminated. A total of 12 animals aborted during the dosing period: 3, 1, 1, and 7 from the control, 0.2, 1, and 2.5 mg/kg groups, respectively. Females aborting were killed the same day and immediate postmortem examinations carried out. The increased occurrence of abortions in the highest-dose group was considered to be a secondary effect of maternal toxicity. No clinical findings in the groups given 0.2 or 1 mg/kg were considered to be the result of TBTO treatment. There was a statistically significant mean body weight loss in females dosed at 2.5 mg/kg per day compared to controls between days 6 and 18 of gestation (the period of actual dosing). Doses of 0.2 and 1.0 mg/kg per day had no effect on growth or survival of fetuses. There was a slight (statistically non-significant) decrease in mean fetal weight in the group dosed with 2.5 mg/kg per day. This may represent minor fetotoxicity. There were no differences in the types or frequency of fetal malformations related to treatment and the conclusion was that TBTO was not teratogenic. Postmortem examination of the mother rabbits indicated no changes associated with treatment, and 1 mg/kg per day was considered to be the NOEL for maternal toxicity and toxicity to the fetus.

When Crofton et al. (1989) treated pregnant Long-Evans rats with TBTO by gastric intubation at 0 to 16 mg/kg per day body weight from day 6 to day 20 of gestation, litter size and pup weight were significantly reduced by doses of 10, 12, or 16 mg/kg per day but no effect was seen at doses of 2.5 and 5 mg/kg per day. Maternal weight gain was affected by the same dose levels that affected litter size and pup weight. Pup survival was further reduced in the first 3 days after birth. Litter size was reduced by 50%, 73%, and 96% at dose levels of 10, 12, and 16 mg/kg per day, respectively, on day 1 post partum and by 63%, 88%, and 100% on day 3 post partum. Pup weight on day 1 post partum was reduced by 45%, 45%, and 68% at the three dose levels. Two out of 71 pups born had cleft palate, but no controls showed any abnormalities. These two pups were both born dead. The five pups born to rats given 16 mg/kg per day showed no malformations, but all died within 3 days. The authors concluded that it was impossible to distinguish between possible fetotoxicity and maternal toxicity, since all effects on offspring occurred at TBTO dose rates that also affected the weight of the mother. They also showed that pregnant female rats were more sensitive to TBTO than non-pregnant females; the MTD (maximum tolerated dose) for non-pregnant females was 16 mg/kg per day, whereas pregnant females showed an MTD of between 5 and 10 mg/kg per day. Most effects on pups were transitory in that survivors to adulthood showed only reductions in body weight and brain weight compared to controls even at the highest dose rates. Motor activity of offspring was monitored in a maze fitted with photoelectric detectors. During the pre-weaning period there was a significant age/treatment interaction, but only on post-natal day 14 was there a significant response per individual day. All doses of TBTO produced a significant decrease in activity on that day. Post-weaning activity was reduced on postnatal days 47 and 62 ($p < 0.01$) but only at a level of 10 mg/kg per day. There was no clear effect on acoustic startle response.

In a two-generation reproduction study, TBTO was given to rats at dietary concentrations of 0, 0.5, 5, and 50 mg/kg. The parental (F_0) generation (30 males and 30 females per group) was exposed for 10 weeks before mating, whereas the pre-mating treatment period for the F_1 adults (30 of each sex per group) was 15 weeks. Culling of litters was performed on day 4 in the F_1 and F_2 generations. Preliminary data (Biodynamics, 1989b) on mortality, body weight development, fertility indices, litter data, and organ weights have been reported. There was no evidence of compound-related mortality, and body weight development was normal in the F_0 generation. At 50 mg/kg diet, the pup weights were decreased on days 14 and 21 in the F_1 generation and on days 7, 14, and 21 in the F_2 generation. Among the F_1 parents, at 50 mg/kg, lower body weights were noted in males throughout the pre-mating period and in females during the first 3 weeks only. No effects on mating, pregnancy, and fertility rates were noted in either generation, and number of pups, litter size, and pup survival were not affected by treatment in either the F_1 or the F_2 generations. Relative and absolute thymus weights were decreased in both sexes at the dietary concentration of 50 mg/kg.

11.5.2 In vitro

Krowke et al. (1986) demonstrated an effect of TBTO on the development of limb buds of mice in organ culture. Clear-cut interference with differentiation was seen at the lowest dose tested (0.03 mg/litre), while at 0.1 mg per litre drastic impairment and abnormal development of the paw skeleton were recorded. The effect was more pronounced still at the highest dose tested (0.3 mg/litre). In view of their failure to show effects on the embryo *in vivo*, Davis et al. (1987) suggested that there is only very limited movement of TBTO across the placenta of mice.

11.6 Carcinogenicity

Summary

One carcinogenicity study on rats has been reported in which neoplastic changes were observed in endocrine organs at 50 mg/kg diet. The pituitary tumours found at 0.5 mg/kg diet are considered as having no biological significance since there was no dose-response relationship. These tumour types appear usually at high and variable background incidences. The significance is, therefore, questionable. A second study on mice is in progress.

Wester (in press) reported the results of a 106-week study on carcinogenicty in Wistar rats at dietary TBTO doses of 0, 0.5, 5, and 50 mg/kg (0, 0.025, 0.25, and 2.5 mg/kg body weight). At the highest dose level, general toxicological effects were present (see section 11.3). The incidence of benign tumours of the pituitary (mainly prolactinomas) was elevated at 0.5 and 50 mg/kg, but not at 5 mg/kg diet, for both sexes. At 50 mg/kg, a significant increase was noted in the incidence of adrenal medullary tumours (pheochromocytomas) in both sexes and of parathyroid adenomas in male animals, while the incidence of adrenal cortical tumours was significantly decreased at 0.5 and 50 mg/kg diet in males only. Isolated occurrence of pancreatic carcinoma was found in treated female rats. These were not considered to be compound related since there was no dose dependency and the incidence rates were low.

12. EFFECTS ON HUMANS

Summary

TBTO is a skin and eye irritant and severe dermatitis has been reported after direct contact with the skin. The potential problem is made worse by the lack of an immediate skin response.

12.1 Ingestion

There have been no reported cases of poisoning from ingestion of TBTO or other TBT salts.

12.2 Inhalation

Seventy percent of the workers in a rubber factory using TBTO in the vulcanizing process reported irritation of the upper respiratory tract (and eyes). About 20% also experienced lower chest symptoms (irritation, tightness, and pain), but in all cases pulmonary function was unaffected. The extent of the exposure was not recorded (WHO/FAO, 1985).

12.3 Dermal exposure

Lyle (1958) described skin lesions in workers occupationally exposed to dibutyl and tributyl tin compounds. Skin burns were most commonly caused by small splashes of liquid dibutyl or tributyl tin chlorides. Since the irritancy of these compounds was not immediately apparent (taking at least an hour to be perceived), small splashes were frequently ignored by workers. More severe lesions on the hands were caused by leaking gloves or failure to wear hand protection. Some maintenance staff also suffered burns after kneeling or rubbing against surfaces wet with the chlorides. Clothes wet with these compounds produced burns on the ventral skin and burns were seen immediately above the level of protective boots on the calf of the leg. Two kinds of lesion were seen in workers. The first was an acute burn, which healed relatively quickly, and the second a more diffuse dermatitis (seen in workers wearing contaminated clothes in close contact with the skin), which persisted. Treatment of the back of the hand of volunteers with various undiluted TBT compounds established that the chloride, acetate, laurate, and oxide all produced acute burns. Burns were not caused by dibutyltin esters or oxide or by tetrabutyltin, but were mostly due to dibutyltin chloride or the tributyltin compounds. Reddening of the area treated was seen 2-3 h after treatment with the compounds. Inflammation of the hair follicles was the most obvious symptom, effects being confined to the treated area. On the second day after treatment, minute pustules appeared, which remained discrete and disappeared on the third or fourth day. After a week, all that remained was a faint erythema. The burns were not reported to be painful, either in the case of experimental or occupational exposure. Sufferers complained of itching and "stickiness" of the skin causing adherence of clothes. Proper use of protective clothing, rapid washing of the skin after exposure, and the use of aprons to prevent wetting of overalls were found to be effective in preventing burns, both acute and diffuse.

Baaijens (1987) described cases of accidental exposure to TBTO during the manufacture of organotin compounds. Severe dermatitis developed only where splashes of the material had been retained on the skin for long periods. In one case, a worker had been splashed over the face and neck. He left the work area after the splash and showered. An area behind one ear had not been washed and the dermatitis had developed in this one area. There were no symptoms other than dermatitis. Another worker had been splashed on the arm. He washed his skin but did not change his overalls. Contact was extended and a large blister developed on the arm. Monitoring of the urine tin content showed no difference from normal in these two cases. A third worker, who complained of an intense smell of TBTO, suffered nausea and vomiting after 10 min of exposure. Urine tin levels in this case were elevated for several days. In all cases the symptoms disappeared within a few days. The delayed irritancy of tributyltin was emphasized by the author. It tends to lead to extended exposure since the affected person does not perceive the effect for several hours. The author found no relationship between clinical or haematological parameters and normal occupational exposure to organotin compounds.

Goh (1985) reported irritant effects and dermatitis in painters applying TBTO formulations (0.6% TBTO in acrylic resin-based paints) to buildings. The painters developed rashes 8 to 10 h after exposure. When required to paint ceilings, the men developed more severe symptoms on the face, neck, and trunk, associated with dripping paint. Severe itching, redness, swelling, and blistering were recorded. Hospital examination showed extensive vesiculo-bullous lesions, erythema, and oedema of the face, neck, trunk, arms, and thighs. Although only two patients were examined in detail, most of the workers on the site developed dermatitis. Patch testing of the two reported cases showed erosion 48 and 96 h after patch tests using aqueous solutions of TBTO (0.1 and 0.5 g/litre). Five other volunteer controls were patch-treated with solutions of 0.01 and 0.1 g/litre; these also showed a similar reaction to the patients. No allergenic reaction was found in the patch tests. Replacement of the paint with a preparation having similar constituents other than TBTO prevented further problems amongst the painters.

Lewis & Emmett (1987) describe contact dermatitis in a shipwright resulting from exposure to TBTO-containing antifouling paint. The man had been spray-painting blocks of wood and his skin had been exposed to the spray. There was no immediate sensation, but some irritation was evident within about an hour. Erythema and ulceration of the exposed areas were noted on the second day. There were also some mild pustular lesions on the mucous membrane of the lips, presumed to be the result of wiping the mouth with paint-contaminated arms. The authors conducted patch testing with TBTO at aqueous concentrations of 0.1%, 0.01%, and 0.0015% using the Al test tape method. At the highest dose tested, there were large bullae after 48 h and crusting after 96 h. The other two doses produced no adverse effects. The delayed sensation and effect were highlighted by the authors as being particular problems with TBTO. Great care to prevent any exposure to products containing TBTO at high concentrations was recommended.

Molin & Wahlberg (1975) investigated an outbreak of dermatitis on the feet and ankles of trainee soldiers. Seventy soldiers reported itching and sometimes painful erythematous, vesiculous to bullous, and haemorrhagic lesions after long marches on a hot day. Fifty other soldiers reported less severe symptoms on another occasion. The skin lesions disappeared within 1 or 2 weeks in most cases after treatment with saline compresses and topical steroid creams. In two cases, the skin was red and slightly tender more than 6 months later. The outbreak was traced to a single batch of socks that had been soaked in 7 times the recommended concentration of a disinfectant solution containing TBTO. Recommended use of the disinfectant was calculated to give about 0.001%, whereas the concentration after the accidental over-use would have been about 0.01%. Patch testing of eczema patients not previously exposed to TBTO suggested that the primary irritant concentration for the compound was between 0.1 and 0.01%. Soldiers patch-tested 2 months after their dermatitis had fully healed gave negative results to both 0.001% and 0.01% TBTO. The authors suggested that the effective concentration for TBTO as a disinfectant is too close to the primary irritancy concentration to justify the use of TBTO for disinfecting textiles.

Zedler (1961), on the basis of industrial experience, stated that a concentration of 0.05% TBTO was not harmful to the human skin.

12.4 Miscellaneous effects

Women using a latex spray paint containing TBTO as an additive showed immediate irritant effects on the eye (profuse lacrimation, eye inflammation) and the nasal mucosa. The symptoms worsened over 14 days of spraying, but subsided at the weekends and disappeared completely when addition of TBTO to the paint was discontinued. The extent of exposure in this case was not recorded (WHO/FAO, 1985).

Akatsuka et al. (1959) reported a case of occupational poisoning with butyltin compounds where, along with symptoms of lassitude, slight occipital headaches, and stiffness in the shoulders, there was a marked disturbance of the sense of smell. The authors conducted studies on cats to test whether this effect could be confirmed experimentally. Exposure of the cats to a vapour mixture containing mainly tributyltin bromide revealed a marked loss of the sense of smell.

13. EVALUATION OF HUMAN HEALTH RISKS AND EFFECTS ON THE ENVIRONMENT

13.1 Evaluation of human health risks

Exposure of workers occurs principally during the manufacture and formulation of tributyltin compounds, in the application and removal of TBT paints, and from the use of TBT in wood preservatives. Exposure of the general public may come from the contamination of food, particularly fish and shellfish, and from domestic application of wood preservatives.

On the basis of both animal tests and direct observations on humans, it is clear that TBT compounds are irritant to the skin and eyes and that inhalation of aerosols leads to respiratory irritation.

The handling of treated wood poses no dermal irritant hazard once the wood has dried. However, aerosols of TBT are very hazardous and re-entry to the treatment area should be prohibited until the wood has thoroughly dried.

Acute systemic poisoning has never been reported and clearance of TBT from the body is expected to occur within a few days. Acute toxicity from handling TBT products is, therefore, unlikely if proper precautions are taken.

Short- and long-term effects on experimental animals have been reported in the liver and haematological and endocrine systems. The effects of TBT compounds on the immune system, and particularly on host resistance, have proved the most sensitive parameter of toxicity in the rat, the most sensitive species tested. The no-observed-effect level (NOEL), using the *Trichinella spiralis* host-resistance model, lies between 0.5 and 5.0 mg/kg diet (0.025 and 0.25 mg/kg body weight), whereas using measures of immune function it is 0.6 mg/kg body weight.

Owing to wide variation in the consumption of fish and shellfish and local differences in residues of TBT in seafood, only illustrative estimates relating exposure and NOEL values can be made. It needs to be emphasized that local measurements of residues, local estimates of seafood consumption, and local decisions on acceptable safety margins must be made to assess potential risk of these compounds.

Using fish consumption figures of 15 and 150 g/day, a value of 1 mg/kg for residues in fish, and an average human body weight of 60 kg, the following safety margins based on different immune endpoints are obtained.

Fish consumption (g/day)	Estimated daily intake of TBT (μg/kg)	Safety margin T. spiralis model	Other immune parameters
15	0.25	100-1000	2500
150	2.5	10-100	250

Indiscriminate and irresponsible use of TBT compounds and a failure to follow the recommendations, outlined in this monograph, to reduce exposure of humans could lead to intake of levels of TBT compounds hazardous to human health.

Teratogenic effects have only occurred in experimental animals at doses that caused overt maternal toxicity. The teratogenic potential of TBT is, therefore, considered to be very low.

Based on the results of comprehensive mutagenicity studies, tributyltin compounds are not considered to have mutagenic potential. In a carcinogenicity study on rats with TBTO, an increased incidence was noted for endocrine tumours that occur spontaneously at a high and variable incidence. Therefore, the available evidence does not clearly demonstrate a carcinogenic hazard of TBT compounds for humans.

13.2 Evaluation of effects on the environment

Diffuse input of tributyltin (TBT) into the environment occurs predominantly from the use of TBT in antifouling paint. It could also occur if it were used as a molluscicide. Point source contamination occurs if TBT is used as a biocide in cooling systems, wood pulping, leather processing, wood preservation processes, and textile treatment.

Due to their physico-chemical properties, TBT compounds concentrate in the surface microlayer and in sediments. Abiotic degradation does not appear to be a major mechanism of removal under environmental conditions. Although TBTO is biodegradable in the water column, this process is not rapid enough to prevent the occurrence of elevated TBT levels in some areas. Bioaccumulation occurs in most aquatic organisms, but in laboratory mammals, metabolic degradation is a more efficient process.

TBT is extremely hazardous to some aquatic organisms because it is toxic at very low concentrations in water. Such concentrations have been found in some areas. Adverse effects on non-target invertebrates, particularly molluscs, have been reported in field studies, and these have been sufficiently severe to lead to reproductive failure and population decline. Adverse effects on the commercial production of shellfish have been successfully reversed by restrictions on the use of antifouling paints in some areas, and these restrictions are also leading to the reversal of imposex effects in gastropod populations. The effects on farmed fish indicate that TBT-containing paints should not be used on restraining nets.

The general hazard to the terrestrial environment is likely to be low. TBT-treated wood could pose a hazard to terrestrial organisms living in close contact with it.

The enhancement of TBT concentrations in the surface microlayer may present a hazard to littoral organisms, neustonic species (including benthic invertebrate and fish larvae) and surface-feeding sea-birds and wildfowl. Accumulation and low biodegradation of TBT in sediments may present a hazard to aquatic organisms when these polluted sediments are disturbed by natural processes or dredging activities.

14. RECOMMENDATIONS

14.1 Recommendations for protecting human and environmental health

a) Member countries that have not yet regulated the use of TBT compounds should be encouraged to do so.

b) There is a need for evaluation and, if necessary, regulation of organotin input to the environment from sources other than antifouling paints. For example, this would include evaluation of the potential risk from the application of TBT-contaminated sewage sludge to soil.

c) Improved methods for the safe application, removal, and disposal of organotin paints should be developed.

14.2 Research needs

a) Methods of detection and analysis need to be improved to provide rapid and accurate measurements of butyltin species in pg/litre concentrations. One reason for this recommendation is that a biological effect, i.e. imposex in gastropods, may occur at levels lower than present detection limits.

b) There is a need for research into mechanisms which concentrate rather than disperse TBT and which retard degradation, with particular attention to the fundamental chemistry of TBT and its interaction with biological molecules. More study is needed on the uptake of TBT at all trophic levels.

c) A study of the toxicity of TBT in aquatic organisms is required. This work should investigate metabolism, endocrine effects, and immunological toxicity, where appropriate.

d) A search for other sensitive bioindicator species in other groups, including freshwater species, is required.

e) Models for the assessment of immunotoxicity in mammals need to be validated and no-effect levels for relevant parameters need to be defined more accurately.

f) A long-term toxicity study in a second mammalian species should be undertaken.

g) A tumorigenicity study in a second mammalian species should be undertaken.

h) Information on butyltin residue levels in fish and shellfish for human consumption using speciating methods is needed.

REFERENCES

ABEL, R., HATHAWAY, R.A., KING, N.J., VOSSER, J.L., & WILKINSON, T.G. (1987) Assessment and regulatory actions for TBT in the UK. In: *Proceedings of the Organotin Symposium, Oceans '87 Conference, Halifax, Nova Scotia, Canada, 28 September-1 October, 1987*, New York, The Institute of Electrical and Electronics Engineers, Inc., Vol. 4, pp. 1314-1319.

AKATSUKA, K., MIYAZAWA, J., IGARASHI, I., MORISHITA, M., HANDA, A., KAWAME, N., IWAMOTO, I., MORITO, F., MURAYAMA, K., NAKANO, S., YANAGIBASHI, H., NAGASAKI, T., KOTANI, Y., MATSUTANI, W., FUKUDA, I., & IYO, T. (1959) [Experimental studies on disturbance of sense of smell due to butyltin compounds.] *J. Tokyo med. Coll.*, 17: 1393-1402 (in Japanese).

ALABASTER, J.S. (1969) Survival of fish in 164 herbicides, insecticides, fungicides, wetting agents and miscellaneous substances. *Int. Pest Control*, 11: 29-35.

ALDRIDGE, W.N. (1958) The biochemistry of organotin compounds. Trialkyltins and oxidation phosphorylation. *Biochem. J.*, **69**: 367-376.

ALDRIDGE, W.N. & STREET, B.W. (1964) Oxidative phosphorylation: Biochemical effects and properties of trialkyltins. *Biochem. J.*, **91**: 287-297.

ALDRIDGE, W.N. & STREET, B.W. (1970) Oxidative phosphorylation: The specific binding of trimethyltin and triethyltin to rat liver mitochondria. *Biochem. J.*, **118**: 171-179.

ALDRIDGE, W.N. & STREET, B.W. (1971) Oxidative phosphorylation: The relation between the specific binding of trimethyltin and triethyltin to mitochondria and their effects on various mitochondrial functions. *Biochem. J.*, **124**: 221-234.

ALDRIDGE, W.N., CASIDA, J.E., FISH, R.H., KIMMEL, E.C., & STREET, B.W. (1977) Action on mitochondria and toxicity of metabolites of tri-*n*-butyltin derivatives. *Biochem. Pharmacol.*, **26**: 1997-2000.

ALLEN, A.J., QUITTER, B.M., & RADICK, C.M. (1980) The biocidal mechanism of controlled release bis (tri-n-butyltin) oxide in *Biomphalaria glabrata*. In: Baker, R., ed. *Controlled release of bioactive materials*, New York, London, Academic Press, p. 399.

ALZIEU, C.P. (1981) *Evaluation des risques dus à l'emploi des peintures antisalissures dans les zones conchylicoles*. Nantes, Institut scientifique et technique des Pêches maritimes, 84 pp.

ALZIEU, C. & HERAL, M. (1984) Ecotoxicological effects of organotin compounds on oyster culture. *Ecotoxicol. Test. mar. Environ.*, 2: 187-196.

ALZIEU, C. & PORTMANN, J.E. (1984) *The effect of tributyl tin on the culture of C. gigas. Proceedings of the 15th Annual Shellfish Conference, 15-16 May, 1984*, London, The Shellfish Association of Great Britain, 17 pp.

ALZIEU, C., HERAL, M., THIBAUD, Y., DARDIGNAC, M.-J., & FEUILLET, M. (1982) Influence des peintures antisalissures à base d'organostanniques sur la calcification de la coquille de l'huitre Crassostrea gigas. Rev. Trav. Inst. Pêches Marit., 45: 101-116.

ALZIEU, C., SANJUAN, J., DELTREIL, J.P., & BOREL, M. (1986) Tin contamination in Arcachon Bay: Effects on oyster shell anomalies. Mar. Pollut. Bull., 17: 494-498.

ALZIEU, C., SANJUAN, J., MICHEL, P., BOREL, M., & DRENO, J.P. (1989) Monitoring and assessment of butyltins in Atlantic coastal waters. Mar. Pollut. Bull., 20: 22-26.

ANGER, J.P., ANGER, F., CANO, Y., CHAUVEL, Y., LOUVET, M., & VAN DEN DRIESSCHE, J. (1976) Effets chez le cobaye, d'un aérosol à base d'oxyde de tributylétain (OTBE). Eur. J. Toxicol., 9: 339-346.

ARAKAWA, Y. & WADA, O. (1984) Inhibition of neutrophil chemotaxis by organotin compounds. Biochem. biophys. Res. Commun., 123: 543-548.

ARGAMAN, Y., HUCKS, C.E., & SHELBY, S.E. (1984) The effects of organotin on the activated sludge process. Water Res., 18: 535-542.

AYALA, C.A.C., TOLEDO, J.V., DA SILVA NETTO, J.A., & GILBERT, B. (1980) *The effect of hexabutyldistannoxane (TBTO) and other molluscicides on non-target species*, Geneva, World Health Organization, Parasitic Diseases Programme (Unpublished report).

BAAIJENS, P.A. (1987) Health effect screening and biological monitoring for workers in organotin industries. In: *Toxicology and analytics of the tributyltins: The present status. Proceedings of an ORTEPA workshop, Berlin, 15-16 May, 1986*, Vlissingen-Oost, The Netherlands, ORTEP-Association, pp. 191-208

BACCI, E. & GAGGI, C. (1989) Organotin compounds in harbour and marina waters from the Northern Tyrrhenian Sea. Mar. Pollut. Bull., 20: 290-292.

BAHR, G. & PAWLENKO, S. (1978) Organic tin compounds. In: Bahr, G., Kalinowski, H.-O., & Pawlenko, S., ed. *Organometallic compounds, germanium, tin*, Stuttgart, Georg Thieme Verlag, pp. 512-515 (Methods in Organic Chemistry series).

BAILEY, S.K. & DAVIES, I.M. (1988a) Tributyltin contamination around an oil terminal in Sullom Voe (Shetland). Environ. Pollut., 55: 161-172.

BAILEY, S.K. & DAVIES, I.M. (1988b) Tributyltin contamination in the Firth of Forth (1975-87). Sci. total Environ., 76: 185-192.

BAKER, J.M. & TAYLOR, J.M. (1967) The toxicity of tributyltin oxide to the wood-boring beetles *Lyctus brunneus* Steph. and *Anobium punctatum* (Deg.). Ann. appl. Biol., 60: 181-190.

BALLS, P.W. (1987) Tributyltin (TBT) in the waters of a Scottish sea loch arising from the use of antifoulant treated netting by salmon farms. Aquaculture, 65: 227-237.

References

BARNES, J.M. & STONER, H.B. (1958) Toxic properties of some dialkyl and trialkyl tin salts. *Br. J. ind. Med.,* 15: 15-22.

BARUG, D. (1981) Microbial degradation of bis (tributyltin) oxide. *Chemosphere,* 10: 1145-1154.

BARUG, D. & VONK, J.W. (1980) Studies on the degradation of bis (tributyltin) oxide in soil. *Pestic. Sci.,* 11: 77-82.

BEAUMONT, A.R. & BUDD, M.D. (1984) High mortality of the larvae of the common mussel at low concentrations of tributyltin. *Mar. Pollut. Bull.,* 15: 402-405.

BEAUMONT, A.R. & NEWMAN, P.B. (1986) Low levels of tributyltin reduce growth of marine micro-algae. *Mar. Pollut. Bull.,* 17: 457-461.

BEAUMONT, A.R., NEWMAN, P.B., & WALDOCK, M.J. (1987) *Sand substrate microcosm studies on tributyl tin (TBT) toxicity to marine organisms,* 24 pp (Final report to the UK Department of the Environment, London. Contract No. PECD 7/8/73).

BERRIOS-DURAN, L.A. & RITCHIE, L.S. (1968) Molluscicidal activity of bis(tri-*n*-butyltin) oxide formulated in rubber. *World Health Organ. Bull.,* 39: 310-312.

BIODYNAMICS (1989a) *A three month oral range-finding toxicity study in mice with bis (tri-n-butyltin) oxide (TBTO),* East Millstone, New Jersey, Biodynamics (Final report to Aceto Chemical Corporation, M. + T. Chemicals Inc., and Schering Berlin Inc.) (Unpublished).

BIODYNAMICS (1989b) *A two-generation reproduction study in rats with TBTO,* East Millstone, New Jersey, Biodynamics (Interim report to Aceto Chemical Corporation, M. + T. Chemicals Inc., and Schering Berlin Inc.) (Unpublished).

BJORKLUND, I. (1987a) *[Environmental aspects of ship's bottom paints],* Stockholm, Swedish Chemicals Inspectorate, Investigation Department, 16 pp (in Swedish).

BJORKLUND, I. (1987b) *[Environmental effect of antifouling paints],* Stockholm, Swedish National Environment Protection Board, 17 pp.

BLAIR, W.R., OLSON, G.J., BRINCKMAN, F.E., & IVERSON, W.P. (1982) Accumulation and fate of tri-n-butyltin cation in estuarine bacteria. *Microbiol. Ecol.,* 8: 241-251.

BLAIR, W.R., OLSON, G.J., & BRINCKMAN, F.E. (1986) Speciation measurements of butyltins: Application to controlled release rate determination and production of reference standards. In: *Proceedings of the Organotin Symposium, Oceans '86 Conference, Washington, DC, USA, 23-25 September, 1986,* New York, The Institute of Electrical and Electronics Engineers, Inc., Vol. 4, pp. 1141-1145.

BLUNDEN, S.J. & CHAPMAN, A. (1986) Organotin compounds in the environment. In: Craigh, P.J., ed. *Organometallic compounds in the environment,* Harlow, Essex, Longman Group Ltd, pp. 111-159.

BLUNDEN, S.J., HOBBS, L.A., & SMITH, P.J. (1984) The environmental chemistry of organotin compounds. In: Bowen, H.J.M, Blunden, S.J., Colbeck, I., Harrison, R.M., Hobbs, L.A., Katz, S.A., Simkiss, K., Smith, P.J., & Taylor, M.G., ed. *Environmental chemistry*, London, Royal Society of Chemistry, Vol. 3, pp. 49-77.

BOKRANZ, A. & PLUM, H. (1975) *Industrial manufacture and use of organotin compounds*, Bergkamen, Federal Republic of Germany, Schering AG, 33 pp.

BOORMAN, L.A. (1989) The effects of TBT on two salt marsh plant species, *Aster tripolium* and *Limonium vulgare*. In Preparation.

BOULDIN, T.W., GOINES, N.D., BAGNELL, C.R., & KRIGMAN, M.R. (1981) Pathogenesis of trimethyltin neuronal toxicity. Ultrastructural and cytochemical observations. *Am. J. Pathol.*, **104**: 237-249.

BRAMAN, R.S. & TOMPKINS, M.A. (1979) Separation and determination of nanogram amounts of inorganic and methyltin compounds in the environment. *Anal. Chem.*, **51**: 12-19.

BRESSA, G., CIMA, L., CANOVA, F., & CARAVELLO, G.U. (1984) Bioaccumulation of tin in the fish tissues *(Liza aurata)*. In: *Proceedings of the International Conference on Environmental Contamination, London, July 1984* - Geneva, International Register of Potentially Toxic Chemicals, United Nations Environment Programme, pp. 812-815.

BRIDGES, J.W., DAVIES, D.S., & WILLIAMS, R.T. (1967) The fate of ethyltin and diethyltin derivatives in the rat. *Biochem. J.*, **105**: 1261-1266.

BRINCKMAN, F.E. (1981) Environmental organotin chemistry today: Experiences in the field and laboratory. *J. organomet. Chem. Libr.*, **12**: 343-376.

BRINCKMAN, F.E., JACKSON, J.A., BLAIR, W.R., OLSON, G.J., & IVERSON, W.P. (1983) Ultratrace speciation and biogenesis of methyltin transport species in estuarine waters. In: Trace metals in sea water, New York, Plenum Press, pp. 39-72.

BROWN, R.A., NAZARIO, C.M., DE TIRADO, R.S., CASTRILLON, J., & AGARD, E.T. (1977) A comparison of the half-life of inorganic and organic tin in the mouse. *Environ. Res.*, **13**: 56-61.

BRYAN, G.W., GIBBS, P.E., HUMMERSTONE, L.G., & BURT, G.R. (1986) The decline of the gastropod *Nucella lapillus* around south-west England: Evidence for the effect of tributyltin from antifouling paints. *J. Mar. Biol. Assoc. UK*, **66**: 611-640.

BRYAN, G.W., GIBBS, P.E., HUMMERSTONE, L.G., & BURT, G.R. (1987) Copper, zinc, and organotin as long-term factors governing the distribution of organisms in the Fal estuary in southwest England. *Estuaries*, **10**: 208-219.

BRYAN, G.W., GIBBS, P.E., & BURT, G.R. (1988) A comparison of the effectiveness of tri-n-butyltin chloride and five other organotin compounds in promoting the development of imposex in the dog-whelk *Nucella lapillus*. *J. Mar. Biol. Assoc. UK*, **68**: 733-744.

References

BUSHONG, S.J., HALL, W.S., JOHNSON, W.E., & HALL, L.W. (1987) Toxicity of tributyltin to selected Chesapeake Bay biota. In: *Proceedings of the Organotin Symposium, Oceans '87 Conference, Halifax, Nova Scotia, Canada, 28 September-1 October, 1987*, New York, The Institute of Electrical and Electronics Engineers, Inc., Vol. 4, pp. 1494-1503.

BUSHONG, S.J., HALL, L.W., HALL, W.S., JOHNSON, W.E., & HERMAN, R.L. (1988) Acute toxicity of tributyltin to selected Chesapeake Bay fish and invertebrates. *Water Res.*, 22: 1027-1032.

CALLEY, D.J., GUESS, W.L., & AUTIAN, J. (1967) Hepatotoxicity of a series of organotin esters. *J. pharm. Sci.*, 56: 240-243.

CARDARELLI, N.F. (1973) *Effects of ultralow molluscicide dosages on Biomphalaria glabrata and Lebistes reticulatus in micro ecological systems: Report I*, Akron, Ohio, University of Akron, 15 pp.

CARDARELLI, N.F. (1978) Controlled release organotins as mosquito larvicides. *Mosq. News*, 38: 328-333.

CARDARELLI, N.F. & EVANS, W. (1980) Chemodynamics and environmental toxicology of controlled release organotin molluscicides. In: Baker, R.W., ed. *Controlled release of bioactive materials. Proceedings of the 6th International Meeting of the Controlled Release Society*, New York, London, Academic Press, pp. 357-385.

CASIDA, J.E., KIMMEL, E.C., HOLM, B., & WIDMARK, G. (1971) Oxidative dealkylation of tetra-, tri-, and dialkyltin and tetra- and trialkyleads by liver microsomes. *Acta chem. Scand.*, 25: 1497-1499.

CHAMP, M.A. & PUGH, W.L. (1987) Tributyltin antifouling paints: Introduction and overview. In: *Proceedings of the Organotin Symposium, Oceans '87 Conference, Halifax, Nova Scotia, Canada, 28 September-1 October, 1987*, New York, The Institute of Electrical and Electronics Engineers, Inc., Vol. 4, pp. 1296-1308.

CHAPMAN, A.H. & PRICE, J.W. (1972) Degradation of triphenyltin acetate by ultraviolet light. *Int. Pest Control*, 14: 11-12.

CHENG, Z. & JENSEN, A. (1989) Accumulation of organic and inorganic tin in blue mussel, *Mytilus edulis*, under natural conditions. *Mar. Pollut. Bull.*, 20: 281-286.

CHLIAMOVITCH, Y.-P. & KUHN, C. (1977) Behavioural, haematological and histological studies on acute toxicity of bis(tri-n-butyltin) oxide on *Salmo gairdneri* Richardson and *Tilapia rendalli* Boulenger. *J. Fish Biol.*, 10: 575-585.

CHU, K.Y. (1976) Effects of environmental factors on the molluscicidal activities of slow-release hexabutyldistannoxane and copper sulfate. *Bull. World Health Organ.*, 54: 417-420.

CLARK, J.R., PATRICK, J.M., MOORE, J.C., & LORES, E.M. (1987) Waterborne and sediment-source toxicities of six organic chemicals to grass shrimp *(Palaemonetes pugio)* and amphioxus *(Branchiostoma caribaeum)*. *Arch. environ. Contam. Toxicol.*, 16: 401-407.

CLEARY, J.J. & STEBBING, A.R.D. (1985) Organotin and total tin in coastal waters of southwest England. *Mar. Pollut. Bull.*, 16: 350-355.

CLEARY, J.J. & STEBBING, A.R.D. (1987) Organotin in the surface microlayer and subsurface waters of Southwest England. *Mar. Pollut. Bull.*, 18: 238-246.

CREMER, J.E. (1957) The metabolism *in vitro* of tissue slices from rats given triethyltin compounds. *Biochem. J.*, 67: 87-96.

CROFTON, K.M., DEAN, K.F., BONCEK, V.M., ROSEN, M.B., SHEETS, L.P., CHERNOFF, N., & REITER, L.W. (1989) Prenatal or postnatal exposure to bis(tri-*n*-butyltin)oxide in the rat: Postnatal evaluation of teratology and behavior. *Toxicol. appl. Pharmacol.*, 97: 113-123.

DAVIDSON, B.M., VALKIRS, A.O., & SELIGMAN, P.F. (1986) Acute and chronic effects of tributyltin on the mysid *Acanthomysis sculpta* (Crustacea, Mysidacea). In: *Proceedings of the Organotin Symposium, Oceans '86 Conference, Washington, DC, USA, 23-25 September, 1986,* New York, The Institute of Electrical and Electronics Engineers, Inc., pp. 1219-1225.

DAVIES, R.J., FLETCHER, R.L., & FURTADO, S.E.J. (1984) The effects of tributyltin compounds on spore development in the green alga *Enteromorpha intestinalis* (L) Link. In: *Proceedings of the 6th International Congress on Marine Corrosion and Fouling, Athens, September 1984,* pp. 557-565.

DAVIES, I.M., DRINKWATER, J., MCKIE, J.C., & BALLS, P. (1987a) Effects of the use of tributyltin antifoulants in mariculture. In: *Proceedings of the Organotin Symposium, Oceans '87 Conference, Halifax, Nova Scotia, Canada, 28 September-1 October, 1987,* New York, The Institute of Electrical and Electronics Engineers, Inc., pp. 1477-1481.

DAVIES, I.M., BAILEY, S.K., & MOORE, D.C. (1987b) Tributyltin in Scottish sea Lochs, as indicated by degree of imposex in the dogwhelk, *Nucella lapillus* (L.). *Mar. Pollut. Bull.*, 18: 400-404.

DAVIS, A., BARALE, R., BRUN, G., FORSTER, R., GUNTHER, T., HAUTEFEUILLE, H., VAN DER HEIJDEN, C.A., KNAAP, A.G.A.C., KROWKE, R., KUROKI, T., LOPRIENO, N., MALAVEILLE, C., MERKER, H.J., MONACO, M., MOSESSO, P., NEUBERT, D., NORPPA, H., SORSA, M., VOGEL, E., VOOGD, C.E., UMEDA, M., & BARTSCH, H. (1987) Evaluation of the genetic and embryotoxic effects of bis(tri-*n*-butyltin) oxide (TBTO), a broad-spectrum pesticide, in multiple *in vivo* and *in vitro* short-term tests. *Mutat. Res.*, 188: 65-95.

DESCHIENS, R. & FLOCH, H. (1962) Les propriétés molluscicides du chlorure et de l'acétate de triphénylétain dans le cadre de la prophylaxie des bilharzioses. *C. R. Acad. Sci. Paris,* 255: 1236-1237.

References

DESCHIENS, R. & FLOCH, H. (1968) Action biologique comparée de 6 molluscicides chimique dans le cadre de la prophylaxie des bilharzioses. Conclusions pratiques. *Bull. Soc. Pathol. Exot.*, **61**: 640-650.

DESCHIENS, R., BROTTES, H., & MVOGO, L. (1966) Application sur le terrain, au Cameroun, dans la prophylaxie des bilharzioses de l'action molluscicide de l'oxyde de tributylétain. *Bull. Soc. Pathol. Exot.*, **59**: 968-973.

DE VILLIERS, J.P. & MACKENZIE, J.G. (1963) Organotin and organolead molluscicides, Geneva, World Health Organization, Parasitic Diseases Programme, p. 63 (Unpublished report Mol/Inf/13).

DIXON, D.R. & MCFADZEN, I. (1987) Bis(tributyltin) oxide (TBTO), an antifouling compound, promotes SCE induction in the larvae of the common mussel, *Mytilus edulis*. *Mutagenesis*, **2**: 312.

DIXON, D.R. & PROSSER, H. (1986) An investigation of the genotoxic effects of an organotin antifouling compound (bis(tributyltin) oxide) on the chromosomes of the edible mussel, *Mytilus edulis*. *Aquat. Toxicol.*, **8**: 185-195.

DOJMI DI DELUPIS, G., GUCCI, P.M.B., & VOLTERRA, L. (1987) Toxic effects of bis-tributyltinoxide on phytoplancton. *Main Group Metal Chem.*, **10**: 77-82.

DONARD, O., RAPSOMANIKIS, S., & WEBER, J.H. (1986) Speciation of inorganic tin and alkyltin compounds by atomic absorption spectrometry using electrothermal quartz furnace after hydride generation. *Anal. Chem.*, **58**: 772-777.

EAJ (1988) *Outline of TBT compounds monitored in Japan*, Tokyo, Environment Agency of Japan (OECD Clearing House Project on Organotins).

EBDON, L., EVANS, K., & HILL, S. (1988) The variation of tributyltin levels with time in selected estuaries prior to the introduction of regulations governing the use of tributyltin-based anti-fouling paints. *Sci. total Environ.*, **68**: 207-223.

EBDON, L., EVANS, K., & HILL, S. (1989) The accumulation of organotins in adult and seed oysters from selected estuaries prior to the introduction of U.K. regulations governing the use of tributyltin-based antifouling paints. *Sci. total Environ.*, **83**: 63-84.

ELFERINK, J.G.R., DEIERKAUF, M., & VAN STEVENINCK, J. (1986) Toxicity of organotin compounds for polymorphonuclear leukocytes: the effect on phagocyctosis and exocytosis. *Biochem. Pharmacol.*, **35**: 3727-3732.

ELSEA, J.R. & PAYNTER, O.E. (1958) Toxicological studies on bis(tri-n-butyltin) oxide. *Am. Med. Assoc. Arch. Ind. Health*, **18**: 214-217.

EVANS, C.J. & KARPEL, S. (1985) Organotin compounds in modern technology. *J. organomet. Chem. Libr.*, **16**: 178-217.

EVANS, D.W & LAUGHLIN, R.B. (1984) Accumulation of bis (tributyltin) oxide by the mud crab, *Rhitropanopeus harrisii*. *Chemosphere*, **13**: 213-219.

EVANS, W.H., CARDARELLI, N.F., & SMITH, D.J. (1979) Accumulation and excretion of [1-^{14}C] bis (tri-n-butyltin) oxide in mice. *J. Toxicol. environ. Health*, **5**: 871-877.

FENT, K. (1989a) Organotin speciation in municipal wastewater and sewage slude: Ecotoxicological consequences. *Mar. environ. Res.*, **28**: 477-483.

FENT, K. (1989b) *Teratogenic effects of tributyltin on embryos of the freshwater fish Phoxinus phoxinus.* Presented at the OECD Workshop on Tributyltin: Activities related to Field Studies at Sea, Centre IFREMER, Nantes, 27-29 June, 1989 (Unpublished report).

FENT, K., FASSBIND, R., & SIEGRIST, H. (1989) *Organotins in a municipal wastewater treatment plant. Proceedings of the 1st European Conference on Ecotoxicology, Copenhagen, Denmark, 17-19 October, 1988*, Lyngby, Denmark, The Technical University of Denmark, Laboratory of Environmental Sciences and Ecology.

FERAL, C. & LE GALL, S. (1983) The influence of a pollutant factor (tributyltin) on the neuroendocrine mechanism responsible for the occurrence of a penis in the females of *Ocenebra erinacea*. In: Lever, J. & Boer, H.H., ed. *Molluscan neuroendocrinology. Proceedings of the International Minisymposium on Molluscan Endocrinology*, Amsterdam, North-Holland Publishing Company, pp. 173-175.

FISH, R.H., KIMMEL, E.C., & CASIDA, J.E. (1975) Bioorganotin chemistry: Biological oxidation of tributyltin derivatives. *J. organomet. Chem.*, **93**: C1-C4.

FISH, R.H., KIMMEL, E.C., & CASIDA, J.E. (1976) Bioorganotin chemistry: Biological oxidation of organotin compounds. In: Zuckerman, J.J., ed. *Organotin compounds: New chemistry and applications*, Washington, DC, American Chemical Society, pp. 197-203 (Advances in Chemistry Series No. 157).

FLOCH, H., DESCHIENS, R., & FLOCH, T. (1964) Sur les propriétés molluscicides de l'oxyde et de l'acétate de tributylétain (prophylaxie des bilharzioses). *Bull. Soc. Pathol. Exot.*, **57**: 454-465.

FOSTER, R.B. (1981) Use of Asiatic clam larvae in aquatic hazard evaluations. In: Bates, J.M. & Weber, C.I., ed. *Ecological assessments of effluent impacts on communities of indigenous aquatic organisms*, Philadelphia, American Society for Testing and Materials, pp. 280-288 (ASTM STP No. 730).

FUNAHASHI, N., IWASAKI, I., & IDE, G. (1980) Effects of bis(tri-n-butyltin) oxide on endocrine and lymphoid organs of male rats. *Acta pathol. Jpn.*, **30**: 955-966.

GARDINER, B.G. & POLLER, R.C. (1964) Insecticidal activity and structure of some organotin compounds. *Bull. entomol. Res.*, **55**: 17-21.

GIBBS, P.E. & BRYAN, G.W. (1986) Reproductive failure in populations of the dog-whelk, *Nucella lapillus*, caused by imposex induced by tributyltin from antifouling paints. *J. Mar. Biol. Assoc. UK*, **66**: 767-777.

References

GIBBS, P.E. & BRYAN, G.W. (1987) TBT paints and the demise of the dog-whelk, *Nucella lapillus* (Gastropoda). In: *Proceedings of the Organotin Symposium, Oceans '87 Conference, Halifax, Nova Scotia, Canada, 28 September-1 October, 1987,* New York, The Institute of Electrical and Electronics Engineers, Inc., Vol. 4, pp. 1482-1487.

GIBBS, P.E., BRYAN, G.W., PASCOE, P.L., & BURT, G.R. (1987) The use of the dog-whelk, *Nucella lapillus,* as an indicator of tributyltin (TBT) contamination. *J. Mar. Biol. Assoc. UK,* 67: 507-523.

GIBBS, P.E., PASCOE, P.L., & BURT, G.R. (1988) Sex change in the female dog-whelk, *Nucella lapillus,* induced by tributyltin from antifouling paints. *J. Mar. Biol. Assoc. UK,* 68: 715-731.

GILBERT, B., PAES LEME, L.A., FERREIRA, A.M., BULHOES, M.S., & CASTLETON, C. (1973) Field tests of hexabutyldistannoxane (TBTO) in slow-release formulations against *Biomphalaria* spp. *Bull. World Health Organ.,* 49: 633-636.

GILE, J.D., COLLINS, J.C., & GILLETT, J.W. (1982) Fate and impact of wood preservatives in a terrestrial microcosm. *J. agric. food Chem.,* 30: 295-301.

GILLETT, J.W., GILE, J.D., & RUSSELL, L.K. (1983) Predator-prey (vole-cricket) interactions: the effects of wood preservatives. *Environ. Toxicol. Chem.,* 2: 83-93.

GOH, C.L. (1985) Irritant dermatitis from tri-n-butyl tin oxide in paint. *Contact dermatitis,* 12: 161-163.

GOHLKE, R., LEWA, W., STRACHOVSKY, A., & KOHLER, R. (1969) [Investigations in experimental animals of the inhalatory effects of tributyltin chloride in a subchronic experiment.] *Z. gesamte Hyg. Grenzgeb.,* 15: 97-104 (in German).

GOODMAN, L.R., CRIPE, G.M., MOODY, P.H., & HALSELL, D.G. (1988) Acute toxicity of malathion, tetrabromobisphenol-A, and tributyltin chloride to mysids *(Mysidopsis bahia)* of three ages. *Bull. environ. Contam. Toxicol.,* 41: 746-753.

GROVHOUG, J.G., SELIGMAN, P.F., VAFA, G., & FRANSHAM, R.L. (1986) Baseline measurements of butyltin in U.S. harbors and estuaries. In: *Proceedings of the Organotin Symposium, Oceans '86 Conference, Washington, DC, USA, 23-25 September, 1986,* New York, The Institute of Electrical and Electronics Engineers, Inc., Vol. 4, pp. 1283-1288.

GUARD, H.E., COGBET, A.B., & COLEMAN, W.M. (1981) Methylation of trimethyltin compounds by estuarine sediments. *Science,* 213: 770-771.

HADA, N. (1986) [Studies on the kinetics of tributyltin compounds in the body: With special reference to their biological half times in goldfish and rats as estimated by newly developed analytical method.] *Nichidai Igaku Zasshi,* 45: 1005-1013 (in Japanese).

HALL, L.W., PINKNEY, A.E., ZEGER, S., BURTON, D.T., & LENKEVICH, M.J. (1984) Behavioral responses to two estuarine fish species subjected to bis (tri-*n*-butyltin) oxide. *Water Resour. Bull.*, **20**: 235-239.

HALL, L.W., LENKEVICH, M.J., HALL, W.S., PINKNEY, A.E., & BUSHONG, S.J. (1986) Monitoring organotin concentrations in Maryland waters of Chesapeake Bay. In: *Proceedings of the Organotin Symposium, Oceans '86 Conference, Washington, DC, USA, 23-25 September, 1986*, New York, The Institute of Electrical and Electronics Engineers, Inc., Vol. 4, pp. 1275-1279.

HALL, L.W., BUSHONG, S.J., JOHNSON, W.E., & HALL, W.S. (1988a) Spacial and temporal distribution of butyltin compounds in a Northern Chesapeake Bay marina and river system. *Environ. Monit. Assess.*, **10**: 229-244.

HALL, L.W., BUSHONG, S.J., HALL, W.S., & JOHNSON, W.E. (1988b) Acute and chronic effects of tributyltin on a Chesapeake Bay copepod. *Environ. Toxicol. Chem.*, **7**: 41-46.

HALLAS, L.E., MEANS, J.C., & COONEY, J.J. (1982) Methylation of tin by estuarine microorganisms. *Science*, **215**: 1505-1507.

HARRIS, J.R.W. & CLEARY, J.J. (1987) Particle-water partitioning and organotin dispersal in an estuary. In: *Proceedings of the Organotin Symposium, Oceans '87 Conference, Halifax, Nova Scotia, Canada, 28 September-1 October, 1987*, New York, The Institute of Electrical and Electronics Engineers, Inc., Vol. 4, pp. 1370-1374.

HENDERSON, R.S. (1986) Effects of organotin antifouling paint leachates on Pearl Harbor organisms: a site specific flowthrough bioassay. In: *Proceedings of the Organotin Symposium, Oceans '86 Conference, Washington, DC, USA, 23-25 September, 1986*, New York, The Institute of Electrical and Electronics Engineers, Inc., Vol. 4, pp. 1226-1233.

HENSHAW, B.G., LAIDLAW, R.A., ORSLER, R.J., CAREY, J.K., & SAVORY, J.G. (1978) The permanence of tributyltin oxide in timber. In: *Record of the 1978 Annual Convention of the British Wood Preserving Association, Cambridge, 27-30 June, 1978*, London, British Wood Preserving Association, pp. 19-29.

HINGA, K.R., ADELMAN, D., & PILSON, M.E.Q. (1987) Radiolabeled butyl tin studies in the Merl enclosed ecosystems. In: *Proceedings of the Organotin Symposium, Oceans '87 Conference, Halifax, Nova Scotia, Canada, 28 September-1 October, 1987*, New York, The Institute of Electrical and Electronics Engineers, Inc., Vol. 4, pp. 1416-1420.

HIS, E. & ROBERT, R. (1980) *Action d'un sel organo-métallique, l'acétate de tributylétain sur les oeufs et les larves de* Crassostrea gigas (Thunberg), Copenhagen, International Council for the Exploration of the Sea (ICES) Mariculture Commission, 27 pp (CM 1980/F).

HIS, E. & ROBERT, R. (1985) Développement des véligères de *Crassostrea gigas* dans le Bassin d'Arcachon, études sur les mortalités larvaires. *Rev. Trav. Inst. Pêches Marit.*, **47**: 63-88.

HIS, E., MAURER, D., & ROBERT, R. (1986) Observations complémentaires sur les causes possibles des anomalies de la reproduction de *Crassostrea gigas* (Thunberg) dans le Basin d'Arcachon. *Rev. Trav. Inst. Pêches Marit.*, **48**: 45-54.

HODGE, V.F., SEIDEL, S.L., & GOLDBERG, E.D. (1979) Determination of tin (IV) and organotin compounds in natural waters, coastal sediments, and macro algae by atomic absorption spectrometry. *Anal. Chem.*, **51**: 1256-1259.

HOPF, H.S., DUNCAN, J., BEESLEY, J.S.S., WEBLEY, D.J., & STURROCK, R.F. (1967) Molluscicidal properties of organotin and organolead compounds. *World Health Organ. Bull.*, **36**: 955-961.

HUGGETT, R.J., UNGER, M.A., & WESTBROOK, D.J. (1986) Organotin concentrations in the southern Chesapeake Bay. In: *Proceedings of the Organotin Symposium, Oceans '86 Conference, Washington, DC, USA, 23-25 September, 1986*, New York, The Institute of Electrical and Electronics Engineers, Inc., Vol. 4, pp. 1262-1265.

HUMPEL, M., KUHNE, G., TAUBER, U., & SCHULZE, P.E. (1986) Studies on the kinetics of bis (tris-n-butyl-^{113}tin) oxide (TBTO). In: *Toxicology and analytics of the tributyltins: The present status. Proceedings of an ORTEPA workshop, Berlin, 15-16 May, 1986*, Vlissingen-Oost, The Netherlands, ORTEP-Association, pp. 122-142.

HUMPHREY, B. & HOPE, D. (1987) Analysis of water, sediments and biota for organotin compounds. In: *Proceedings of the Organotin Symposium, Oceans '87 Conference, Halifax, Nova Scotia, Canada, 28 September-1 October, 1987*, New York, The Institute of Electrical and Electronics Engineers, Inc., Vol. 4, pp. 1348-1351.

ICES (1987) *Concentrations of organotin and total tin in open Danish sea areas and in pleasure craft marinas along the sound*. International Council for the Exploration of the Sea (ICES) (TWG 14/9/3-E).

IWAI, H., MANABE, M., MATSUI, H., ONO, T., & WADA, O. (1980) Effects of tributyltin and its metabolites on brain function. *J. toxicol. Sci.*, **5**: 257.

IWASAKI, I., FUNABASHI, N., TOIZUMI, S., & IDE, G. (1976) Histopathological studies on rat's nervous system by oral administration of bis-(tri-n-butyltin) oxide. (I). *J. toxicol. Sci.*, **1**: 99 (abstract).

JENSEN, A. & CHENG, Z. (1987) Total tin and organotin in seawater from pleasure craft marinas along Danish coast of the Sound. In: *Proceedings of the 15th Conference of Baltic Oceanographers (CBO), Copenhagen, 1986*. Charlottenlung, Denmark, Marine Pollution Laboratory, Vol. 1, pp. 289-298.

JEWETT, K.L. & BRINCKMAN, F.E. (1981) Speciation of trace di- and triorganotins in water by ion exchange HPLC-GFAA. *J. chromatogr. Sci.*, **19**: 583.

JOHANSEN, K. & MOHLENBERG, F. (1987) Impairment of egg production in *Acartia tonsa* exposed to tributyltin oxide. *Ophelia*, **27**: 137-141.

JOHNSON, T.L. & KNOWLES, C.O. (1983) Effects of organotins on rat platelets. *Toxicology*, 29: 39-48.

JORDAN, P. (1985) *Schistosomiasis - The St Lucia Project*, Cambridge, Cambridge University Press, 442 pp.

KAKUNO, A. & KIMURA, S. (1987) [Acute toxicity of bis (tributyltin) oxide to girella *(Girella punctata).] Bull. Tokai Reg. Fish. Res. Lab.*, 123: 41-44 (in Japanese).

KALBFUS, W. (1988) *TBT-burden from antifouling paints in different waters.* Presented at the OECD Workshop on Monitoring, Chemical Analysis and Leaching Rates of TBT, Paris, 30 November-2 December, 1988, 11 pp (Unpublished report).

KALNINS, M.A. & DETROY, B.F. (1984) Effect of wood preservative treatment of beehives on honey bees and hive products. *J. agric. food Chem.*, 32: 1176-1180.

KEY, D., NUNNY, R.S., DAVIDSON, P.E., & LEONARD, M.A. (1976) *Abnormal shell growth in the Pacific oyster* Crassostrea gigas. *Some preliminary results from experiments undertaken in 1975*, Copenhagen, International Council for the Exploration of the Sea (ICES), 12 pp. (C. M. 1976/K/11).

KIMMEL, E.C., FISH, R.H., & CASIDA, J.E. (1977) Bioorganotin chemistry: Metabolism of organotin compounds in microsomal monooxygenase system and in mammals. *J. agric. food Chem.*, 25: 1-8.

KLIMMER, O.R. (1969) [The use of organic tin compounds from the viewpoint of experimental toxicology.] *Arzneimittelforschung*, 19: 934-939 (in German).

KNOWLES, C.O. & JOHNSON, T.L. (1986) Influence of organotins on rat platelet aggregation mechanism. *Environ. Res.*, 39: 172-179.

KRAJNC, E.I. (1989) Presentation to OECD working group on TBT immune effects. *In Preparation.*

KRAJNC, E.I., WESTER, P.W., LOEBER, J.G., VAN LEEUWEN, F.X.R., VOS, J.G., VAESSEN, H.A.M.G., & VAN DER HEIJDEN, C.A. (1984) Toxicity of bis(tri-n-butyltin)oxide in the rat. 1. Short-term effects on general parameters and on the endocrine and lymphoid systems. *Toxicol. appl. Pharmacol.*, 75: 363-386.

KRAMPITZ, G., ENGELS, J., & CAZAUX, C. (1976) Biochemical studies on water-soluble proteins and related components of gastropods shells. In: Watabe, N. & Wilbur, K.M., ed. *The mechanisms of mineralization in the invertebrates and plants*, Columbia, University of South Carolina Press, pp. 155-173.

KRAMPITZ, G., DROLSHAGEN, H., & DELTREIL, J.P. (1983) Soluble matrix components in malformed oyster shells. *Experientia (Basel)*, 39: 1105-1106.

KROWKE, R., BLUTH, U., & NEUBERT, D. (1986) *In vitro* studies on the embryotoxic potential of (bis[tri-n-butyltin])oxide in a limb bud culture system. *Arch. Toxicol.*, 58: 125-129.

LANGSTON, W.J., BURT, G.R., & ZHOU, M. (1987) Tin and organotin in water, sediments, and benthic organisms of Poole Harbour. *Mar. Pollut. Bull.,* **18**: 634-639.

LAUGHLIN, R.B. & FRENCH, W.J. (1980) Comparative study of the acute toxicity of a homologous series of trialkyltins to larval shore crabs, *Hemigrapsus nudus,* and lobster, *Homarus americanus. Bull. environ. Contam. Toxicol.,* **25**: 802-809.

LAUGHLIN, R. & LINDEN, O. (1982) Sublethal responses of the tadpoles of the European frog *Rana temporaria* to two tributyltin compounds. *Bull. environ. Contam. Toxicol.,* **28**: 494-499.

LAUGHLIN, R., FRENCH, W., & GUARD, H.E. (1983) Acute and sublethal toxicity of tributyltin oxide (TBTO) and its putative environmental product, tributyltin sulfide (TBTS) to zoeal mud crabs, *Rhithropanopeus harrisii. Water Air Soil Pollut.,* **20**: 69-79.

LAUGHLIN, R., NORDLUND, K., & LINDEN, O. (1984) Long-term effects of tributyltin compounds on the baltic amphipod, *Gammarus oceanicus. Mar. environ. Res.,* **12**: 243-271.

LAUGHLIN, R.B., JOHANNESEN, R.B., FRENCH, W., GUARD, H., & BRINKMAN, F.E. (1985) Structure-activity relationships for organotin compounds. *Environ. Toxicol. Chem.,* **4**: 343-351.

LAUGHLIN, R.B., GUARD, H.E., & COLEMAN, W.M. (1986a) Tributyltin in seawater: Speciation and octanol-water partition coefficient. *Environ. Sci. Technol.,* **20**: 201-204.

LAUGHLIN, R.B., FRENCH, W., & GUARD, H.E. (1986b) Accumulation of bis (tributyltin) oxide by the marine mussel *Mytilus edulis. Environ. Sci. Technol.,* **20**: 884-890.

LAUGHLIN, R.B., PENDOLEY, P., & GUSTAFSON, R.G. (1987) Sublethal effects of tributyltin on the hard shell clam, *Mercenaria mercenaria.* In: *Proceedings of the Organotin Symposium, Oceans '87 Conference, Halifax, Nova Scotia, Canada, 28 September-1 October, 1987,* New York, The Institute of Electrical and Electronics Engineers, Inc., Vol. 4, pp. 1494-1498.

LAUGHLIN, R.B., GUSTAFSON, R., & PENDOLEY, P. (1988) Chronic embryo-larval toxicity of tributyltin (TBT) to the hard shell clam *Mercenaria mercenaria. Mar. Ecol. Prog. Ser.,* **48**: 29-36.

LAWLER, I.F. & ALDRICH, J.C. (1987) Sublethal effects of bis(tri-*n*-butyltin)oxide on *Crassostrea gigas* spat. *Mar. Pollut. Bull.,* **18**: 274-278.

LEE, R.F. (1985) Metabolism of tributyltin oxide by crabs, oysters and fish. *Mar. environ. Res.,* **17**: 145-148.

LEE, R.F. (1986) Metabolism of bis (tributyltin) oxide by estuarine animals. In: *Proceedings of the Organotin Symposium, Oceans '86 Conference, Washington, DC, USA, 23-25 September, 1986,* New York, The Institute of Electrical and Electronics Engineers, Inc., Vol. 4, pp. 1182-1188.

LEE, R.F., VALKIRS, A.O., & SELIGMAN, P. (1987) Fate of tributyltin in estuarine waters. In: *Proceedings of the Organotin Symposium, Oceans '87 Conference, Halifax, Nova Scotia, Canada, 28 September-1 October, 1987*, New York, The Institute of Electrical and Electronics Engineers, Inc., Vol. 4, pp. 1411-1415.

LEWIS, P.G. & EMMETT, E.A. (1987) Irritant dermatitis from tri-butyl tin oxide and contact allergy from chlorocresol. *Contact dermatitis*, 17: 129-132.

LINDEN, O. (1987) The scope of the organotin issue in Scandinavia. In: *Proceedings of the Organotin Symposium, Oceans '87 Conference, Halifax, Nova Scotia, Canada, 28 September-1 October, 1987*, New York, The Institute of Electrical and Electronics Engineers, Inc., Vol. 4, pp. 1320-1323.

LINDEN, E., BENGTSSON, B.-E., SVANBERG, O., & SUNDSTROM, G. (1979) The acute toxicity of 78 chemicals and pesticide formulations against two brackish water organisms, the bleak *(Alburnus alburnus)* and the harpacticoid *Nitocra spinipes*. *Chemosphere*, 8: 843-851.

LYLE, W.H. (1958) Lesions of the skin in process workers caused by contact with butyl tin compounds. *Br. J. ind. Med.*, 15: 193-196.

MCCULLOUGH, F.S., GAYRAL, P., DUNCAN, J., & CHRISTIE, J.D. (1980) Molluscicides in schistosomiasis control. *World Health Organ. Bull.*, 58: 681-689.

MACKLAD, F., TAMAN, F., & EL SEBAE, A.K. (1983) Toxicity of tributyltin fluoride and copper sulfate in slow release formulation to *Biomphalaria alexandrina* snails. *Bull. High Inst. Public Health*, 14: 1-12.

MAFF/HSE (1988) *Pesticides 1988: Pesticides approved under the control of pesticides regulations 1986*, London, UK Ministry of Agriculture, Fisheries and Food (MAFF) and UK Health and Safety Executive (HSE), 399 pp (Reference Book HMSO 500).

MAFF/HSE (1989) *Pesticides 1989: Pesticides approved under the control of pesticides regulations 1986*, London, UK Ministry of Agriculture, Fisheries and Food (MAFF) and UK Health and Safety Executive (HSE), 407 pp (Reference Book HMSO 500).

MAGUIRE, R.J. (1984) Butyltin compounds and inorganic tin in sediments in Ontario. *Environ. Sci. Technol.*, 18: 291-294.

MAGUIRE, R.J. (1987) Review: Environmental aspects of tributyltin. *Appl. organomet. Chem.*, 1: 475-498.

MAGUIRE, R.J. & HUNEAULT, H. (1981) Determination of butyltin species in water by gas chromatography with flame photometric detection. *J. Chromatogr.*, 209: 458-462.

MAGUIRE, R.J. & TKACZ, R.J. (1983) Analysis of butyltin compounds by gas chromatography. Comparison of flame photometric and atomic absorption spectrophotometric detectors. *J. Chromatogr.*, 268: 99-101.

References

MAGUIRE, R.J. & TKACZ, R.J. (1985) Degradation of the tri-n-butyltin species in water and sediment from Toronto Harbor. *J. agric. food Chem.*, 33: 947-953.

MAGUIRE, R.J. & TKACZ, R.J. (1987) Concentration of tributyltin in the microlayer of natural waters. *Water Pollut. Res. J. Can.*, 22: 227-233.

MAGUIRE, R.J., CHAU, Y.K., BENGERT, G.A., HALE, E.J., WONG, P.T.S., & KRAMAR, O. (1982) Occurrence of organotin compounds in Ontario lakes and rivers. *Environ. Sci. Technol.*, 16: 698-702.

MAGUIRE, R.J., CAREY, J.H., & HALE, E.J. (1983) Degradation of the tri-*n*-butyltin species in water. *J. agric. food Chem.*, 31: 1060-1065.

MAGUIRE, R.J., WONG, P.T.S., & RHAMEY, J.S. (1984) Accumulation and metabolism of tri-*n*-butyltin cation by a green alga, *Ankistrodesmus falcatus*. *Can. J. Fish. aquat. Sci.*, 41: 537-540.

MAGUIRE, R.J., TKACZ, R.J., & SARTOR, D.L. (1985) Butyltin species and inorganic tin in water and sediment of the Detroit and St. Clair rivers. *J. Great Lakes Res.*, 11: 320-327.

MAGUIRE, R.J., TKACZ, R.J., CHAU, Y.K., BENGERT, G.A., & WONG, P.T.S. (1986) Occurrence of organotin compounds in water and sediment in Canada. *Chemosphere*, 15: 253-274.

MATSUI, H., WADA, O., MANABE, S., ONO, T., IWAI, H., & FUJIKURA, T. (1982) [Properties and mechanism of hyperlipidemia induced in rabbits by tributyltin fluoride.] *Jpn. J. ind. Health*, 24: 163-171 (in Japanese).

MATTHIAS, C.L., BELLAMA, J.M., & BRINCKMAN, F.E. (1986a) Determination of ultra-trace concentrations of butyltin compounds in water by simultaneous hydridization/extraction with GC/FPD detection. In: *Proceedings of the Organotin Symposium, Oceans '86 Conference, Washington, DC, USA, 23-25 September, 1986*, New York, The Institute of Electrical and Electronics Engineers, Inc., Vol. 4, pp. 1146-1151.

MATTHIAS, C.L., OLSON, G.J., BELLAMA, J.M., & BRINCKMAN, F.E. (1986b) Comprehensive method for determination of aquatic butyltin and butylmethyltin species at ultratrace levels using simultaneous hydridization/extraction with GC/FPD detection. *Environ. Sci. Technol.*, 20: 609-615.

MATTHIESSEN, P. (1974) *Some effects of slow-release bis (tri-n-butyl tin) oxide on the tropical fish, Tilapia mossambica Peters.* Controlled Release Pesticide Symposium, Akron, Ohio, University of Akron, Community Technical College, Engineering and Science Division, pp. 25.1-25.16.

MATTHIESSEN, P. & THAIN, J.E. (in press) A method for studying the impact of polluted marine sediments on colonising organisms; tests with diesel-based drilling mud and tributyltin antifouling paint. *Hydrobiologia*.

MAURER, D., HERAL, M., HIS, E., & RAZET, D. (1985) Influence d'une peinture antisalissure à base de sels organométalliques de l'étain sur le captage en milieu naturel de l'huitre *Crassostrea gigas*. *Rev. Trav. Inst. Pêches Marit.*, 47: 241-250.

MEADOR, J.P. (1986) An analysis of photobehavior of *Daphnia magna* exposed to tributyltin. In: *Proceedings of the Organotin Symposium, Oceans '86 Conference, Washington, DC, USA, 23-25 September, 1986*, New York, The Institute of Electrical and Electronics Engineers, Inc., Vol. 4, pp. 1213-1218.

MEINEMA, H.A., BURGER-WIERSMA, T., VERSLUIS DE HAAN, G., & GEVERS, E.C. (1978) Determination of trace amounts of butyltin compounds in aqueous systems by gas chromatography/mass spectrometry. *Environ. Sci. Technol.*, 12: 288-293.

MICHEL, P. (1987) Automatization of a hydride generation/A.A.S. system - an improvement for organotin analysis. In: *Proceedings of the Organotin Symposium, Oceans '87 Conference, Halifax, Nova Scotia, Canada, 28 September-1 October, 1987*, New York, The Institute of Electrical and Electronics Engineers, Inc., Vol. 4, pp. 1340-1343.

MIDDLETON, M.C. & PRATT, I. (1977) Skin water content as a quantitative index of the vascular and histologic changes produced in rat skin by di-n-butyltin and tri-n-butyltin. *J. invest. Dermatol.*, 68: 379-384.

MIDDLETON, M.C. & PRATT, I. (1978) Changes in incorporation of [^{3}H]thymidine into DNA of rat skin following cutaneous application of dibutyltin, tributyltin and 1-chloro-2:4-dinitrobenzene and the relationship of these changes to a morphological assessment of the cellular damage. *J. invest. Dermatol.*, 71: 305-310.

MINCHIN, D., DUGGAN, C.B., & KING, W. (1987) Possible effects of organotins on scallop recruitment. *Mar. Pollut. Bull.*, 18: 604-608.

MOLIN, L. & WAHLBERG, J.E. (1975) Toxic skin reactions caused by tributyltin oxide (TBTO) in socks. *Berufs-dermatosen*, 4: 138-142.

MORI, Y., IESATO, K., UEDA, S., MORI, T., IWASAKI, I., OHNISHI, K., SEINO, Y., WAKASHIM, Y., WAKASHIN, M., & OKUDA, K. (1984) Renal tubular disturbances induced by tributyl-tin oxide in guinea pigs: a secondary Fanconi syndrome. *Clin. Nephrol.*, 21: 118-125.

MULLER, H.A. (1987) Determination of tributyltin oxide in air. In: *Toxicology and analytics of the tributyltins: The present status. Proceedings of an ORTEPA workshop, Berlin, 15-16 May, 1986*, Vlissingen-Oost, The Netherlands, ORTEP Association, pp. 162-172.

MULLER, M.D. (1984) Tributyltin detection at trace levels in water and sediments using GC with flame-photometric detection and GC-MS. *Fresenius Z. anal. Chem.*, 317: 32-36.

MULLER, M.D. (1987b) Comprehensive trace level determination of organotin compounds in environmental samples using high-resolution gas chromatography with flame photometric detection. *Anal. Chem.*, 59: 617-623.

MUSHAK, P., KRIGMAN, M.R., & MAILMAN, R.B. (1982) Comparative organotin toxicity in the developing rat: somatic and morphological changes and relationship to accumulation of total tin. *Neurobehav. Toxicol. Teratol.*, 4: 209-215.

References

NEMEC, M.D. (1987) *A teratology study in rabbits with TBTO: Final Report*, Wil Research Laboratories Inc., 210 pp (Report No. WIL-B0002) (Confidential report to the Tributyl Tin Oxide Consortium).

NEWTON, F., THUM, A., DAVIDSON, B., VALKIRS, A., & SELIGMAN, P. (1985) *Effects on the growth and survival of eggs and embryos of the California grunion* (Leuresthes tenuis) *exposed to trace levels of tributyltin*, San Diego, California, Naval Ocean Systems Center, 15 pp (Technical Report No. 1040).

NIVA (1986) *[Organic tin compounds in fjord areas]*, Oslo, Norwegian Institute for Water Research (NIVA) (in Norwegian).

O'CALLAGHAN, J.P. & MILLER, D.B. (1988) Acute exposure of the neonatal rat to tributyltin results in decreases in biochemical indicators of synaptogenesis and myelinogenesis. *Pharmacol. exp. Ther.*, 246: 394-402.

OKOSHI, K., MORI, K., & NONURA, T. (1987) Characteristics of shell chamber formation between the two races in Japanese oyster, *Crassostrea gigas*. *Aquaculture*, 67: 313-320.

OLSON, G.J. & BRINCKMAN, F.E. (1986) Biodegradation of tributyltin by Chesapeake Bay microorganisms. In: *Proceedings of the Organotin Symposium, Oceans '86 Conference, Washington, DC, USA, 23-25 September, 1986*, New York, The Institute of Electrical and Electronics Engineers, Inc., Vol. 4, pp. 1196-1201.

OSBORN, D. & LEACH, D.V. (1987) *Organotin in birds: Pilot study*, Huntingdon, Institute of Terrestrial Ecology, 15 pp (Final report to the UK Department of the Environment. Contract No. F3CR/27/D4/01).

PAGE, D.S. (1989) An analytical method for butyltin species in shellfish. *Mar. Pollut. Bull.*, 20: 129-133.

PAUL, J.D. & DAVIES, I.M. (1986) Effects of copper- and tin-based anti-fouling compounds on the growth of scallops *(Pecten maximus)* and oysters *(Crassostrea gigas)*. *Aquaculture*, 54: 191-203.

PAULINI, E. (1964) *Laboratory experiments with some organotin compounds*, Geneva, World Health Organization, Parasitic Diseases Programme, pp. 1-3 (Unpublished report Mol/Inf/16).

PAULINI, E. & DE SOUZA, C.P. (1970) *Influence of different suspended solids in the water upon molluscicide activity*, Geneva, World Health Organization, Parasitic Diseases Programme, pp. 1-10 (Unpublished report PD/Mol/70.12).

PELIKAN, Z. (1969) Effects of bis(tri-n-butyltin) oxide on the eyes of rabbits. *Br. J. ind. Med.*, 26: 165-170.

PELIKAN, Z. & CERNY, E. (1968) [The toxic effects of tri-n-butyltin compounds on white mice.] *Arch. Toxikol.*, 23: 283-292 (in German).

PELIKAN, Z. & CERNY, E. (1969) Toxic effects of bis (tributyltin) oxide (TBTO) on the skin of rats. *Berufs-dermatosen*, 17: 305-316.

PICKWELL, G.V. & STEINERT, S.A. (1988) Accumulation and effects of organotin compounds in oysters and mussels: correlation with serum biochemical and cytological factors and tissue burdens. *Mar. environ. Res.*, 24: 215-218.

PIETERS, R.H., KAMPINGA, J., BOL-SCHOENMAKERS, M., LAMB, B.W., PENNINKS, A.H., & SEINEN, W. (1989) Organotin-induced thymus atrophy concerns the OX-44+ immature thymocytes: Relation to the interaction between early thymocytes and thymic epithelial cells? *Thymus*, 14(1-3): 79-88.

PINKNEY, A.E., HALL, L.W., LENKEVICH, M.J., BURTON, D.T., & ZEGER, S. (1985) Comparison of avoidance responses of an estuarine fish, *Fundulus heteroclitus*, and crustacean, *Palaemonetes pugio*, to bis (tri-*n*-butyltin) oxide. *Water Air Soil Pollut.*, 25: 33-40.

PINKNEY, A.E., MATTESON, L.L., & WRIGHT, D.A. (1988) Effects of tributyltin on survival, growth, morphometry and RNA-DNA ratio of larval striped bass, Morone saxatilis. In: *Proceedings of the Organotin Symposium, Oceans '88 Conference*, New York, The Institute of Electrical and Electronics Engineers, Inc., Vol. 4, pp. 987-991.

PLUM, H. (1981) Comportement des composés organostanniques vis-à-vis de l'environnement. *Inf. chim.*, 220: 135-139.

POITOU, P., MARIGNAC, B., CERTIN, C., & GRADISKI, D. (1978) Etude de l'effet sur le système nerveux central et du pouvoir sensibilisant de l'oxyde de tributylétain. *Ann. Pharm. fr.*, 36: 569-572.

POLSTER, M. & HALACKA, K. (1971) [9. Contributions to the health-toxic problems of some anti-microbially used organo-tin compounds.] *Ernährungsforschung*, 16: 527-535 (in German).

RACEY, P.A. & SWIFT, S.M. (1986) The residual effects of remedial timber treatments on bats. *Biol. Conserv.*, 35: 205-214.

RANDALL, L., DONARD, O.F.X., & WEBER, J.H. (1986) Speciation of n-butyltin compounds by atomic absorption spectrophotometry using electro-thermal quartz furnace after hydride generation. *Anal. Chim. Acta.*, 184: 197-203.

REIMANN, R. & LANG, R. (1987) Mutagenicity studies with tributyltin compounds. In: *Toxicology and analytics of the tributyltins: The present status. Proceedings of an ORTEPA workshop, Berlin, 15-16 May, 1986*, Vlissingen-Oost, The Netherlands, ORTEP Association, pp. 66-90.

REINHARDT, C.A., SCHAWALDER, H., & ZBINDEN, G. (1982) Cell detachment and cloning efficiency as parameters for cytotoxicity. *Toxicology*, 25: 47-52.

RICE, C.D., ESPOURTEILLE, F.A., & HUGGETT, R.J. (1987) Analysis of tributyltin in estuarine sediments and oyster tissue, *Crassostrea virginica*. *Appl. organomet. Chem.*, 1: 541-544.

RITCHIE, L.S., BERRIOS-DURAN, L.A., FRICK, L.P., & FOX, I. (1964) Molluscicidal time-concentration relationships of organo-tin compounds. *World Health Organ. Bull.*, 31: 147-149.

References

RITCHIE, L.S., LOPEZ, V.A., & CORA, J.M. (1974) Prolonged applications of an organotin against *Biomphalaria glabrata* and *Schistosoma mansoni*. In: *Molluscicides in schistosomiasis control*, New York, London, Academic Press, pp. 77-88.

RIVM (1989) In: Mathijssen-Spiekman, E.A.M., Canton, J.H., & Roghair, C.J., ed. *[Investigation into the toxicity of TBTO for a number of freshwater organisms]*, Bilthoven, National Institute of Public Health and Environmental Hygiene, 48 pp (Report No. 668118.001) (in Dutch).

ROBERTS, M.H. (1987) Acute toxicity of tributyltin chloride to embryos and larvae of two bivalve mollusks, *Crassostrea virginica* and *Mercenaria mercenaria*. *Bull. environ. Contam. Toxicol.*, 39: 1012-1019.

ROBERTS, M.H., BENDER, M.E., DE LISLE, P.F., SUTTON, H.C., & WILLIAMS, R.L. (1987) Sex ratio and gamete production in American oysters exposed to tributyltin in the laboratory. In: *Proceedings of the Organotin Symposium, Oceans '87 Conference, Halifax, Nova Scotia, Canada, 28 September-1 October, 1987*, New York, The Institute of Electrical and Electronics Engineers, Inc., Vol. 4, pp. 1471-1476.

ROBINSON, I.N. (1969) Effects of some organotin compounds on tissue amine levels in rats. *Food Cosmet. Toxicol.*, 7: 47-52.

ROSENBERG, D.W. & DRUMMOND, G.S. (1983) Direct *in vitro* effects of bis (tributyl) tin oxide on hepatic cytochrome P-450. *Biochem. Pharmacol.*, 32: 3823-3829.

ROSENBERG, D.W., DRUMMOND, G.S., CORNISH, H.C., & KAPPAS, A. (1980) Prolonged induction of hepatic haem oxygenase and decreases in cytochrome P-450 content by organotin compounds. *Biochem. J.*, 190: 465-468.

ROSENBERG, D.W., DRUMMOND, G.S., & KAPPAS, A. (1981) The influence of organometals on heme metabolism. *In vivo* and *in vitro* studies with organotins. *Mol. Pharmacol.*, 21: 150-158.

ROSENBERG, D.W., ANDERSON, K.E., & KAPPAS, A. (1984) The potent induction of intestinal heme oxygenase by the organotin compound, bis(tri-n-butyltin) oxide. *Biochem. biophys. Res. Commun.*, 119: 1022-1027.

SALAZAR, S.M. (1985) *The effects of bis(tri-n-butyltin) oxide on three species of marine phytoplankton*, San Diego, California, Naval Ocean Systems Center, 16 pp (Technical Report No. 1039).

SALAZAR, M.H. & SALAZAR, S.M. (1985) *Ecological evaluation of organotin-contaminated sediment*, San Diego, California, Naval Ocean Systems Center, 21 pp (Technical Report No. 1050).

SALAZAR, M.H. & SALAZAR, S.M. (1987) Tributyltin effects on juvenile mussel growth. In: *Proceedings of the Organotin Symposium, Oceans '87 Conference, Halifax, Nova Scotia, Canada, 28 September-1 October, 1987*, New York, The Institute of Electrical and Electronics Engineers, Inc., Vol. 4, pp. 1504-1510.

SALAZAR, S.M., DAVIDSON, B.M., SALAZAR, M.H., STANG, P.M., & MEYERS-SCHULTE, K.J. (1987) Effects of TBT on marine organisms: Field assessment of a new site-specific bioassay system. In: *Proceedings of the Organotin Symposium, Oceans '87 Conference, Halifax, Nova Scotia, Canada, 28 September-1 October, 1987*, New York, The Institute of Electrical and Electronics Engineers, Inc., Vol. 4, pp. 1461-1470.

SAXENA, P.N. & CROWE, A.J. (1988) An investigation of the efficacy of organotin compounds for the control of the cotton stainer, *Dysdercus cingulatus*, the mosquito, *Anopheles stephensi*, and the common house fly, *Musca domestica*. Appl. organomet. Chem., 2: 185-187.

SCHAFER, E.W. & BOWLES, W.A. (1985) Acute oral toxicity and repellency of 933 chemicals to house and deer mice. Arch. environ. Contam. Toxicol., 14: 111-129.

SCHERING (1983) *Repeated dose inhalation study of ZK21.995 in the rat for 29-32 days (21-24 exposures)*, Bergkamen, Federal Republic of Germany, Schering Inc. (Report No. IC 1/83. Study No. TX81.177).

SCHERING (1986) *Re-evaluation of a "mouse micronucleus test on TBTO"*, Bergkamen, Federal Republic of Germany, Schering Inc. (Confidential report No. IC 7186 prepared by the Institute of Occupational Health, Helsinki, Finland, September 1984).

SCHERING (1989a) *TBTO - 4 week oral (dietary administration) toxicity study in the rat*, Bergkamen, Federal Republic of Germany, Schering Inc. (Report No. 280118 by Hazelton, France. Study No. 14/502).

SCHERING (1989b) *TBTO - Plaque forming assay following a 5 week oral toxicity study in the rat*, Bergkamen, Federal Republic of Germany, Schering Inc. (Report No. 283118 by Hazelton, France. Study No. 14/503).

SCHERING (1989c) *TBTO - Resistance to Listeria monocytogene infection following a 34 day oral toxicity study in the rat*, Bergkamen, Federal Republic of Germany, Schering Inc. (Report No. 282118 by Hazelton, France. Study No. 14/505).

SCHERING (1989d) *TBTO - Delayed type hypersensitivity test following a 37 day oral toxicity study in the rat*, Bergkamen, Federal Republic of Germany, Schering Inc. (Report No. 281118 by Hazelton, France).

SCHERING (1989e) *TBTO - Systemic toxicity study in beagle dogs with daily oral (intragastric) administration over a total of 18-19 weeks*, Bergkamen, Federal Republic of Germany, Schering Inc. (Report No. IC6/88).

SCHWEINFURTH, H. (1985) Toxicology of tributyltin compounds. Tin Uses, 143: 9-12.

SEIFFER, E.A. & SCHOOF, H.F. (1967) Tests of 15 experimental molluscicides against *Australorbis glabratus*. Public Health Rep., 82: 833-839.

SEINEN, W., HELDER, T., VERNIJ, H., PENNINKS, A., & LEEUWANGH, P. (1981) Short term toxicity of tri-n-butyltinchloride in rainbow trout *(Salmo gairdneri* Richardson) yolk sac fry. *Sci. total Environ.,* **19**: 155-166.

SELIGMAN, P.F., VALKIRS, A.O., & LEE, R.F. (1986a) Degradation of tributyltin in marine and estuarine waters. In: *Proceedings of the Organotin Symposium, Oceans '86 Conference, Washington, DC, USA, 23-25 September, 1986,* New York, The Institute of Electrical and Electronics Engineers, Inc., Vol. 4, pp. 1189-1195.

SELIGMAN, P.F., GROVHOUG, J.G. & RICHTER, K.E. (1986b) Measurement of butyltins in San Diego Bay, CA: A monitoring strategy. In: *Proceedings of the Organotin Symposium, Oceans '86 Conference, Washington, DC, USA, 23-25 September, 1986,* New York, The Institute of Electrical and Electronics Engineers, Inc., Vol. 4, pp. 1289-1296.

SELIGMAN, P.F., GROVHOUG, J.G., VALKIRS, A.O., STANG, P.M., FRANSHAM, R., STALLARD, M.O., DAVIDSON, B., & LEE, R.F. (1989) Distribution and fate of tributyltin in the United States marine environment. *Appl. organomet. Chem.,* (in press).

SHELDON, A.W. (1975) Effects of organotin anti-fouling coatings on man and his environment. *J. Paint Technol.,* **47**: 54-58.

SHERMAN, L.R. & CARLSON, T.L. (1980) A modified phenylfluorone method for determining organotin compounds in the ppb and sub-ppb range. *J. anal. Toxicol.,* **4**: 31-33.

SHIFF, C.J., YIANNAKIS, C., & EVANS, A.C. (1975) Further trials with TBTO and other slow release molluscicides in Rhodesia. In: *Proceedings of the Controlled Release Pesticide Symposium, Wright State University, Dayton, Ohio, 8-10 September, 1975,* pp. 177-188.

SHIMIZU, A. & KIMURA, S. (1987) [Effect of bis (tributyltin) oxide on gonadal development of a salt-water goby, *Chasmichthys dolichognathus:* Exposure during maturing period.] *Bull. Tokai Reg. Fish. Res. Lab.,* **123**: 45-49 (in Japanese).

SHORT, J.W. & THROWER, F.P. (1986) Accumulation of butyltins in muscle tissue of chinook salmon reared in sea pens treated with tri-n-butyltin. In: *Proceedings of the Organotin Symposium, Oceans '86 Conference, Washington, DC, USA, 23-25 September, 1986,* New York, The Institute of Electrical and Electronics Engineers, Inc., Vol. 4, pp. 1177-1181.

SHORT, J.W. & THROWER, F.P. (1987) Toxicity of tri-n-butyl-tin to chinook salmon, *Oncorhynchus tshawytscha,* adapted to seawater. *Aquaculture,* **61**: 193-200.

SLESINGER, A.E. & DRESSER, I. (1978) The environmental chemistry of three organotin chemicals. In: Good, M., ed. *Report of the Organotin Workshop, New Orleans, Louisiana, 17-19 February, 1978,* pp. 115-162.

SMITH, B.S. (1981a) Male characteristics on female mud snails caused by antifouling paints. *J. appl. Toxicol.,* **1**: 22-25.

SMITH, B.S. (1981b) Tributyltin compounds induce male characteristics on female mud snails *Nassarius obsoletus* = *Ilyanassa obsoleta*. *J. appl. Toxicol.*, 1: 141-144.

SMITH, B.S. (1981c) Male characteristics in female Nassarius obsoletus: Variations related to locality, season and year. *Veliger*, 23: 212-216.

SMITH, D.R., STEPHENSON, M.D., GOETZL, J., ICHIKAWA, G., & MARTIN, M. (1987) The use of transplanted juvenile oysters to monitor the toxic effects of tributyltin in California waters. In: *Proceedings of the Organotin Symposium, Oceans '87 Conference, Halifax, Nova Scotia, Canada, 28 September-1 October, 1987*, New York, The Institute of Electrical and Electronics Engineers, Inc., Vol. 4, pp. 1511-1516.

SMITH, P.J., CROWE, A.J., ALLEN, D.W., BROOKS, J.S., & FORMSTONE, R. (1977) Study by 119m Sn Mossbauer spectroscopy of bis(tri-n-butyltin) oxide adsorbed on cellulosic materials. *Chem. Ind.*, 23: 874-875.

SNOEIJ, N.J. (1987) *Triorganotin compounds in immunotoxicology and biochemistry*, Utrecht, The Netherlands, University of Utrecht, 170 pp (Ph.D. Thesis).

SNOEIJ, N.J., VAN IERSEL, A.A.J., PENNINKS, A.H., & SEINEN, W. (1985) Toxicity of triorganotin compounds: Comparative *in vivo* studies with a series of trialkyltin compounds and triphenyltin chloride in male rats. *Toxicol. appl. Pharmacol.*, 81: 274-286.

SNOEIJ, N.J., PUNT, P.M., PENNINKS, A.H., & SEINEN, W. (1986a) Effects of tri-n-butyltin chloride on energy metabolism, macromolecular synthesis, precursor uptake and cyclic AMP production in isolated rat thymocytes. *Biochim. Biophys. Acta*, 852: 234-243.

SNOEIJ, N.J., VAN IERSEL, A.A.J., PENNINKS, A.H., & SEINEN, W. (1986b) Triorganotin-induced cytotoxicity to rat thymus, bone marrow and red blood cells as determined by several *in vitro* assays. *Toxicology*, 39: 71-83.

SNOEIJ, N.J., PIETERS, R.H.H., PENNINKS, A.H., & SEINEN, W. (1987) Toxicity of triorganotin compounds: Orally administered tri-n-butyltin compounds are rapidly dealkylated in the rat. In: *Triorganotincompounds in immunology and biochemistry*, Utrecht, The Netherlands, University of Utrecht, Chapter 4, pp. 73-93 (Snoeij, N.J., Ph.D. Thesis).

SNOEIJ, N.J., BOL-SCHOENMAKERS, M., PENNINKS, A.H., & SEINEN, W. (1988a) Differential effects of tri-n-butyltin chloride on macromolecular synthesis and ATP levels of rat thymocyte subpopulations obtained by centrifugal elutriation. *Int. J. Immunopharmacol.*, 10: 29-37.

SNOEIJ, N.J., PENNINKS, A.H., & SEINEN, W. (1988b) Dibutyltin and tributyltin compounds induce thymus atrophy in rats due to a selective action on thymic lymphoblasts. *Int. J. Immunopharmacol.*, 10: 891-899.

SORACCO, R.J. & POPE, D.H. (1983) Bacteriostatic and bactericidal modes of action of bis (tributlytin) oxide on *Legionella pneumophila*. *Appl. environ. Microbiol.*, 45: 48-57.

References

STALLARD, M., HODGE, V., & GOLDBERG, E.D. (1987) TBT in California coastal waters: Monitoring and assessment. *Environ. Monit. Assess.*, **9**: 195-220.

STANG, P.M. & SELIGMAN, P.F. (1986) Distribution and fate of butyltin compounds in the sediment of San Diego Bay. In: *Proceedings of the Organotin Symposium, Oceans '86 Conference, Washington, DC, USA, 23-25 September, 1986*, New York, The Institute of Electrical and Electronics Engineers, Inc., Vol. 4, pp. 1256-1261.

STANG, P.M. & SELIGMAN, P.F. (1987) In situ adsorption and desorption of butyltin compounds from Pearl Harbor, Hawaii, sediment. In: *Proceedings of the Organotin Symposium, Oceans '87 Conference, Halifax, Nova Scotia, Canada, 28 September-1 October, 1987*, New York, The Institute of Electrical and Electronics Engineers, Inc., Vol. 4, pp. 1386-1391.

STEIN, T. & KUSTER, K. (1982) Der biologische abbau von tributylzinnoxid (TBTO) in einer belebtschlammanlage. *Z. Wasser Abwasser Forsch.*, **15**: 178-180.

STEPHENSON, M.D., SMITH, D.R., GOETZL, J., ICHIKAWA, G., & MARTIN, M. (1986) Growth abnormalities in mussels and oysters from areas with high levels of tributyltin in San Diego Bay. In: *Proceedings of the Organotin Symposium, Oceans '86 Conference, Washington, DC, USA, 23-25 September, 1986*, New York, The Institute of Electrical and Electronics Engineers, Inc., Vol. 4, pp. 1246-1251.

STEPHENSON, M.D., SMITH, D.R., HALL, L.W., JOHNSON, W.E., MICHEL, P., SHORT, J., WALDOCK, M., HUGGETT, R.J., SELIGMAN, P., & KOLA, S. (1987) An international intercomparison of butyltin determinations in mussel tissue and sediments. In: *Proceedings of the Organotin Symposium, Oceans '87 Conference, Halifax, Nova Scotia, Canada, 28 September-1 October, 1987*, New York, The Institute of Electrical and Electronics Engineers, Inc., Vol. 4, pp. 1334-1338.

STROMGREN, T. & BONGARD, T. (1987) The effect of tributyltin oxide on growth of *Mytilus edulis*. *Mar. Pollut. Bull.*, **18**: 30-31.

TEMMINK, J.H.M. & EVERTS, J.W. (1987) Comparative toxicity of tributyltin-oxide (TBTO) for fish and snail. In: *Proceedings of the Seventh World Meeting of the ORTEP-Association, Amsterdam, 7-8 May, 1987*, Vlissingen-Oost, The Netherlands, ORTEP-Association, pp. 6-20.

THAIN, J.E. (1983) *The acute toxicity of bis (tributyl tin) oxide to the adults and larvae of some marine organisms*, Copenhagen, International Council for the Exploration of the Sea (ICES), 5 pp (Report No. C. M. 1983/E.13).

THAIN, J.E. (1986) Toxicity of TBT to bivalves: Effects on reproduction, growth and survival. In: *Proceedings of the Organotin Symposium, Oceans '86 Conference, Washington, DC, USA, 23-25 September, 1986*, New York, The Institute of Electrical and Electronics Engineers, Inc., Vol. 4, pp. 1306-1313.

THAIN, J.E. & WALDOCK, M.J. (1985) *The growth of bivalve spat exposed to organotin leachates from antifouling paints*, Copenhagen, International Council for the Exploration of the Sea (ICES), 10 pp (Report No. C. M. 1985/E.28).

THAIN, J.E. & WALDOCK, M.J. (1986) The impact of tributyl tin (TBT) antifouling paints on molluscan fisheries. *Water Sci. Technol.*, **18**: 193-202.

THAIN, J.E., WALDOCK, M.J., & WAITE, M.E. (1987) Toxicity and degradation studies of tributyltin (TBT) and dibutyltin (DBT) in the aquatic environment. In: *Proceedings of the Organotin Symposium, Oceans '87 Conference, Halifax, Nova Scotia, Canada, 28 September-1 October, 1987*, New York, The Institute of Electrical and Electronics Engineers, Inc., Vol. 4, pp. 1398-1404.

THOMAS, T.E. & ROBINSON, M.G. (1986) The physiological effects of the leachates from a self-polishing organotin antifouling paint on marine diatoms. *Mar. environ. Res.*, **18**: 215-229.

THOMAS, T.E. & ROBINSON, M.G. (1987) Initial characterization of the mechanisms responsible for the tolerance of Amphora coffeaeformis to copper and tributyltin. *Bot. mar.*, **30**: 47-53.

THOMPSON, J.A.J., SHEFFER, M.G., PIERCE, R.C., CHAU, Y.K., COONEY, J.J., CULLEN, W.R., & MAGUIRE, R.J. (1985) *Organotin compounds in the aquatic environment: Scientific criteria for assessing their effects on environmental quality*, Ottawa, National Research Council Canada, 284 pp (NRCC No. 22494).

TOLEDO, J.V., MONTEIRO DA SILVA, C.S., BULHOES, M.S., PAES LEME, L.A., DA SILVA NETTO, J.A., & GILBERT, B. (1976) Snail control in urban sites in Brazil with slow-release hexabutyldistannoxane and pentachlorophenol. *World Health Organ. Bull.*, **54**: 421-425.

TRUHAUT, R., CHAUVEL, Y., ANGER, J.-P., PHU LICH N., VAN DEN DRIESSCHE, J., GUESNIER, L.R., & MORIN, N. (1976) Contribution à l'étude toxicologique et pharmacologique de l'oxyde de tributylétain (OTBE). *Eur. J. Toxicol.*, **9**: 31-40.

TRUHAUT, R., ANGER, J.P., REYMANN, J.M., CHAUVEL, Y., & VAN DEN DRIESSCHE, J. (1979) Influence de l'oxyde de tributylétain (OTBE) en aérosol sur le comportement exploratoire chez la souris. *Toxicol. Eur. Res.*, **11**: 181-186.

TRUHAUT, R., ANGER, J.P., ANGER, F., BRAULT, A., BRUNET, P., CANO, Y., LOUVET, M., SACCAVINI, J.C., VAN DEN DRIESSCHE, J., JANSON, C., & SUBLET, Y. (1981) Dégradation thermique de l'oxyde de tributylétain (OTBE) et toxicité pulmonaire des produits de combustion chez la souris et le cobaye. *Toxicol. Eur. Res.*, **111**: 35-44.

TSUDA, T., NAKANISHI, H., AOKI, S., & TAKEBAYASHI, J. (1986) Bioconcentration of butyltin compounds by round crucian carp. *Toxicol. environ. Chem.*, **12**: 137-143.

TSUDA, T., NAKANISHI, H., AOKI, S., & TAKEBAYASHI, J. (1987) Bioconcentration and metabolism of phenyl tin chlorides in carp. *Water Res.*, **21**: 949-953.

TSUDA, T., NAKANISHI, H., AOKI, S., & TAKEBAYASHI, J. (1988) Bioconcentration and metabolism of butyltin compounds in carp. *Water Res.*, **22**: 647-651.

References

TWG (1988a) *Uses and production of organotin compounds*. Presented by the Federal Republic of Germany at the Convention for the Prevention of Marine Pollution from Land-based Sources (15th Meeting of the Technical Working Group), Brussels, 7-11 March, 1988, 6 pp (Report No. TWG 15/5/1-E).

TWG (1988b) *Tributyl tin compounds in antifouling paints*. Presented by the Federal Republic of Germany at the Convention for the Prevention of Marine Pollution from Land-based Sources (15th Meeting of the Technical Working Group, Brussels, 7-11 March, 1988, 2 pp, (Report No. TWG 15/5/2-E).

TWG (1988c) *Organotins in the Netherlands*. Presented by the Netherlands at the Convention for the Prevention of Marine Pollution from Land-based Sources (15th Meeting of the Technical Working Group, Brussels, 7-11 March, 1988, 11 pp (Report No. TWG 15/5/4-E).

UHL, S. (1986) *[Population exposure to the environmental chemical pentachlorophenol (PCP) and bis (tri-n-butyltin)oxide (TBTO)]*, Zurich, Maus Offsetdruck Konstanz, 145 pp (ETH Thesis No. 8014, University of Gottingen) (in German).

UNEP (1989) *Mediterranean Action Plan. Assessment of organotin compounds as marine pollutants in the Mediterranean*, Athens, United Nations Environment Programme (MAP Technical Report Series, No. 33).

UNITED KINGDOM DEPARTMENT OF THE ENVIRONMENT (1986) *Organotin in antifouling paints environmental considerations*, London, UK Department of the Environment, 82 pp (Pollution Paper No. 25).

UNITED KINGDOM DEPARTMENT OF THE ENVIRONMENT (1989) *Water and the environment*, London, UK Department of the Environment, p. 26 (Circular No. 7/89).

UPATHAM, E.S., KOURA, M., AHMED, M.D., & AWAD, A.H. (1980) Laboratory trials of controlled release molluscicides on *Bulinus (Ph.) abyssinicus*, the intermediate host of *Schistosoma haematobium* in Somalia. In: Baker, R.W., ed. *Controlled release of bioactive materials. Proceedings of the 6th International Meeting of the controlled Release Society*, New York, London, Academic Press, pp. 461-469.

U'REN, S.C. (1983) Acute toxicity of bis(tributyltin) oxide to a marine copepod. *Mar. Pollut. Bull.*, 14: 303-306.

VALKIRS, A.O., SELIGMAN, P.F., STANG, P.M., HOMER, V., LIEBERMAN, S.H., VAFA, G., & DOOLEY, C.A. (1986) Measurement of butyltin compounds in San Diego Bay. *Mar. Pollut. Bull.*, 17: 319-324.

VALKIRS, A.O., DAVIDSON, B.M., & SELIGMAN, P.F. (1987) Sublethal growth effects and mortality to marine bivalves from long-term exposure to tributyltin. *Chemosphere*, 16: 201-220.

VIGHI, M. & CALAMARI, D. (1985) QSARs for organotin compounds on *Daphnia magna*. *Chemosphere*, 14: 1925-1932.

VIYANANT, V., THIRACHANTRA, S., & SORNMANI, S. (1982) The effect of controlled release copper sulphate and tributyltin fluoride on the mortality and infectivity of *Schistosoma mansoni* cercariae. *J. Helminthol.*, 56: 85-92.

VOS, J.G., DE KLERC, A., KRAJNC, E.I., KRUIZINGA, W., VAN OMMEN, B., & ROZING, J. (1984) Toxicity of bis(tri-*n*-butyltin)oxide in the rat. II. Suppression of thymus-dependent immune responses and of parameters of non-specific resistance after short-term exposure. *Toxicol. appl. Pharmacol.*, 75: 387-408.

VOS, J.G., KRAJNC, E.I., & WESTER, P.W. (1985) Immunotoxicity of bis (tri-*n*-butyltin) oxide. In: Dean, J., ed. *Immunotoxicology and immunopharmacology*, New York, Raven Press, pp. 327-340.

WADE, T.L., GARCIA-ROMERO, B., & BROOKS, J.M. (1988) Tributyltin contamination in bivalves from U.S. coastal estuaries. *Environ. Sci. Technol.*, 22: 1488-1493.

WALDOCK, M.J. (1989) Organotin concentrations in the Rivers Bure and Yare, Norfolk Broads, England *(Unpublished report of the Ministry of Agriculture, Fisheries and Food, Fisheries Laboratory, Burnham-on-Crouch, Essex, UK)*.

WALDOCK, M.J. & MILLER, D. (1983) *The determination of total and tributyl tin in seawater and oysters in areas of high pleasure craft activity*, Copenhagen, International Council for the Exploration of the Sea (ICES), 18 pp (Report No. C. M. 1983/E.12).

WALDOCK, M.J. & THAIN, J.E. (1983) Shell thickening in *Crassostrea gigas:* Organotin antifouling or sediment induced? *Mar. Pollut. Bull.*, 14: 411-415.

WALDOCK, M.J. & THAIN, J.E. (1985) *The comparative leach rates and toxicity of two fish net antifouling preparations*, Copenhagen, International Council for the Exploration of the Sea (ICES), 5 pp (Report No. C. M. 1985/E.29).

WALDOCK, M.J., THAIN, J.E. & MILLER, D. (1983) *The accumulation and depuration of bis (tributyl tin) oxide in oysters: A comparison between the Pacific oyster* (Crassostrea gigas) *and the European flat oyster* (Ostrea edulis), Copenhagen, International Council for the Exploration of the Sea (ICES), 6 pp (Report No. C. M. 1983/E.52).

WALDOCK, M.J., WAITE, M.E., & THAIN, J.E. (1987a) Changes in concentrations of organotins in U.K. rivers and estuaries following legislation in 1986. In: *Proceedings of the Organotin Symposium, Oceans '87 Conference, Halifax, Nova Scotia, Canada, 28 September-1 October, 1987*, New York, The Institute of Electrical and Electronics Engineers, Inc., Vol. 4, pp. 1352-1356.

WALDOCK, M.J., THAIN, J.E., & WAITE, M.E. (1987b) The distribution and potential toxic effects of TBT in UK estuaries during 1986. *Appl. organomet. Chem.*, 1: 287-301.

References

WALDOCK, M.J., WAITE, M.E., & THAIN, J.E. (1988) Inputs of TBT to the marine environment from shipping activity in the U.K. *Environ. Technol. Lett.,* 9: 999-1010.

WALNE, P.R. & HELM, M.M. (1979) Introduction of *Crassostrea gigas* into the United Kingdom. In: Mann, R., ed. *Proceedings of a Symposium on Exotic Species in Mariculture: Case histories of the Japanese Oyster* Crassostrea gigas *(Thunberg), with implications for other fisheries, Woods Hole, Massachusetts, USA, 18-20 September, 1978,* Cambridge, London, MIT Press, pp. 83-105.

WALSH, G.E. (1986) Organotin toxicity studies conducted with selected marine organisms at EPA's environmental research laboratory, Gulf Breeze, Florida. In: *Proceedings of the Organotin Symposium, Oceans '86 Conference, Washington, DC, USA, 23-25 September, 1986,* New York, The Institute of Electrical and Electronics Engineers, Inc., Vol. 4, pp. 1210-1212.

WALSH, G.E., MCLAUGHLAN, L.L., LORES, E.M., LOUIE, M.K., & DEANS, C.H. (1985) Effects of organotins on growth and survival of two marine diatoms, *Skeletonema costatum* and *Thalassiosira pseudonana. Chemosphere,* 14: 383-392.

WALSH, G.E., LOUIE, M.K., MCLAUGHLIN, L.L., & LORES, E.M. (1986a) Lugworm *(Arenicola cristata)* larvae in toxicity tests: Survival and development when exposed to organotins. *Environ. Toxicol. Chem.,* 5: 749-754.

WALSH, G.E., MCLAUGHLIN, L.L., LOUIE, M.K., DEANS, C.H., & LORES, E.M. (1986b) Inhibition of arm regeneration by *Ophioderma brevispina* (Echinodermata, Ophiuroidea) by tributyltin oxide and triphenyltin oxide. *Ecotoxicol. environ. Saf.,* 12: 95-100.

WALTON, R., ADEMA, C.M., & SELIGMAN, P.F. (1986) Mathematical modeling of the transport and fate of organotin in harbors. In: *Proceedings of the Organotin Symposium, Oceans '86 Conference, Washington, DC, USA, 23-25 September, 1986,* New York, The Institute of Electrical and Electronics Engineers, Inc., Vol. 4, pp. 1297-1301.

WARD, G.S., CRAMM, G.C., PARRISH, P.R., TRACHMAN, H., & SLESINGER, A. (1981) Bioaccumulation and chronic toxicity of bis(tributyltin) oxide (TBTO): Tests with a saltwater fish. In: Branson, D.R. & Dickson, K.L., ed. *Proceedings of the Fourth Conference on Aquatic Toxicology and Hazard Assessment,* Philadelphia, American Society for Testing and Materials, pp. 183-200 (ASTM STP No. 737).

WEBBE, G. (1963) Laboratory tests of some new molluscicides (organotin compounds), Geneva, World Health Organization, Parasitic Diseases Programme, pp. 1-2 (Unpublished report Mol/Inf/14).

WEBER, J.H., DONARD, O.F.X., RANDALL, I., & HAN, J.S. (1986) Speciation of methyl and butyltin compounds in the Great Bay estuary (N.H.). In: *Proceedings of the Organotin Symposium, Oceans '86 Conference, Washington, DC, USA, 23-25 September, 1986,* New York, The Institute of Electrical and Electronics Engineers, Inc., Vol. 4, pp. 1280-1282.

WEIS, J.S., WEIS, P., & WANG, F. (1987a) Developmental effects of tributyltin on the fiddler crab, *Uca pugilator*, and the killifish, *Fundulus heteroclitus*. In: *Proceedings of the Organotin Symposium, Oceans '87 Conference, Halifax, Nova Scotia, Canada, 28 September-1 October, 1987*, New York, The Institute of Electrical and Electronics Engineers, Inc., Vol. 4, pp. 1456-1460.

WEIS, J.S., GOTTLIEB, J., & KWIATKOWSKI, J. (1987b) Tributyltin retards regeneration and produces deformities of limbs in the fiddler crab, *Uca pugilator*. *Arch. environ. Contam. Toxicol.*, 16: 321-326.

WESTER, P.W., CANTON, J.H., VAN IERSAL, A.A.J., KRANJC, E.I., & VAESSEN, H.A.M.G. (1988) *The toxicity of bis(tri-n-butyltin)oxide (TBTO) and di-n-butyltindichloride (DBTC) in the small fish species Orysias latipes (medaka) and Poecilia reticulata (guppy)*, Utrecht, The Netherlands, University of Utrecht (Wester, P.W., Ph.D. Thesis).

WESTER, P.W. (in press) Chronic toxicity and carcinogenicity of bis (tri-n-butyltin) oxide in the rat. *Food Chem. Toxicol.*

WHO/FAO (1984) *Data sheet on pesticides No. 65: Bis (tributyltin)oxide*, Geneva, World Health Organization (VBC/PDS/DS/85.65).

WOLNIAKOWSKI, K.U., STEPHENSON, M.D., & ICHIKAWA, G.S. (1987) Tributyltin concentrations and Pacific oyster deformations in Coos Bay, Oregon. In: *Proceedings of the Organotin Symposium, Oceans '87 Conference, Halifax, Nova Scotia, Canada, 28 September-1 October, 1987*, New York, The Institute of Electrical and Electronics Engineers, Inc., Vol. 4, pp. 1438-1442.

WONG, P.T.S., CHAU, Y.K., KRAMAR, O., & BENGERT, G.A. (1982) Structure-toxicity relationship of tin compounds on algae. *Can. J. Fish. aquat. Sci.*, 39: 483-488.

WOOTEN, R., DAVIES, I.M., MCKIE, J.C., & BRUNO, D.W. (1986) *Chemical and histopathological changes in salmon exposed to low concentrations of tributyltin in seawater*, Aberdeen, Department of Agriculture and Fisheries for Scotland, 3 pp (Working Paper No. 15/86).

YLA-MONONEN, L. (1988) *Finnish studies on the use, occurrence and effects of organic tin compounds*. Presented at the OECD Workshop on Monitoring, Chemical Analysis and Leaching Rates of TBT, Paris, 30 November-2 December, 1988, 9 pp (Unpublished report).

YOUNG, D.R., SCHATZBERG, P., BRINCKMAN, F.E., CHAMP, M.A., HOLM, S.E., & LANDY, R.B. (1986) Summary report - Interagency workshop on aquatic sampling and analysis for organotin compounds. In: *Proceedings of the Organotin Symposium, Oceans '86 Conference, Washington, DC, USA, 23-25 September, 1986*, New York, The Institute of Electrical and Electronics Engineers, Inc., Vol. 4, pp. 1135-1140.

ZEDLER, R.J. (1961) Organotin as industrial biochemicals. *Tin Uses*, 53: 7-11.

References

ZIMMERLI, B. & ZIMMERMANN, H. (1980) Gas-chromatische bestimmung von spuren von n-butylzinnverbindungen (tetra-, tri-, di-). *Fresenius Z. anal. Chem.*, **304**: 23-27.

ZUCKERMAN, J.J., REISDORF, R.P., ELLIS, H.V., & WILKINSON, R.R. (1978) Organotins in biology and the environment. In: Brinkman, F.E. & Bellama, J.M., ed. *Organometals and organometalloids, occurrence and fate in the environment*, Washington, DC, American Chemical Society, pp. 388-424 (ACS Symposium Series No. 82).

RESUME

1. Identité, propriétés physiques et chimiques

Les dérivés du tributylétain (TBT) sont des dérivés organiques de l'étain tétravalent. Ils se caractérisent par la présence de liaisons covalentes entre des atomes de carbone et un atome d'étain et leur formule générale est la suivante: $(n-C_4H_9)_3$ Sn-X (dans laquelle X désigne un anion). La pureté de l'oxyde de tributylétain du commerce est généralement supérieure à 96%; les principales impuretés sont le dibutylétain et dans une moindre mesure le tétrabutylétain et d'autres trialkylétains. L'oxyde de tributylétain est un liquide incolore d'odeur caractéristique et de densité comprise entre 1,17 et 1,18. Il est peu soluble dans l'eau (solubilité comprise entre moins de 1,0 et plus de 100 mg/litre selon le pH, la température et les anions présents dans l'eau qui déterminent l'espèce chimique en cause). Dans l'eau de mer et dans les conditions normales, on rencontre trois dérivés du tributylétain: l'hydroxyde, le chlorure et le carbonate, qui sont en équilibre. Aux pH inférieurs à 7,0 les formes prédominantes sont $Bu_3SnOH_2^+$ et Bu_3SnCl; à pH 8 ce sont Bu_3SnCl, Bu_3SnOH et $Bu_3SnCO_3^-$; au-delà de 10, ce sont Bu_3SnOH et $Bu_3SnCO_3^-$ qui prédominent.

Le coefficient de partage octanol/eau (log de P_{ow}) est compris entre 3,18 et 3,84 pour l'eau distillée et il est égal à 3,54 pour l'eau de mer. L'oxyde de tributylétain s'adsorbe fortement aux matières particulaires, puisque les coefficients d'absorption indiqués dans la littérature vont de 110 à 55 000. La tension de vapeur est faible mais les valeurs publiées sont extrêmement variables. On n'a constaté aucune perte d'oxyde de tributylétain à partir d'une solution de 1 mg/litre en 62 jours, toutefois 20% de l'eau avait disparu par évaporation.

2. Méthodes d'analyse

On utilise plusieurs méthodes pour le dosage des dérivés du tributylétain dans l'eau, les sédiments ou les biotes. La plus communément utilisée est la spectrométrie d'absorption atomique. La spectrométrie d'absorption atomique avec flamme a une limite de détection de 0,1 mg/litre. Sans flamme, avec atomisation dans un four électrique à graphite, elle est plus sensible et ses limites de détection varient entre 0 et 1,0 µg/litre d'eau. Il existe plusieurs méthodes d'extraction et de préparation de dérivés volatils. La séparation de ces dérivés s'effectue habituellement par piégeage ou par chromatographie en phase gazeuse. Les limites de détection se situent entre 0,5 et 5,0 µg/kg dans le cas des sédiments et des biotes.

3. Sources de pollution de l'environnement

Les dérivés du tributylétain sont homologués comme molluscicides, comme produits antisalissures pour la préservation des coques de bateaux, des appontements, des bouées, des casiers à crabes, des filets et des cages, comme enduits de protection du bois, comme alguicides dans le bâtiment, comme désinfectants et comme biocides dans les systèmes de réfrigération, les tours de réfrigération des centrales électriques, les usines de pâte à papier, les brasseries, les tanneries et les usines textiles. Les premières peintures antisalissures à base de TBT contenaient ce produit sous une forme qui en permettait la libération sans entrave. Plus récemment, sont apparues des peintures dans lesquelles l'incorporation du TBT dans une matrice en copolymère permet d'en limiter la libération. On a également mis au point des matrices caoutchouteuses qui permettent une libération lente et durable et assurent aux peintures antisalissures et aux molluscicides une efficacité prolongée. Le TBT n'est pas utilisé en agriculture en raison de sa forte phytotoxicité.

4. Réglementation

De nombreux pays ont restreint l'utilisation des peintures antisalissures à base de TBT du fait de l'action de cette substance sur les fruits de mer. Les détails de la réglementation varient d'un pays à l'autre mais la plupart interdisent l'emploi de peintures à base de TBT sur les navires de moins de 25 mètres. Dans certains pays, les navires à coque d'aluminium ne sont pas visés par cette interdiction. En outre, certaines réglementations limitent la teneur des peintures en TBT ou la lixiviation de cette substance à partir des peintures qui en contiennent (4 à 5 $\mu g/cm^2$ par jour sur une longue période).

5. Concentrations dans l'environnement

On a trouvé de fortes concentrations de TBT dans l'eau, les sédiments et les biotes à proximité de zones de plaisance, plus particulièrement de marinas, de chantiers navals et de bassins de radoub, de filets et de cages traités au moyen de peintures antisalissures et de systèmes de réfrigération. Ces concentrations de TBT dépendent également de la submersion par la marée et de la turbidité de l'eau.

On a observé que les concentrations de TBT pouvaient atteindre 1,58 μg/litre dans l'eau de mer et les estuaires, 7,1 μg/litre dans l'eau douce, 26 300 $\mu g/kg$ dans les sédiments littoraux, 3700 $\mu g/kg$ dans les sédiments d'eau douce, 6,39 mg/kg dans les bivalves, 1,92 mg/kg dans les gastéropodes et 11 mg/kg dans le poisson. Il ne faut pas considérer cependant ces concentrations maximales comme caractéristiques car un certain nombre de facteurs peuvent donner lieu à des teneurs anormalement élevées (par exemple la présence de particules de peinture dans les échantillons d'eau et de sédiments). On a constaté que les concentrations de TBT dans la micro-couche de surface des eaux douces et des eaux de mer étaient jusqu'à 100 fois plus élevées que celles qu'on pouvait mesurer juste en dessous de la surface. Toutefois, il convient de noter que la concentration en TBT dans la micro-couche de surface peut dépendre dans une très large mesure de la technique d'échantillonnage.

Il se peut que les données anciennes ne soient pas comparables aux données récentes en raison des améliorations apportées aux méthodes de dosage du TBT dans l'eau, les sédiments et les tissus.

6. Transport et transformation dans l'environnement

Du fait de sa faible solubilité dans l'eau et de son caractère lipophile, le TBT s'adsorbe facilement aux particules. On estime que 10 à 95% de l'oxyde de tributylétain qui pénètrent dans l'eau s'adsorbent ainsi sur les

Résumé

particules. La disparition progressive du TBT absorbé n'est pas due à sa désorption mais à sa dégradation. Le degré d'adsorption dépend de la salinité, de la nature et de la taille des particules en suspension, de la quantité de matières en suspension, de la température et de la présence de matières organiques dissoutes.

La dégradation de l'oxyde de tributylétain s'effectue par rupture de la liaison carbone-étain. Celle-ci peut résulter de divers mécanismes qui se produisent simultanément dans l'environnement et notamment des mécanismes physico-chimiques (hydrolyse et photodécomposition) ou biologiques (dégradation par des micro-organismes et métabolisation par des organismes supérieurs). L'hydrolyse des dérivés organostanniques se produit à des valeurs extrêmes du pH mais n'apparaît guère dans les conditions qui règnent normalement dans l'environnement. La photodécomposition se produit par exposition en laboratoire de solutions à un rayonnement ultra-violet de 300 nm (et à un moindre degré, à un rayonnement de 350 nm). Dans le milieu naturel, la photolyse est limitée par la longueur d'onde du rayonnement solaire et par la pénétration du rayonnement ultra-violet dans l'eau. La présence de substances photosensibilisatrices peut accélérer la photodécomposition. La biodégradation dépend de l'état du milieu, et de caractéristiques telles que sa température, son oxygénation, son pH, sa teneur en éléments minéraux, la présence de substances organiques facilement biodégradables pouvant subir une co-métabolisation ainsi que la nature de la micro-flore et sa capacité à s'adapter. Elle ne peut également avoir lieu que si la concentration en oxyde de tributylétain est inférieure à la concentration létale ou inhibitrice pour les bactéries. Comme dans le cas de la décomposition abiotique, la dégradation biologique du TBT comporte une débutylation oxydante progressive avec rupture de la liaison carbone-étain. Il se forme des dérivés dibutylés dont la dégradation est plus facile que celle du tributylétain. Les monobutylétains sont lentement minéralisés. Il se produit également une dégradation anaérobie mais son importance reste discutée. Certains chercheurs estiment que la dégradation en anaérobiose est lente alors que d'autres la jugent plus rapide que la dégradation aérobie. On a identifié des espèces de bactéries, d'algues et de champignons attaquant le bois qui sont capables de dégrader l'oxyde de tributylétain. Les estimations de la demi-vie du TBT dans l'environnement varient dans d'importantes proportions.

Le TBT s'accumule dans les organismes du fait de sa solubilité dans les graisses. Des recherches en laboratoire portant sur des mollusques et des poissons ont donné, pour les facteurs de bioconcentration, des valeurs allant jusqu'à 7000 mais des valeurs encore plus élevées ont été observées lors d'études sur le terrain. L'absorption à partir de la nourriture est plus importante qu'à partir de l'eau. Les facteurs de concentration plus élevés observés chez les micro-organismes (entre 100 et 30 000) peuvent s'expliquer par une adsorption plutôt que par une absorption intracellulaire. Rien n'indique que le TBT puisse passer dans les organismes terrestres par l'intermédiaire de la chaîne alimentaire.

7. Cinétique et métabolisme

Le tributylétain est absorbé au niveau intestinal (20 à 50% selon le véhicule) ainsi que par voie percutanée chez les mammifères (dans la proportion d'environ 10%). Il peut traverser la barrière hémo-méningée et passer du placenta dans le foetus. Une fois absorbé, il est rapidement et largement diffusé dans l'organisme (principalement au niveau du foie et des reins).

Chez les mammifères, la métabolisation du TBT est rapide; on peut déceler les métabolites dans le sang dans les 3 heures suivant l'administration. Des études *in vitro* ont montré que le TBT servait de substrat aux oxydases à fonction mixte mais qu'il inhibait ces enzymes à très forte concentration.

L'élimination du TBT s'effectue plus ou moins rapidement selon la nature du tissu et les estimations de la demi-vie biologique chez les mammifères varient de 23 à environ 30 jours.

Les organismes inférieurs métabolisent également le TBT mais le processus est plus lent - en particulier chez les mollusques - que chez les mammifères. La capacité de bioaccumulation est donc beaucoup plus importante que chez les mammifères.

Résumé

Les tributylétains inhibent la phosphorylation oxydative et modifient la structure et la fonction des mitochondries. Le TBT empêche la calcification de la coquille des huîtres (espèces du genre *Crassostrea*).

8. Effets sur les micro-organismes

Le TBT est toxique pour les micro-organismes et on le vend comme bactéricide et algicide. Les concentrations toxiques varient considérablement selon les espèces. Le TBT est plus toxique pour les bactéries gram-positives avec une concentration minimale inhibitrice (CMI) allant de 0,2 à 0,8 mg/litre que pour les bactéries gram-négatives (CMI des 3 mg/litre). La CMI de l'acétate de TBT pour les champignons est de 0,5 à 1 mg/litre et celle de l'oxyde de tributylétain est de 0,5 mg/litre pour l'algue verte *Chlorella pyrenoidosa*. La productivité primaire d'une communauté naturelle d'algues d'eau douce a été réduite de 5% par une concentration d'oxyde de tributylétain de 3 µg/litre. On a récemment établi la dose sans effet observable pour 2 espèces d'algues; elle est respectivement de 18 et 32 µg/litre. La toxicité pour les microorganismes marins varie également selon les espèces et selon les études; il est difficile d'établir la valeur de la dose sans effet observable mais on pense qu'elle est inférieure à 0,1 µg/litre pour certaines espèces. Les concentrations algicides vont de moins de 1,5 µg/litre à plus de 1000 µg/litre selon les espèces.

9. Effets sur les organismes aquatiques

9.1 Effets sur les organismes marins et estuariels

La Figure 1 donne un diagramme récapitulatif des effets létaux et sublétaux que peuvent produire les concentrations de TBT relevées en mer et dans les estuaires. Des concentrations supérieures à celles qui produisent les effets létaux aigus ont été observées en différents points du globe, notamment là où se déroulent des activités de plaisance.

Ce sont les spores mobiles d'une algue verte géante qui se sont révélés les plus sensibles au TBT (CE_{50} à 5 jours: 0,001 µg/litre). On a constaté une réduction de

EHC 116: *Tributyltin Compounds*

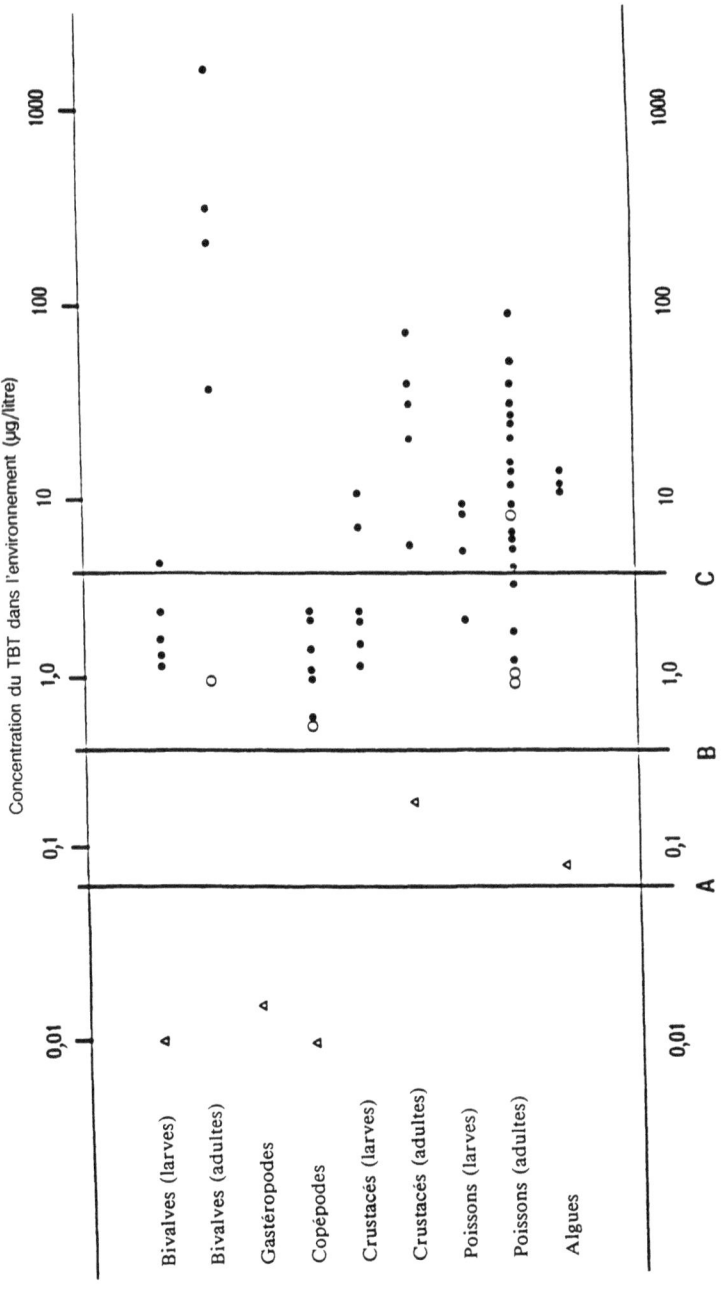

Fig. 1. Toxicité du tributylétain pour les organismes marins

● CL_{50} après exposition inférieure ou égale à 96 heures;   o CL_{50} après exposition de plus de 96 heures;   △ Concentration la plus faible produisant un effet sublétal;   A = Concentration la plus forte mesurée
* On a consacré une rubrique spéciale aux copépodes en raison de leur sensibilité plus forte que celle des autres crustacés;   A = Concentration la plus forte mesurée dans les marinas.
en haute mer;   B = Concentration la plus forte mesurée en plein estuaire;   C = Concentration la plus forte mesurée dans les marinas.

233

Résumé

la croissance d'un angiosperme marin à des concentrations de TBT de 1 mg/kg de sédiments, aucun effet n'étant noté à 0,1 mg/kg.

Le tributylétain est très toxique pour les mollusques marins. On a montré expérimentalement qu'il perturbait la formation de la coquille, le développement des gonades et la différenciation sexuelle des huîtres adultes, leur fixation et leur croissance; en outre on a noté une mortalité des larves d'huîtres et d'autres bivalves et l'apparition de caractères mâles chez les gastéropodes femelles. La dose sans effet observable serait de 20 ng/litre pour le naissain de l'espèce d'huître la plus sensible, l'huître japonaise *(Crassostrea gigas)*. Chez les adultes, il se produit également une déformation de la coquille qui est liée à la dose. Expérimentalement, on n'a pas observé d'effets sur la morphologie coquillière à des concentrations de TBT de 2 ng/litre. La dose sans effet observable correspondant à l'apparition de caractères mâles chez les mollusques femelles du genre *Thais* est inférieure à 1,5 ng/litre. Les formes larvaires sont généralement plus sensibles que les adultes; la différence est particulièrement marquée dans le cas des huîtres.

Les copépodes sont plus sensibles que les autres crustacés aux effets létaux aigus du TBT, avec des valeurs de la CL_{50} pour des périodes allant jusqu'à 96 heures comprises entre 0,6 et 2,2 µg/litre. Ces valeurs sont comparables à celles qui s'appliquent aux larves les plus sensibles des autres groupes de crustacés. Le TBT réduit la capacité de reproduction, la survie néonatale et la vitesse de croissance des crustacés. Dans le cas de la crevette *Acanthomysis sculpta,* un mysidé, la dose sans effet observable sur la reproduction serait de 0,09 µg/litre. La crevette ne cherche pas à éviter le TBT au-dessous de 30 µg/litre.

La toxicité du tributylétain pour les poissons de mer est très variable, les valeurs de la CL_{50} à 96 heures allant de 1,5 à 36 µg/litre. Les stades larvaires sont plus sensibles que les adultes (Figure 1). Il semblerait que les poissons de mer évitent l'oxyde de tributylétain à partir de 1 µg/litre.

9.2 Effets sur les organismes d'eau douce

Un diagramme récapitulatif concernant les effets létaux et sublétaux des concentrations de TBT mesurées dans l'eau douce est donné à la Figure 2. On a observé la présence de concentrations supérieures à celles qui produisent des effets sublétaux, notamment dans les zones de navigation de plaisance.

Une concentration d'oxyde de tributylétain de 0,5 mg/litre a été mortelle pour des angiospermes d'eau douce et leur croissance était inhibée dès 0,06 mg/litre.

On ne dispose que de peu de données sur les invertébrés d'eau douce, tout au plus sur trois espèces autres que les organismes cibles. Pour divers sels de tributylétain on a obtenu des valeurs de la CL_{50} à 48 heures de 2,3-70 µg/litre pour la daphnie et de 5,5-33 µg par litre pour les vers de vase. La dose sans effet observable pour la daphnie est évaluée à 0,5 µg/litre, le critère choisi étant la réapparition d'une réaction normale à la lumière. En ce qui concerne la palourde d'Asie, on indique une CL_{50} à 24 heures de 2100 µg/litre, les valeurs corrrespondantes allant de 30 à 400 µg/litre pour les mollusques adultes que l'on cherche à détruire dans les opérations de lutte contre la schistosomiase.

On a montré que le tributylétain était toxique pour les larves de schistosome à leur stade aquatique; la CL_{50} du fluorure de tributylétain est de 16,8 µg par litre pour une exposition d'une heure. Une dose de TBT comprise en 2 et 6 µg/litre supprime à hauteur de 99 à 100% l'infectiosité des cercaires pour la souris.

La sensibilité des mollusques au TBT diminue avec l'âge mais les oeufs sont plus résistants que les jeunes ou les adultes. La ponte est notablement affectée à une concentration en oxyde de tributylétainde 0,001 µg/litre.

La toxicité aiguë du TBT pour les poissons d'eau douce s'est située, pour des périodes allant jusqu'à 168 heures, dans les limites de 13 à 240 µg/litre, valeurs correspondant à la CL_{50}. Dans le cas du guppy, la dose sans effet histopathologique observable a été estimée à 0,01 µg/litre.

Après exposition de grenouilles *Rana temporaria* à des concentrations inférieures ou égales 3 µg/litre, on n'a

Résumé

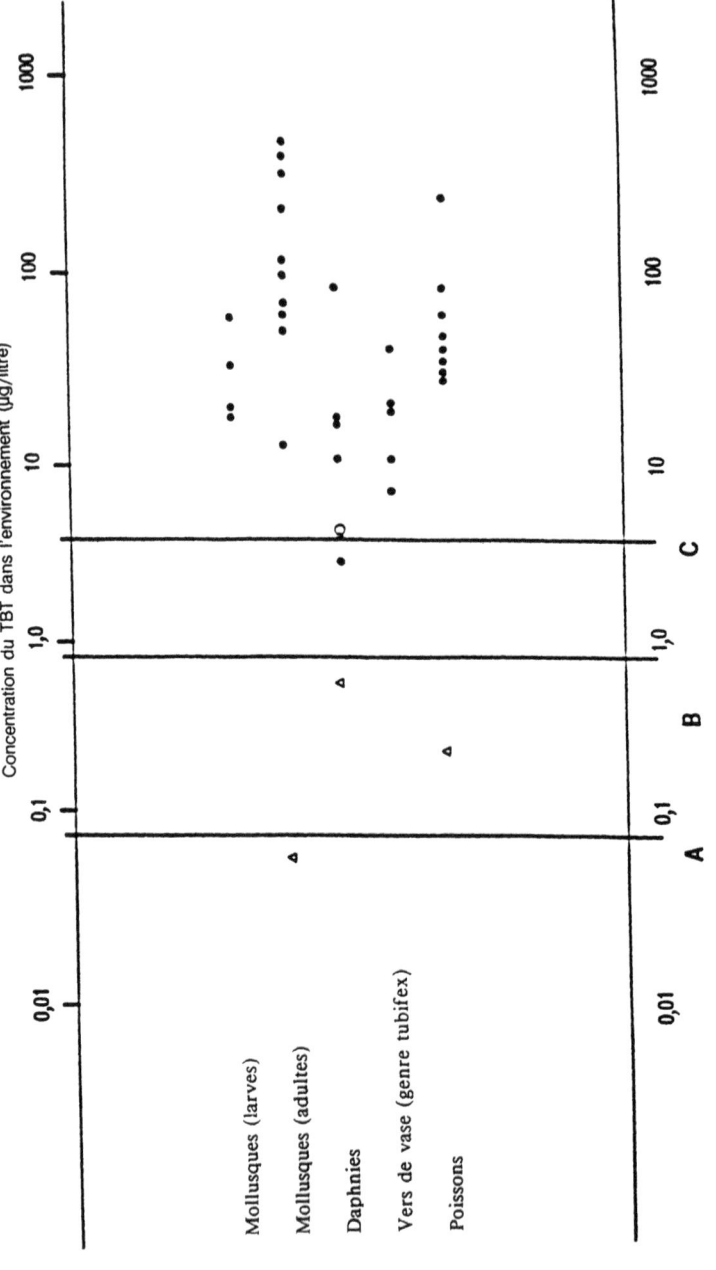

Fig. 2. Toxicité du tributylétain pour les organismes d'eau douce

● CL_{50} après exposition inférieure ou égale à 96 heures; ○ CL_{50} après exposition de plus de 96 heures; △ Concentration la plus faible produisant un effet sublétal;
A = Concentration la plus forte mesurée en amont d'une marina; B = Concentration la plus forte mesurée en aval d'une marina; C = Concentration la plus forte mesurée dans une marina.

observé aucun effet sur la survie des oeufs ni des larves; en revanche, à la concentration de 30 µg/litre on a noté une mortalité sensible.

9.3 Etudes de microcosme

En vue de la modélisation des écosystèmes marins on a effectué des études de microcosme consistant à introduire dans ces milieux certains organismes et en se plaçant dans des conditions où un apport d'eau de mer permettait la colonisation du milieu par d'autres biotes. On a constaté qu'à des concentrations d'oxyde de tributylétain comprises entre 0,06 et 3 µg/litre, il y avait réduction du nombre d'individus et une moindre diversité des espèces.

Les résultats obtenus par modélisation d'écosystèmes d'eau douce montrent que les doses qui tuent les mollusques sont également nocives pour d'autres espèces, notamment les poissons.

10. Effets sur les organismes terrestres

L'exposition des organismes terrestres au TBT découlent essentiellement de l'utilisation de ces substances pour la protection du bois. L'oxyde de tributylétain est toxique pour la population des ruches dont le bois de construction a été traité au TBT. Une étude, d'ailleurs unique, a montré que le TBT était toxique pour les chauves-souris mais le résultat ne peut pas être considéré comme statistiquement significatif en raison de la forte mortalité des témoins. Les dérivés du tributylétain sont toxiques pour les insectes exposés, soit topiquement soit par suite de xylophagie. Pour les souris de type sauvage, la toxicité aiguë du TBT est moyenne; les valeurs de la CL_{50} par voie alimentaire, calculées d'après la consommation de semences traitées et soumises à des épreuves de répulsivité, vont de 37 à 240 mg/kg par jour.

11. Effets sur l'aquaculture

Les observations effectuées dans des zones d'aquaculture ont permis d'attribuer à la présence de fortes concentrations de tributylétain, un certain nombre d'effets nocifs observés sur des bivalves tels que: mortalité, incapacité à se fixer, moindre croissance, épaississement de la coquille et autres malformations notamment chez les huîtres, apparition de caractères mâles chez les gastéropodes (avec diminution simultanée des populations) ainsi que chez les mollusques du genre *Thais*. C'est en France que pour la première fois on a attribué à la présence de TBT dans l'eau, l'anéantissement total de parcs à huîtres, observations qui ont été faites ensuite dans d'autres pays. Les effets étaient particulièrement marqués dans les secteurs proches de marinas destinées aux navires de plaisance. La réglementation de l'usage des peintures antisalissures à base TBT sur les petits navires a permis aux huîtres de retrouver leur capacité de reproduction et de croissance. Toutefois la concentration du TBT dans l'eau reste suffisamment forte dans certains secteurs pour nuire aux gastéropodes marins. On utilise la croissance de la coquille et son gaufrage chez les huîtres japonaises ainsi que l'apparition de caractères mâles chez les mollusques du genre *Thais* comme indicateurs biologiques d'une contamination par du tributylétain.

Peu d'études ont été consacrées aux effets du TBT sédimentaire sur la faune marine mais on pense qu'il peut être absorbé par les organismes fouisseurs et provoquer une certaine mortalité.

Des effets toxiques macroscopiques et des altérations histopathologiques ont été observés dans des élevages de poissons de mer, les filets délimitant les bassins ayant été traités au moyen de peintures aintisalissures à base de TBT.

On a proposé d'utiliser du TBT comme molluscicides pour détruire les mollusques d'eau douce qui transmettent la bilharziose (bilharzies). Un certain nombre d'essais ont été effectués sur le terrain, dont il ressort que le TBT est difficile à utiliser sans préjudice pour les organismes non visés.

12. Toxicité pour les mammifères de laboratoire

12.1 Toxicité aiguë

Le tributylétain est moyennement à fortement toxique pour les mammifères de laboratoire, avec des valeurs de la

DL_{50} par voie orale allant de 94 à 234 mg/kg de poids corporel chez le rat et de 44 à 230 mg/kg de poids corporel chez la souris. Pour le cobaye et le lapin, les valeurs sont du même ordre de grandeur. Les variations enregistrées sont dues aux différents anions entrant dans la composition du sel de tributylétain. Ces composés entraînent une mortalité plus forte lorsqu'ils sont administrés par voie parentérale plutôt que par voie orale, probablement du fait qu'ils ne sont que partiellement absorbés au niveau intestinal.

Parmi les autres effets toxiques aigus on peut citer des anomalies concernant les taux de lipide sanguins, le système endocrinien, le foie, la rate et un déficit passager dans le développement cérébral. La portée toxicologique réelle de ces effets, qui n'ont été observés qu'après administration de doses uniques élevées de ces composés, reste discutable et la cause effective de la mort n'est pas véritablement connue.

Par voie percutanée, la toxicité aiguë est faible, la DL_{50} étant supérieure à 9000 mg/kg de poids corporel chez le lapin. Chez le rat, après inhalation purement nasale, la DL_{50} à 4 heures se situait à 77 mg/m^3 (65 mg/m^3 si l'on ne tient compte que des particules respirables). Des mélanges d'air et de vapeurs de tributylétain ne produisent pas d'effets toxiques observables, même à saturation. Toutefois le TBT est très dangereux sous forme d'aérosol lorsqu'il est inhalé et il produit alors une irritation et un oedème des poumons.

Le TBT est très irritant pour la peau et extrêmement irritant pour l'oeil. L'oxyde de tributylétain n'a pas d'effet sensibilisateur cutané.

12.2 Toxicité à court terme

Les composés du tributylétain ont été très étudiés chez le rat (toutes les données présentées dans ce qui suit concernent cet animal, sauf indication contraire).

On a observé un fort taux de mortalité après une durée d'exposition de plus de quatre semaines à des doses dans l'alimentation de 320 mg/kg (environ 25 mg/kg de poids corporel). Acune mortalité n'a été observée à la dose de 100 mg/kg de nourriture (10 mg/kg de poids corporel) ni

Résumé

---

après l'administration par gavage d'une dose correspondant à 12 mg de TBT/kg de poids corporel. Administrée à des ratons peu après leur naissance, une dose de 3 mg/kg de poids corporel a augmenté la mortalité. Les principaux symptômes observés après administration de doses mortelles consistaient en perte d'appétit, faiblesse et émaciation.

On a observé des effets marginaux sur la croissance aux doses de 50 mg/kg de nourriture (6 mg/kg de poids corporel) et de 6 mg/kg de poids corporel (administrées par gavage). Les souris sont moins sensibles, ces effets n'étant observés qu'à partir de 150 à 200 mg/kg de nourriture (22 à 29 mg/kg de poids corporel).

Des effets structuraux ont été observés sur les organes endocrines, essentiellement l'hypophyse et la thyroïde, lors d'études à court et à long terme. Lors des études à court terme, on a observé des anomalies dans la concentration des hormones circulantes ainsi que dans la réponse aux stimuli physiologiques (trophines hypophysaires); toutefois après une exposition de longue durée, la plupart de ces anomalies avaient disparu. Le mécanisme sous-jacent n'est pas connu.

L'exposition à un aérosol d'oxyde de tributylétain à la dose de 2,8 mg/m^3 a déterminé une forte mortalité, une détresse respiratoire, une réaction inflammatoire au niveau des voies respiratoires et des anomalies histopathologiques des organes lymphatiques. En revanche, l'exposition à des vapeurs à la concentration la plus forte possible (0,16 mg/m^3) à la température ambiante, n'a produit aucun effet.

On a signalé des effets toxiques au niveau du foie et des canaux biliaires chez ces trois espèces de mammifères. Ainsi une nécrose des cellules hépatiques et des altérations inflammatoires du canal cholédoque ont été observées chez des rats qui avaient reçu de l'oxyde de tributylétain à raison de 320 mg/kg de nourriture (soit approximativement 25 mg/kg de poids corporel) pendant quatre semaines et des souris qui en avaient reçu 80 mg/kg de nourriture (soit approximativement 12 mg/kg de poids corporel) pendant trois mois. Chez des chiens soumis à une dose de 10 mg/kg de poids corporel pendant huit à neuf semaines, on a observé une vacuolisation des hépatocytes de la région périportale. Ces altérations s'accompagnaient occasionnellement d'un accroissement du poids du foie et d'une augmentation de l'activité sérique des enzymes hépatiques.

La réduction de la concentration d'hémoglobine et de l'hématocrite chez le rat, à la suite de l'administration d'une dose correspondant à 80 mg/kg de nourriture (soit 8 mg/kg de poids corporel), montre qu'il y a un effet sur la synthèse de l'hémoglobine qui conduit à une anémie hypochrome microcytaire. La réduction des taux d'hémosidérine splénique donne à penser qu'il y a action au niveau des réserves martiales. Une anémie a également été observée chez la souris.

La formation de rosettes érythrocytaires au niveau des ganglions lymphatiques mésentériques a été observée lors de certaines études à court terme mais pas lors d'études à long terme. La portée biologique de cette observation (vraisemblablement passagère) reste obscure.

L'oxyde de tributylétain exerce un effet toxique caractéristique sur le système immunitaire; du fait de son action sur le thymus, il perturbe les fonctions immunitaires à médiation cellulaire. Le mode d'action demeure inconnu mais il pourrait y avoir conversion métabolique en dibutylétain. La résistance non spécifique est également amoindrie.

Un certain nombre d'études sur rats et chiens mais à l'exclusion des souris, ont été effectuées avec de l'oxyde de tributylétain et ont révélé l'existence d'effets généraux sur le système immunitaire (par exemple poids et morphologie des tissus lymphoïdes, numération des lymphocytes périphériques, concentration totale des immunoglobulines sériques), à des doses largement toxiques (des effets ont été observés chez la souris à des doses de 150 mg/kg de chlorure de tributylétain). Seul le rat manifeste des effets généraux sur le système immunitaire sans autres signes patents de toxicité et il se révèle indiscutablement être l'espèce la plus sensible. Des études à court terme sur le rat ont permis d'établir que la dose sans effet observable était de 5 mg/kg de nourriture (soit 0,6 mg/kg de poids corporel). Lors des études portant sur le chlorure de tributylétain, on a observé des effets analogues au niveau du thymus. Ces effets disparaissaient rapidement lorsqu'on cessait d'administrer

Résumé

la substance. On a montré que l'oxyde de tributylétain, étudié dans le cadre de travaux sur la résistance de l'hôte, perturbait les fonctions immunitaires spécifiques du rat. L'organisme de cet animal présentait une moindre aptitude à éliminer les *Listeria monocytogenes* après exposition à une dose de 50 mg/kg de nourriture (dose sans effet observable: 5 mg/kg et par jour), et une moindre résistance à *Trichinella spiralis* a été observée aux doses respectives de 50 et 5 mg/kg de nourriture, cet effet disparaissant à la dose de 0,5 mg/kg de nourriture (ce qui correspond à des doses quotidiennes respectives de 2,5, 0,25 et 0,025 mg/kg de poids corporel). Des effets analogues ont été observés chez des animaux âgés mais ils étaient moins marqués.

Dans l'état actuel des connaissances, les effets sur la résistance de l'hôte sont probablement très utiles pour évaluer les risques pour la santé humaine, mais l'on ne possède pas une expérience suffisante de ces systèmes d'épreuve pour tirer des conclusions définitives des résultats obtenus. Il reste que l'observation de rats glabres athymiques soumis à une inoculation de *T. spiralis* virulentes a permis l'interprétation des résultats obtenus sur le modèle *T. spiralis*. En effet, l'absence totale d'immunité thymo-dépendante a multiplié par 10 à 20 le nombre de larves présentes dans les muscles; par contre l'exposition à des concentrations d'oxyde de tributylétain respectivement égales à 5 et 50 mg/kg de nourriture a multiplié par 2 et 4 respectivement le nombre de ces larves.

Il existe quelques données concernant les effets du tributylétain sur le système immunitaire en développement mais sans aucune information sur la résistance de l'hôte.

Pour évaluer les dangers potentiels pour l'homme, il serait plus prudent de prendre en considération les effets produits sur l'espèce la plus sensible. On a observé des effets sur la résistance de l'hôte à *T. spiralis* à des concentrations dans l'alimentation ne dépassant pas 5 mg/kg (soit l'équivalent de 0,25 mg/kg de poids corporel par jour), la dose sans effet observable étant égale à 0,25 mg/kg (ce qui correspond à 0,025 mg/kg par jour). Toutefois, l'interprétation de ces résultats en vue d'une évaluation du risque pour l'homme reste controversée.

Toutes les études qui ont été effectuées font ressortir que la dose quotidienne sans effet observable pour ce qui est des effets généraux ou spécifiques sur le système immunitaire se situe à 5 mg/kg de nourriture (soit l'équivalent de 0,5 mg/kg de poids corporel selon les études à court terme).

12.3 Toxicité à long terme

Une étude de longue durée chez le rat a montré que le tributylétain a une effet marginal sur les paramètres toxicologiques généraux (sans grande signification toxicologique) à la dose de 5 mg/kg de nourriture (soit 0,25 mg/kg de poids corporel).

12.4 Génotoxicité

La génotoxicité de l'oxyde de tributylétain a fait l'objet d'études approfondies. La plupart de ces études ont donné des résultats négatifs et rien n'indique de façon convaincante que ce produit puisse présenter le moindre risque mutagène.

12.5 Toxicité vis-à-vis de la fonction de reproduction

On a évalué l'embryotoxicité potentielle de l'oxyde de tributylétain sur trois espèces de mammifères (souris, rat et lapin), après administration de la substance par voie orale à la mère. La principale malformation observée chez les foetus de rat et de souris était une fissure congénitale du palais osseux mais il est vrai qu'elle ne se produisait qu'à des doses manifestement toxiques pour la mère. On ne peut pas considérer que ces résultats témoignent d'une activité tératogène aux doses inférieures à celles qui sont toxiques pour la mère. La dose minimale sans effet observable pour ce qui est de l'embryotoxicité et de la foetotoxicité chez ces trois espèces se situait à 1,0 mg/kg de poids corporel.

12.6 Cancérogénicité

Une étude de cancérogénicité a été effectuée sur des rats et on a observé à cette occasion des modifications néoplasiques au niveau des organes endocrines à la dose de

Résumé

50 mg/kg de poids corporel. Les tumeurs hypophysaires observées à la dose de 0,5 mg/kg de nourriture ne semblent pas avoir d'importance biologique car il n'y a pas de relation précise dose-réponse. Ces types de tumeurs apparaissent en général chez les témoins à des fréquences élevées et variables et leur signification reste donc discutable. Une autre étude de cancérogénicité est en cours sur des souris.

13. Effets sur l'homme

On a constaté que l'exposition professionnelle d'ouvriers à des dérivés du tributylétain produisait une irritation des voies respiratoires supérieures. Ces substances sont dangereuses pour l'homme lorsqu'elles sont sous la forme d'aérosols. L'oxyde de tributylétain est irritant pour la peau et les muqueuses oculaires et il a été fait état de dermatites graves à la suite d'un contact direct avec la peau. Le risque est d'autant plus grave que la réaction cutanée n'est pas immédiate.

EVALUATION DES RISQUES POUR LA SANTE HUMAINE ET EFFETS SUR L'ENVIRONNEMENT

1. Evaluation des risques pour l'homme

Les travailleurs sont principalement exposés lors de la préparation et de la formulation des dérivés du tributylétain, de l'application ou de l'élimination de peintures à base de TBT et de l'utilisation de produits de protection du bois à base de ces substances. Quant à la population dans son ensemble, elle peut être exposée par contamination de la nourriture, en particulier des poissons et des coquillages, et lors de l'utilisation de produits de protection du bois à usage ménager.

Si l'on s'appuie sur l'expérimentation animale et l'observation directe sur l'homme, il est clair que les dérivés du tributylétain sont irritants pour la peau et les yeux et que l'inhalation d'aérosols conduit à une irritation des voies respiratoires.

La manipulation de bois traités n'entraîne aucune irritation de l'épiderme une fois que le produit a séché. Cependant les aérosols de TBT sont extrêmement dangereux et il ne faut pas revenir dans le local où le bois a été traité avant séchage complet.

On n'a jamais fait état d'intoxications aiguës généralisées par le TBT qui en principe doit s'éliminer de l'organisme en l'espace de quelques jours. Il est donc peu probable que l'on puisse s'exposer à des intoxications aiguës par la manipulation de produits à base de tributylétain si l'on prend les précautions voulues.

On a fait état d'effets à court et à long terme chez des animaux de laboratoire, sur le foie, le sang et les glandes endocrines. Chez le rat, qui est l'espèce la plus sensible, c'est l'effet au niveau du système immunitaire et en particulier sur la résistance de l'hôte, qui constitue le paramètre le plus sensible de la toxicité de ces produits. En utilisant comme modèle la résistance de l'hôte à l'infestation par *Trichinella spiralis*, on obtient une dose sans effet observable qui se situe entre 0,5 et 5 mg/kg de nourriture (c'est-à-dire 0,025 et 0,25 mg/kg de poids corporel) alors que si l'on se rapporte à

Evaluation

l'action sur la fonction immunitaire, la dose est égale à 0,6 mg/kg de poids corporel.

En raison des grandes variations dans la consommation de poissons et de coquillages ainsi que dans les teneurs locales des fruits de mer en résidus de TBT, on ne peut donner que quelques exemples pour illustrer l'exposition résultante et les valeurs des doses sans effet observable. Il importe de souligner que pour déterminer le risque résultant de la présence de ces composés, il faut procéder sur place à des mesures de résidus dans les denrées, évaluer la consommation locale de fruits de mer et définir une marge de sécurité acceptable.

En retenant pour la consommation de poisson les chiffres de 15 et 150 grammes par jour, de 1 mg/kg pour les résidus de TBT dans le poisson et un poids corporel moyen de 60 kg, on obtient pour l'homme les marges suivantes de sécurité selon les divers paramètres immunitaires.

Consommation de poisson (g/jour)	Apport estimatif journalier de TBT (μg/kg)	Marge de sécurité	
		Modèle T. Spiralis	Autres paramètres immunitaires
15	0,25	100-1000	2500
150	2,5	10-100	250

Utiliser des dérivés du TBT à tort et à travers et de manière irresponsable sans suivre les recommandations qui figurent dans la présente monographie pour réduire l'exposition humaine peut conduire à l'ingestion de quantités de TBT dangereuses pour la santé humaine.

On a noté jusqu'ici d'effets tératogènes, chez l'animal de laboratoire, qu'à des doses manifestement toxiques pour la mère. On peut donc considérer que l'activité tératogène du TBT est très faible.

En s'appuyant sur les résultats d'études très complètes de mutagénicité, on estime que les dérivés du tributylétain n'ont aucun pouvoir mutagène. Une étude de cancérogénicité chez le rat, portant sur l'oxyde de tributylétain, a fait apparaître une incidence accrue de tumeurs endocriniennes; mais il s'agissait de tumeurs spontanées dont l'incidence, généralement élevée, est très variable. Ces résultats ne constituent donc pas un argument bien net en faveur d'un risque cancérogène pour l'homme.

2. Evaluation du risque écologique

La pénétration diffuse du tributylétain (TBT) dans l'environnement a principalement pour origine l'utilisation de peintures antisalissures qui en contiennent. Une contamination ponctuelle peut se produire lorsqu'on utilise du TBT comme biocide dans les systèmes de réfrigération, lors du traitement de la pulpe de bois, le tannage du cuir, la préservation du bois et le traitement des textiles.

Du fait de leurs prioriétés physico-chimiques, les dérivés du TBT se concentrent dans la micro-couche de surface ainsi que dans les sédiments. Il ne semble pas que le principal mécanisme d'élimination de ces substances dans les conditions naturelles soit une dégradation abiotique. L'oxyde de tributylétain est biodégradable dans l'eau mais le processus n'est pas suffisamment rapide pour empêcher la présence dans certaines zones de concentrations élevées en TBT. Une bioaccumulation se produit dans la plupart des organismes aquatiques mais chez les mammifères de laboratoire, la dégradation métabolique est plus efficace.

Le TBT est extrêment dangereux pour certains organismes aquatiques, du fait de sa toxicité à très faibles concentrations dans l'eau. On le rencontre à ces concentrations dans certaines zones. On a signalé la présence d'effets nocifs sur des invertébrés non visés, en particulier des mollusques et ces effets sont suffisamment graves pour bloquer la reproduction et entraîner un déclin des populations de mollusques. Ces effets néfastes pour la conchyliculture ont pu être combattus avec succès grâce à des restrictions imposées à l'utilisation des peintures antisalissures dans certains secteurs, restrictions qui ont également permis d'éviter l'apparition de caractères mâles chez les gastéropodes femelles. En ce qui concerne

Evaluation

le pisciculture, il convient de ne pas utiliser de peintures à base de TBT sur les filets qui limitent les bassins.

D'une manière générale, le risque pour l'environnement terrestre est vraisemblablement faible. Cependant le traitement du bois par ces substances pourrait se révéler dangereux pour les organismes qui vivent à son contact.

L'augmentation de la teneur en TBT de la micro-couche superficielle pourrait se révéler dangereuse pour la faune côtière, pour les neustons (y compris les invertébrés benthiques et les larves de poissons) ainsi que pour les oiseaux de mer et le gibier d'eau qui se nourrissent en surface. L'accumulation et le faible taux de biodégradation du TBT dans les sédiments peut présenter un risque pour les organismes aquatiques lorsque des sédiments pollués sont soulevés par des processus naturels ou des activités de dragage.

RECOMMANDATIONS

1. **Recommandations pour la protection de la santé humaine et de l'environnement**

   a) Les pays membres qui jusqu'ici n'ont pas réglementé l'utilisation des dérivés du TBT devraient être invités à le faire.

   b) Il est nécessaire d'évaluer la pénétration des dérivés organo-stanniques dans l'environnement à partir de sources autres que les peintures antisalissures et, si besoin est, d'édicter une réglementation à ce sujet. Il faut en particulier évaluer le risque résultant du déversement sur le sol de boues d'égouts contaminés par du tributylétain.

   c) Il faudrait améliorer, du point de vue de la sécurité, les techniques d'application, d'élimination et d'évacuation des peintures à base d'organo-stanniques.

2. **Recherches à effectuer**

   a) Il faut améliorer les méthodes de recherche et de dosage du butylétain afin d'avoir une estimation rapide et exacte des concentrations de l'ordre de pg/litre. Une des raisons de cette recommandation tient à un effet biologique, à savoir l'apparition de caractères mâles chez les gastéropodes femelles, qui est susceptible de se produire à des concentrations plus basses que les limites actuelles de détection.

   b) Il faut effectuer des recherches sur les mécanimes par lesquels le TBT se concentre au lieu de se disperser et qui retardent sa décomposition; à cet effet on étudiera avec une attention particulière la chimie fondamentale du tributylétain et ses interactions avec les molécules biologiques. Il faut étudier davantage la fixation du TBT à tous les niveaux de la chaîne alimentaire.

   c) Il est nécessaire d'entreprendre des études sur la toxicité du TBT pour les organismes aquatiques. On étudiera en particulier le métabolisme, les effets endocriniens et immunologiques, selon le cas.

Recommandations

d) Il est nécessaire de rechercher d'autres espèces sensibles capables de servir d'indicateurs biologiques, notamment parmi les espèces d'eau douce.

e) Il faut valider les modèles permettant l'évaluation de l'immunotoxicité chez les mammifères et définir de façon plus précise les doses sans effet toxique correspondant aux paramètres pertinents.

f) Etude de toxicité chronique à entreprendre sur une deuxième espèce de mammifères.

g) Etude de tumorigénicité à entreprendre sur une deuxième espèce de mammifères.

h) Données sur les résidus de butylétain dans le poisson et les coquillages destinés à la consommation humaine en distinguant les différentes espèces.

RESUMEN

1. Propiedades físicas y químicas

Los compuestos de tributilestaño (TBE) son derivados orgánicos del estaño tetravalente. Caracterizados por la presencia de enlaces covalentes entre átomos de carbono y un átomo de estaño, tienen la siguiente fórmula general: $(n-C_4H_9)_3$ Sn-X, en la que X es un anión. En general, la pureza del óxido de tributilestaño (OTBE) comercial pasa del 96%; las principales impurezas están constituidas por derivados del dibutilestaño y, en menor grado, por compuestos de tetrabutilestaño y otros compuestos trialquílicos de ese elemento. El OTBE es un líquido incoloro con olor característico y una densidad relativa de 1,17 a 1,18. La solubilidad en el agua es baja, variando entre < 1,0 y > 100 mg/litro según el pH, la temperatura, y los aniones presentes en el agua (que determinan la especificidad). En el agua del mar y en condiciones normales, el TBE aparece en tres formas o especies (hidróxido, cloruro y carbonato), que se mantienen en equilibrio. En valores de pH inferiores a 7,0, las formas predominantes son $Bu_3SnOH_2^+$ y Bu_3SnCl, a pH 8 son Bu_3SnCl, Bu_3SnOH y $Bu_3SnCO_3^-$, mientras que cuando el pH pasa de 10 predominan Bu_3SnOH y $Bu_3SnCO_3^-$.

El coeficiente de partición octanol/agua (log P_{oa}) varía entre 3,19 y 3,84 para el agua destilada y es de 3,54 para el agua del mar. El OTBE adsorbe intensamente las partículas, con coeficientes de adsorción comprendidos entre 110 y 55 000 según los informes publicados. La presión de vapor es baja, pero los valores publicados acusan variaciones considerables. En una solución de 1 mg/litro no se observó disminución alguna del OTBE durante 62 días, pero el 20% del agua se perdió por evaporación.

2. Métodos analíticos

Se utilizan diversos métodos para medir los derivados tributilestánnicos en el agua, en el sedimento o en la flora y la fauna (biota). El más usado es la espectrometría de absorción atómica (AA). La espectrometría de AA con llama permite alcanzar un límite de detección de 0,1

Resumen

mg/litro. Resulta más sensible la AA sin llama, basada en la atomización en un horno eléctrico con grafito, cuyos límites de detección están comprendidos entre 0,1 y 1,0 µg/litro de agua. Existen diferentes métodos de extracción y para formar derivados volátiles. La separación de estos derivados suele hacerse por "purga y captura" o cromatografía de gases. Los límites de detección son de 0,5 y 5,0 µg/kg para el sedimento y la biota.

3. Fuentes de contaminación ambiental

Se han registrado diversos compuestos de tributilestaño como molusquicidas, productos antiincrustantes en botes y otras embarcaciones, muelles, boyas, jaulas de langostas, redes de pesca y nasas, como conservadores de la madera, como "productos anti-cieno" en los trabajos de albañilería, como desinfectantes y como biocidas en los sistemas de refrigeración, las torres de refrigeración de las centrales electrógenas, las fábricas de pulpa y de papel, las cervecerías, las industrias del cuero y los telares. En las pinturas antiincrustantes, el TBE se comercializó al principio bajo una forma que permitía la liberación sin trabas del compuesto. En fecha más reciente se han puesto a la venta pinturas de liberación controlada en las que el TBE se incorpora a una matriz copolimérica. También se han ideado matrices de caucho para hacer más lenta y retrasar la liberación del compuesto, con la consiguiente prolongación de la eficacia de las pinturas antiincrustantes y de los molusquicidas. El TBE no se utiliza en la agricultura por su elevada fitotoxicidad.

4. Reglamentación del empleo

Muchos países han restringido el empleo de pinturas antiincrustantes con TBE por los efectos de éste sobre los mariscos. Los reglamentos varían en detalle de unos países a otros, pero casi siempre prohíben el uso de pinturas de TBE en las embarcaciones de 24 metros de longitud o menos. Algunos países han excluido de esta prohibición a las embarcaciones con casco de aluminio. Además, en algunos reglamentos se restringe el contenido de TBE en las pinturas o el ritmo con que se libera este compuesto de las mismas (a 4 o 5 µg/cm^2 por día, a largo plazo).

5. Concentraciones en el medio ambiente

Se han encontrado concentraciones elevadas de TBE en el agua, los sedimentos y la biota próximos a las zonas de navegación de recreo, especialmente en "marinas" o fondeaderos de yates, embarcaderos, diques secos, redes de pesca y nasas tratadas con pinturas antiincrustantes, así como en los sistemas de refrigeración. La intensidad de las mareas y la turbiedad del agua influyen en las concentraciones de TBE.

Se ha visto que las concentraciones de TBE pueden llegar a 1,58 μg/litro en el agua del mar y en los estuarios, a 7,1 μ/litro en el agua dulce, a 26 300 μg/kg en los sedimentos costeros, a 3700 μg/kg en los sedimentos de agua dulce, a 6,39 mg/kg en los bivalvos, a 1,92 mg/kg en los gasterópodos y a 11 mg/kg en los peces. Ahora bien, no hay que considerar como representativas esas concentraciones máximas de TBE, toda vez que diversos factores pueden dar lugar a valores anormalmente elevados (por ejemplo, las partículas de pintura en las muestras de agua y de sedimentos). Se ha comprobado que en las concentraciones de TBE en la microcapa superficial del agua, tanto dulce como salada, pueden ser dos veces más altas que las medidas inmediatamente por debajo de la superficie. Sin embargo, conviene tener en cuenta que los valores registrados de TBE en las microcapas superficiales pueden verse muy afectados por el método de muestreo.

Es posible que los datos antiguos no sean comparables con los más recientes a causa del perfeccionamiento de los métodos analíticos disponibles para determinar el TBE en el agua, los sedimentos y los tejidos.

6. Transporte y transformación en el medio ambiente

A consecuencia de su baja hidrosolubilidad y de su carácter lipofílico, el TBE se adsorbe fácilmente en las partículas. Se calcula que entre el 10% y el 95% del OTBE introducido en el agua se adsorbe de ese modo. La desaparición progresiva del TBE adsorbido no se debe a la desorción sino a la degradación. El grado de adsorción depende de la salinidad, de la naturaleza y el tamaño de las partículas en suspensión, de la cantidad de material

Resumen

suspendido, de la temperatura y de la presencia de materia orgánica disuelta.

La degradación del OTBE entraña la escisión del enlace carbono-estaño. Este fenómeno puede deberse a diversos mecanismos que intervienen simultáneamente en el medio ambiente, unos fisicoquímicos (hidrólisis y fotodegradación) y otros biológicos (degradación por microorganismos y metabolización por organismos superiores). Mientras que en condiciones extremas de pH se produce una hidrólisis de los compuestos de estaño orgánico, ésta es apenas evidente en condiciones ambientales normales. En el laboratorio se observa fotodegradación cuando se exponen soluciones a una irradiación ultravioleta de 300 nm (y, en menor grado, de 350 nm). En condiciones naturales, la fotólisis está limitada por la gama de longitudes de onda de la luz solar y por la escasa penetración de la luz ultravioleta en el agua. La presencia de sustancias fotosensibilizadoras puede acelerar la fotodegradación. La biodegradación depende de condiciones ambientales tales como la temperatura, la oxigenación, el pH, el nivel de elementos minerales, la presencia de sustancias orgánicas fácilmente biodegradables a efectos de cometabolismo y la naturaleza de la microflora y su capacidad de adaptación. También depende de que la concentración de OTBE sea más baja que el umbral letal o inhibitorio para las bacterias. Como en la degradación abiótica, la ruptura biótica del TBE es un proceso progresivo de debutilización oxidativa fundado en la escisión del enlace carbono-estaño, en el que se forman derivados dibutílicos que se degradan más fácilmente que el tributilestaño. Los monobutilestaños se mineralizan lentamente. Aunque existe degradación anaerobia, no se ha llegado a un acuerdo sobre su importancia. Algunos autores estiman que es lenta, mientras que otros piensan que es más rápida que la degradación aerobia. Se han identificado varias especies de bacterias, algas y hongos nocivos para la madera que pueden degradar el OTBE. Las estimaciones de la semivida del TBE en el medio ambiente acusan grandes variaciones.

El TBE se bioacumula en los organismos a causa de su solubilidad en las grasas. En investigaciones de laboratorio con moluscos y peces se han visto que los factores de bioconcentración pueden llegar a un valor de 7000, y aun se han obtenido valores más altos en los estudios sobre el terreno. La absorción a partir de los alimentos es más importante que la que se efectúa directamente a partir del agua. La presencia de factores de concentración más altos en los microorganismos (entre 100 y 30 000) puede deberse más a adsorción que a absorción intracelular. No hay ninguna indicación de que el TBE se transfiera a los microorganismos terrestres a través de las cadenas alimentarias.

7. Cinética y metabolismo

El tributilestaño se absorbe a través del intestino (20-50%, según el vehículo) y de la piel en los mamíferos (10% aproximadamente), pudiendo atravesar la barrera hematoencefálica y pasar de la placenta al feto. El material absorbido se distribuye rápida y ampliamente por los tejidos (principalmente el hígado y el riñón).

En los mamíferos, el metabolismo del TBE es rápido: a las 3 h de administrar TBE pueden ya descubrirse metabolitos en la sangre. Los estudios in vitro han revelado que el TBE es un sustrato para ciertas oxidasas de función mixta, pero las concentraciones muy altas de TBE inhiben esas enzimas.

La velocidad de desaparición del TBE difiere de unos tejidos a otros; las estimaciones de la semivida biológica en los mamíferos van desde 23 hasta unos 30 días.

La metabolización del TBE se observa también en los organismos inferiores, pero es más lenta (particularmente en los moluscos) que en los mamíferos. La capacidad de bioacumulación, por consiguiente, es mucho mayor que en éstos.

Los compuestos de TBE inhiben la fosforilización oxidativa y alteran la estructura y las funciones de las mitocondrias. El TBE interfiere en la calcificación de la concha de las ostras (*Crassostrea* spp).

8. Efectos en los microorganismos

El TBE es tóxico para los microorganismos y se ha utilizado comercialmente como bactericida y alguicida. Las concentraciones que provocan efectos tóxicos varían mucho de unas especies a otras. El TBE es más tóxico para las bacterias gram-positivas (concentración inhibitoria mínima (CIM): entre 0,2 y 0,8 mg/litro) que para las gram-negativas (CIM: 3 mg/litro). La CIM del acetato de TBE para los hongos es de 0,5-1 mg/litro y la CIM del OTBE para el alga verde *Chlorella pyrenoidosa* es de 0,5 mg/litro. La productividad primaria de una comunidad natural de algas de agua dulce se redujo en un 50% con una concentración de OTBE de 3 µg/litro. En fecha reciente se han determinado en dos especies de algas niveles de efecto no observado (NENO) de 18 y 32 µg/litro. De igual modo, la toxicidad para los microorganismos marinos varía de unas especies a otras y de unos estudios a otros; los NENO son difíciles de establecer pero no llegan a 0,1 µg/litro en algunas especies. Las concentraciones alguicidas varían entre < 1,5 µg/litro y > 1000 µg por litro según las especies.

9. Efectos en los organismos acuáticos

9.1 Efectos en los organismos de agua salada (mar y estuarios)

En la figura 1 se resumen en un diagrama las relaciones entre los efectos letales y subletales y las concentraciones de TBE medidas en diversos organismos del mar y de los estuarios. En todo el mundo, especialmente en los lugares relacionados con actividades náuticas recreativas, se han encontrado concentraciones superiores a las que producen efectos letales.

El desarrollo de las esporas móviles de una macroalga verde se ha revelado como el índice evolutivo más sensible al TBE (CE_{50} de 5 días: 0,001 µg/litro). El crecimiento de una angiosperma marina se redujo en concentraciones de TBE de un mg/kg de sedimento, pero no se observó ningún efecto a 0,1 mg/kg.

El tributilestaño es sumamente tóxico para los moluscos marinos. Experimentalmente se ha demostrado que altera la formación de la concha en las ostras en crecimiento, así como el desarrollo gonadal y el sexo de las ostras adultas, la formación de colonias, el crecimiento y la mortalidad de las ostras y otros bivalvos en la fase larvaria, y que causa "imposex" (desarrollo de características masculinas) en los gasterópodos hembras. Se ha obtenido un valor NENO de 20 ng/litro para la freza de la

EHC 116: Tributyltin Compounds

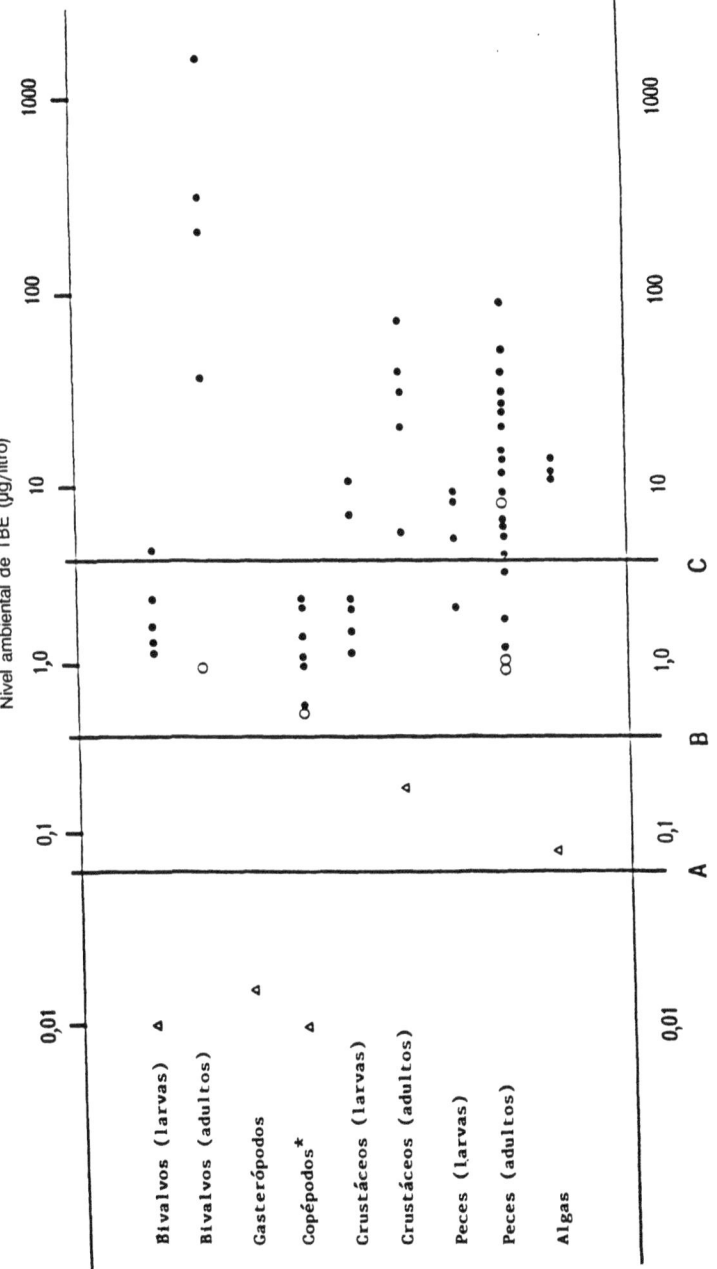

Fig. 1. Toxicidad del tributilestaño para los organismos marinos

● CL$_{50}$ tras la exposición durante 96 h o menos;   o CL$_{50}$ tras la exposición durante más de 96 h;   △ mínima concentración que causa un efecto subletal;   B = máxima concentración medida en mar abierto;
* los copépodos son objeto de mención especial por ser más sensibles que los demás crustáceos;   A = máxima concentración medida en mar abierto;   C = máxima concentración medida en estuario abierto;   C = máxima concentración medida en marinas.

especie de ostra más sensible *(Crassostrea gigas)*. El TBE provoca una deformación de la concha de las ostras adultas más o menos acentuada según la dosis. No se ha observado experimentalmente ningún efecto sobre la morfología de la concha con concentraciones de TBE de 2 ng/litro. En las hembras de buccino, el valor NENO para el imposex no llega a 1,5 ng/litro. En general, las formas larvarias son más sensibles que los adultos, siendo esta diferencia especialmente marcada en el caso de las ostras.

Los copépodos son más sensibles que otros grupos de crustáceos al efecto letal agudo del TBE; los valores de CL_{50} para periodos de exposición de hasta 96 h van de 0,6 a 2,2 µg/litro. Estas cifras son comparables a las obtenidas en las larvas más sensibles de otros grupos de crustáceos. El TBE reduce el rendimiento reproductor, la supervivencia de los recién nacidos y la tasa de crecimiento juvenil en los crustáceos. En el camarón mísido *Acanthomysis sculpta* el valor NENO para la reproducción parece ser de 0,09 µg/litro. Otro camarón, el llamado por los anglosajones "grass shrimp", no evita el TBE a concentraciones que pueden llegar hasta 30 µg/litro.

La toxicidad del tributilestaño para los peces marinos es sumamente variable; los valores de la CL_{50} a 96 h van desde 1,5 hasta 36 µg/litro. Las fases larvarias son más sensibles que los adultos (fig. 1). Hay indicios de que los peces marinos evitan las concentraciones de OTBE de 1 µg/litro o más.

9.2 Efectos en los organismos de agua dulce

En la figura 2 se resumen en un diagrama las relaciones entre los efectos letales y subletales y las concentraciones de TBE medidas en agua dulce. Se han observado concentraciones mayores que las que provocan efectos subletales en diversos sitios, especialmente en relación con actividades náuticas recreativas.

Una concentración OTBE de 0,5 mg/litro produjo la muerte de las angioespermas de agua dulce, mientras que el crecimiento se inhibió a 0,06 mg/litro o más.

Los datos sobre los invertebrados de agua dulce son escasos y no comprenden más que tres especies, además de los organismos tomados como objetivo. Con diferentes sales

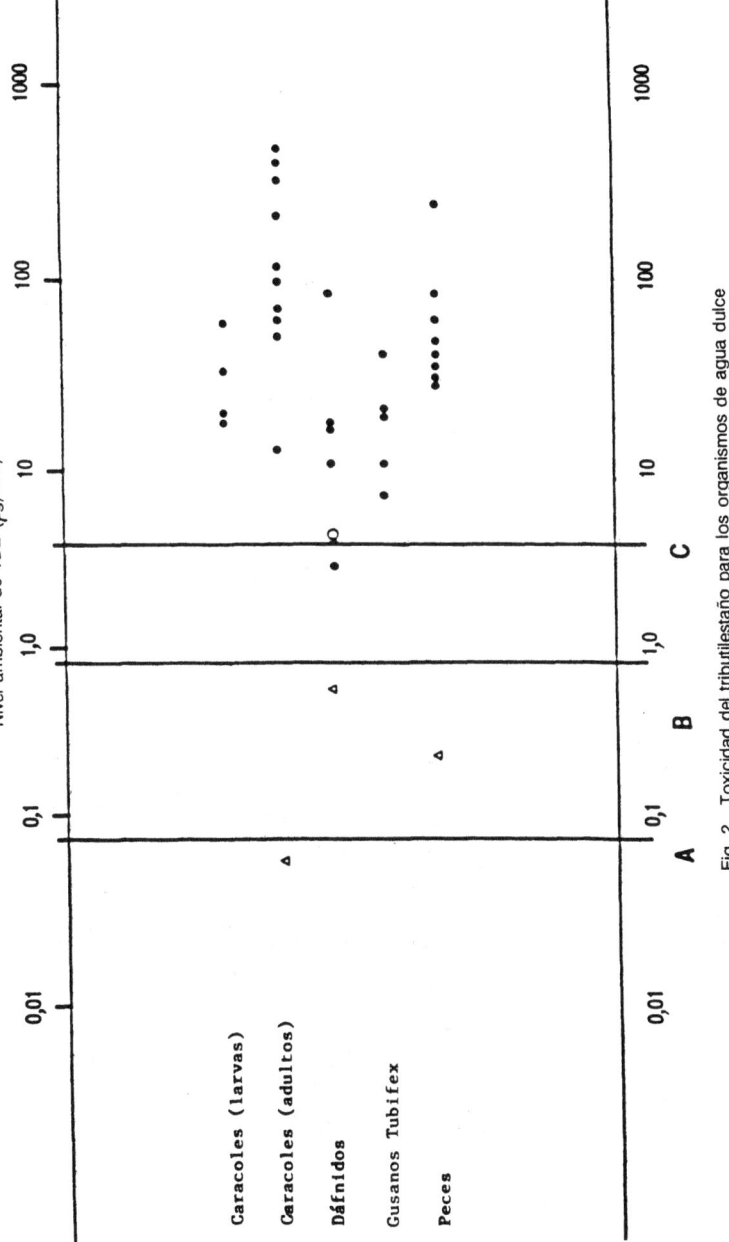

Fig. 2. Toxicidad del tributilestaño para los organismos de agua dulce

o CL$_{50}$ tras la exposición durante 96 h o menos;   o CL$_{50}$ tras la exposición durante más de 96 h;   Δ mínima concentración que causa un efecto subletal;
A = máxima concentración medida aguas arriba de una marina;   B = máxima concentración medida aguas abajo de una marina;   C = máxima concentración medida en una marina.

Resumen

de TBE se han obtenido valores de CL_{50} en 48 h para *Daphnia* de 2,3-70 µg/litro y para *Tubifex* de 5,5-33 µg/litro. Basándose en la reversión de la respuesta normal a la luz, se ha calculado que el NENO para *Daphnia* es de 0,5 µg/litro. La CL_{50} de 24 h para la almeja asiática parece ser, según se ha señalado, de 2100 µg por litro, mientras que para los moluscos adultos contra los que se dirige la lucha antiesquistosomiásica los valores correspondientes son de 30-400 µg/litro.

Se ha demostrado que el tributilestaño es tóxico para las larvas de esquistosoma en las fases acuáticas; la CL_{50} (fluoruro de TBE) parece ser, según los cálculos realizados, de 16,8 µg/litro en el caso de una exposición de 1 h. La dosis de TBE que suprime el 99-100% de la infectividad de las cercarias para el ratón está comprendida entre 2 y 6 µg/litro.

La sensibilidad de los moluscos al TBE disminuye con la edad, pero los huevos son más resistentes que los individuos jóvenes y adultos. La puesta de huevos se ve considerablemente afectada a una concentración de OTBE de 0,001 µg/litro.

En las pruebas de CL_{50} con exposiciones de hasta 168 h, la toxicidad aguda del TBE para los peces de agua dulce varía entre 13 y 240 µg/litro. Basándose en los efectos histopatológicos, se ha calculado que el valor NENO para el "guppy" es de 0,01 µg/litro.

No se ha observado ningún efecto sobre la supervivencia tras la exposición de huevos y larvas de la rana *Rana temporaria* a concentraciones de TBE de 3 µg por litro o menos; en cambio, la mortalidad fue significativa a 30 µg/litro.

9.3 Estudios microcósmicos

Se han realizado algunos "estudios microcósmicos" utilizando como modelo ecosistemas marinos en los que se habían introducido organismos y en los que la entrada de agua de mar facilitaba la colonización por otros organismos. Los resultados obtenidos muestran que tanto el número de individuos como la diversidad de las especies disminuyen cuando la concentración de OTBE en el agua se sitúa entre 0,06 y 3 µg/litro.

Los resultados obtenidos con modelos de ecosistemas de agua dulce hacen pensar que las dosis que matan los caracoles afectan también a otras especies, en particular los peces.

10. Efectos en los organismos terrestres

La exposición de organismos terrestres al TBE proviene sobre todo del uso de este compuesto como conservador de la madera. El OTBE es tóxico para las abejas que viven en colmenas de madera tratadas con TBE. Este producto se mostró tóxico para los murciélagos en un estudio aislado, pero la elevada mortalidad de los testigos resta significación estadística a este resultado. Los compuestos de TBE son tóxicos para los insectos que están en contacto o se alimentan con madera tratada. El TBE tiene una toxicidad aguda moderada para los ratones en libertad y, basándose en el consumo de semillas tratadas en las pruebas de repelentes, se calcula que los valores de CL_{50} en la dieta se sitúan entre 37 y 240 mg/kg al día.

11. Efectos en organismos estudiados sobre el terreno

Las observaciones sobre el terreno han permitido establecer una relación entre las concentraciones elevadas de tributilestaño y la mortalidad de las larvas de bivalvos, la incapacidad de las mismas para constituir colonias, el retraso del crecimiento, el engrosamiento de la concha y otras malformaciones de las ostras en desarrollo, el imposex en los caracoles de suelos cenagosos y el imposex (con disminución concurrente de la población) en el buccino. En Francia inicialmente, y más tarde en otros países, se ha identificado y atribuido la destrucción completa de los criaderos de ostras a la presencia de TBE en el agua. Los efectos son más acusados en las zonas próximas a los centros de deportes náuticos. Al dejar de emplear pinturas antiincrustantes a base de TBE en las pequeñas embarcaciones se restablecieron la reproducción y el crecimiento de las ostras. Sin embargo, en algunas zonas las concentraciones de TBE en el agua siguen siendo bastante elevadas para afectar a los gasterópodos marinos.

Tanto el desarrollo y formación de la concha en las ostras del Pacífico como el imposex en el buccino se han utilizado como indicadores biológicos de contaminación por TBE.

Aunque se han hecho pocos estudios sobre los efectos en los organismos del TBE presente en los sedimentos, hay indicios de que este compuesto puede llegar a los animales que viven en madrigueras y producir mortalidad en condiciones prácticas.

Se han observado efectos tóxicos macroscópicos y alteraciones histopatológicas en los criaderos de pesca marítima expuestos al TBE por el uso de pinturas antiincrustantes en las redes de contención.

Se ha propuesto la utilización de TBE como molusquicida contra los caracoles de agua dulce que transmiten la esquistosomiasis (bilharziasis). Varios ensayos prácticos han demostrado que es difícil aplicar el TBE sin que resulten perjudicados otros organismos distintos de los tomados como objetivo.

12. Toxicidad para los mamíferos de laboratorio

12.1 Toxicidad aguda

El tributilestaño tiene una toxicidad entre moderada y alta para los mamíferos de laboratorio; los valores de la DL_{50} oral aguda varían desde 94 a 234 mg/kg de peso corporal para la rata y desde 44 hasta 230 mg/kg de peso corporal para el ratón. La toxicidad aguda para el cobayo y el conejo es del mismo orden. La variación se debe al componente aniónico de la sal de tributilestaño. Estos compuestos tienen un potencial letal mayor por vía parenteral que por vía oral, probablemente porque la absorción intestinal es incompleta.

Entre otros efectos de la exposición aguda cabe citar alteraciones de las cifras de lípidos sanguíneos, el sistema endocrino, el hígado y el bazo, así como un déficit transitorio del desarrollo cerebral. La importancia toxicológica de estos efectos, observados tras la administración de una fuerte dosis única del compuesto, es discutible y sigue ignorándose cuál es la causa de la muerte.

La toxicidad aguda por vía dérmica es baja; la DL_{50} es > 9000 mg/kg de peso corporal para el conejo.

La DL_{50} por inhalación exclusivamente nasal (4 h) es de 77 mg/m³ (65 mg/m³ cuando sólo se tienen en cuenta las partículas inhalables) para la rata. Las mezclas de aire y vapores de TBE no producen efectos tóxicos observables, ni siquiera en el punto de saturación. Sin embargo, el TBE es muy peligroso cuando se inhala en forma de aerosol, produciendo irritación y edema de los pulmones.

El TBE es muy irritante para la piel y sumamente irritante para los ojos. El OTBE no produce sensibilización cutánea.

12.2 Toxicidad a corto plazo

Los compuestos de TBE han sido muy estudiados en la rata, hasta el punto de que todos los datos expuestos en esta sección se refieren a ese animal a menos que se indique otra cosa.

Con dosis de 320 mg/kg (unos 25 mg/kg de peso corporal) en la dieta se han obtenido altas tasas de mortalidad cuando la exposición se prolonga más de 4 semanas. No se observaron muertes con 100 mg/kg en la dieta (10 mg/kg de peso corporal) ni tras la administración forzada de 12 mg/kg de peso corporal al día. En las ratas tratadas en sus primeros días de vida, la mortalidad aumentó con una dosis de 3 mg/kg de peso corporal. Los principales síntomas causados por las dosis letales fueron inapetencia, debilidad y emaciación.

Se han observado efectos "limítrofes" en el crecimiento de la rata con dosis de 50 mg/kg (6 mg/kg de peso corporal) en la dieta y de 6 mg/kg de peso corporal en estudios de administración forzada. Los ratones se muestran menos sensibles, observándose los efectos del compuesto con dosis de 150 a 200 mg/kg (22 a 29 mg/kg de peso corporal) en la dieta.

Tanto los estudios a corto plazo como en los prolongados se han observado efectos estructurales sobre los órganos endocrinos, principalmente la hipófisis y el tiroides. Las pruebas a corto plazo pusieron de manifiesto alteraciones en la concentración de las hormonas circulantes y en la respuesta a los estímulos fisiológicos (hormonas tróficas hipofisarias), pero tras la exposición prolongada desaparecieron casi todas esas alteraciones. El mecanismo de acción es desconocido.

Resumen

La exposición a un aerosol de OTBE a razón de 2,8 mg/m³ produjo un aumento de la mortalidad, así como dificultades respiratorias, inflamación del tracto respiratorio y alteraciones histopatológicas de los órganos linfáticos. En cambio, la exposición a la máxima concentración de vapor accesible (0,16 mg/m³) a la temperatura del local no produjo ningún efecto.

En tres especies de mamíferos se han señalado efectos tóxicos en el hígado y los conductos biliares. En ratas a las que se administró OTBE en la dieta a razón de 320 mg/kg (unos 25 mg/kg de peso corporal) durante 4 semanas y en ratones tratados con 80 mg/kg (unos 12 mg/kg de peso corporal) en la dieta durante 90 días se produjo una necrosis hepatocelular con alteraciones inflamatorias del árbol biliar. En perros que recibieron una dosis de 10 mg/kg de peso corporal durante 8 o 9 semanas se observó una vacuolización de los hepatocitos periportales. Estos cambios se acompañaban a veces de un aumento del peso del hígado y de la actividad sérica de las enzimas hepáticas.

El descenso de la concentración de hemoglobina y del volumen eritrocítico en la rata, causado por la administración de 80 mg/kg (8 mg/kg de peso corporal) en la dieta, traduce un efecto en la síntesis de la hemoglobina que da lugar a una anemia hipocrómica microcítica. El descenso de las cifras de hemosiderina esplénica sugiere una alteración del equilibrio del hierro. En los ratones se ha observado también anemia.

En ciertas investigaciones a corto plazo, pero no en los estudios prolongados, se ha observado formación de rosetas de hematíes en los ganglios linfáticos del mesenterio. No está clara la significación biológica de este fenómeno (posiblemente transitorio).

El efecto tóxico característico del OTBE tiene lugar en el sistema inmunitario: a causa de los efectos en el timo, la inmunidad celular se menoscaba. Aunque se desconoce el mecanismo de acción, es posible que esté relacionado con la conversión metabólica en compuestos de dibutilestaño. También resulta afectada la resistencia inespecífica.

Asimismo se han observado efectos generales en el sistema inmunitario (por ejemplo, en el peso y la morfología de los tejidos linfoides, los recuentos de linfocitos periféricos y las concentraciones totales de inmunoglobulinas séricas) en diferentes estudios con OTBE realizados en ratas y perros, pero no en ratones, mediante dosis claramente tóxicas (en el ratón se han registrado efectos con dosis de cloruro de tributilestaño de 150 mg/kg). Solamente la rata presenta signos de toxicidad y, evidentemente, es la especie más sensible. En los estudios a corto plazo, el NENO para esta especie fue de 5 mg/kg (0,6 mg/kg de peso corporal) en la dieta. En los estudios con cloruro de tributilestaño se han observado efectos análogos en el timo, rápidamente reversibles tan pronto como se interrumpía la administración. Según se ha observado en estudios in vivo de resistencia del huésped, el OTBE pone en peligro la función inmunitaria específica en la rata. Tras la exposición a un nivel de 50 mg/kg en la dieta (siendo el valor NENO de 5 mg/kg al día), se observó una disminución del "aclaramiento" de *Listeria monocytogenes*, mientras que con 50 y 5 mg/kg en la dieta, pero no con 0,5 mg/kg (2,5, 0,25 y 0,025 mg/kg de peso corporal al día, respectivamente) se produjo un descenso de la resistencia a *Trichinella spiralis*. Los mismos efectos, aunque menos pronunciados, se observaron en animales de más edad.

Según los conocimientos actuales, los efectos en la resistencia del huésped se deben probablemente a una evaluación más adecuada de los posibles riesgos para el hombre; sin embargo, no se tiene suficiente experiencia con los sistemas de prueba para apreciar bien su importancia. En cualquier caso, las observaciones en ratas atímicas "desnudas", estimuladas en las condiciones ordinarias, proporcionan algunos datos para interpretar el modelo de *T. spiralis*. En estos estudios, la ausencia completa de inmunidad timodependiente aumentó de 10 a 20 veces los recuentos de larvas en el músculo; en cambio, la exposición a concentraciones de OTBE de 5 y 50 mg/kg en la dieta duplicó y cuadruplicó, respectivamente, la cifra inicial.

Aunque ahora se dispone de algunos datos sobre los efectos de los compuestos de tributilestaño en el desarrollo del sistema inmunitario, carecemos de información sobre la resistencia del huésped.

Resumen

Lo prudente sería evaluar los posibles riesgos para el hombre en función de los datos obtenidos en la especie más sensible. Los efectos sobre la resistencia del huésped a *T. spiralis* se han observado ya con niveles en la dieta de 5 mg/kg (equivalentes a 0,25 mg/kg de peso corporal al día), por lo que el valor NENO es de 0,5 mg/kg (equivalente a 0,025 mg/kg al día). Sin embargo, no existe acuerdo sobre el significado de estos datos para evaluar los riesgos en el hombre. En todos los demás estudios, una concentración de 5 mg/kg al día en la dieta (equivalente a 0,5 mg/kg de peso corporal, sobre la base de los estudios a corto plazo) correspondía al valor NENO con respecto a los efectos en el sistema inmunitario, tanto generales como específicos.

12.3 Toxicidad a largo plazo

Un estudio a largo plazo en las ratas sugiere un efecto marginal del TBE en los parámetros toxicológicos generales (cuya significación toxicológica es limitada) a una concentración de 5 mg/kg (0,25 mg/kg de peso corporal) en la dieta.

12.4 Genotoxicidad

La genotoxicidad del OTBE ha sido objeto de detenidas investigaciones. En la gran mayoría de los estudios se han obtenido resultados negativos, y no hay ninguna prueba convincente de que el OTBE tenga propiedades mutagénicas.

12.5 Toxicidad en el sistema reproductor

En tres especies de mamíferos (ratón, rata y conejo) se ha evaluado la posible embriotoxicidad del OTBE tras administrarlo por vía oral a la madre. La principal malformación observada en los fetos de rata y de ratón fue la fisura palatina, pero este efecto sólo se registró con dosis claramente tóxicas para las madres. Tal resultado no se ha considerado como indicio de efectos teratogénicos del OTBE en dosis inferiores a las que producen toxicidad materna. El NENO más bajo en lo relativo a la embriotoxicidad y la fetotoxicidad para todos las especies fue de 1,0 mg/kg de peso corporal.

12.6 Carcinogenicidad

En las ratas se ha realizado un estudio de carcinogenicidad en el que se obtuvieron alteraciones neoplásicas de los órganos endocrinos con 50 mg/kg en la dieta. En cuanto a los tumores hipofisarios registrados con 0,5 mg/kg en la dieta, se consideró que no tenían significación biológica por no existir relación dosis-respuesta. Estos tipos de tumores suelen aparecer con una incidencia general elevada y variable, por lo que su significación parece discutible. Está en curso un estudio de carcinogenicidad en el ratón.

13. Efectos en el ser humano

Se ha observado que la exposición profesional de los trabajadores al tributilestaño provoca irritación de las vías respiratorias superiores. En forma de aerosol, el TBE entraña un riesgo para las personas. El OTBE ejerce un efecto irritante en la piel y en los ojos, habiéndose observado casos de dermatitis grave a consecuencia del contacto directo con la piel. El problema se agrava por la falta de una respuesta cutánea inmediata.

EVALUACION DE LOS RIESGOS PARA LA SALUD HUMANA Y DE LOS EFECTOS SOBRE EL MEDIO AMBIENTE

1. Evaluación del riesgo para las personas

La exposición de los trabajadores se produce sobre todo en las actividades de fabricación y formulación de compuestos de tributilestaño, durante la aplicación y la eliminación de pinturas a base de TBE y a consecuencia del empleo de TBE como conservador de la madera. La exposición del público en general puede deberse a la contaminación de los alimentos, particularmente el pescado y los mariscos, así como a la aplicación doméstica de productos de protección de la madera.

A juzgar por las pruebas realizadas en animales y por la observación directa de las personas, parece evidente que los compuestos de TBE ejercen efectos irritantes en la piel y en los ojos y que la inhalación de los aerosoles provoca irritación respiratoria.

La manipulación de madera tratada no entraña riesgos de irritación dérmica si se ha secado el material. En cambio, los aerosoles de TBE son muy peligrosos y no debe permitirse que la madera vuelva a entrar en la zona de tratamiento hasta que esté perfectamente seca.

No se ha señalado ningún caso de intoxicación sistémica aguda y, probablemente, el TBE se elimina del organismo al cabo de pocos días. Por consiguiente, no es de temer que el manejo de productos de TBE entrañe peligro de toxicidad aguda si se toman las precauciones adecuadas.

En los animales de laboratorio se han observado efectos a corto y a largo plazo en el hígado y en los sistemas hematológico y endocrino. Los efectos de los compuestos de TBE en el sistema inmunitario, y especialmente en la resistencia del huésped, han resultado ser el parámetro más sensible de toxicidad en la rata, que es la especie más sensible de todas las estudiadas. Cuando se utiliza *Trichinella spiralis* como modelo de resistencia del huésped, el nivel de efecto no observado (NENO) se sitúa entre 0,5 y 5,0 mg/kg (0,025 y 0,25 mg/kg de peso corporal) en la dieta, mientras que si se utilizan índices de función inmunitaria es de 0,6 mg/kg de peso corporal.

Debido a las grandes variaciones en el consumo de pescado y mariscos y a las diferencias locales de la cantidad de residuos de TBE presentes en la fauna marina, sólo a título de orientación pueden hacerse estimaciones de los valores de exposición y del NENO. Conviene tener en cuenta que para evaluar el riesgo potencial de estos compuestos hay que proceder en el plano local a determinar los residuos, calcular el consumo de pescado y mariscos y fijar los límites aceptables de seguridad.

Partiendo de cifras de consumo de pescado de 15 y 150 g/día, de un valor de residuos en el pescado de 1 mg/kg y de un peso medio de las personas de 60 kilos, se han obtenido los siguientes márgenes de seguridad basados en diferentes puntos finales inmunológicos.

Consumo de pescado (g/día)	Ingestión diaria estimada de TBE (μg/kg)	Margen de seguridad	
		Modelo de T. spiralis	Otros parámetros inmunológicos
15	0,25	100-1000	2500
150	2,5	10-100	250

El empleo indiscriminado e irresponsable de compuesto de TBE y la observancia de las recomendaciones esbozadas en la presente monografía para reducir la exposición de las personas puede dar lugar a la ingestión de concentraciones de compuesto de TBE peligrosas para la salud humana.

En los animales de experimentación sólo de han observado efectos teratogénicos con dosis que causan signos patentes de toxicidad materna. Por consiguiente, se considera que el potencial teratogénico de TBE es muy bajo.

Basándose en los resultados de detallados estudios de mutagenicidad, se considera que los compuestos de tributilestaño no tienen potencial mutagénico. En un estudio de carcinogenicidad realizada en la rata con OTBE, se observó un aumento de la incidencia de ciertos tumores endocrinos que aparecen espontáneamente con una incidencia elevada y variable. Por consiguiente, los datos disponibles no indican claramente que los compuestos de TBE entrañen riesgos carcinogénicos para las personas.

2. Evaluación de los riesgos ambientales

La difusión del tributilestaño (TBE) en el medio ambiente se debe sobre todo al empleo de ese compuesto en las pinturas antiincrustantes. También puede deberse al empleo de TBE como molusquicida. La contaminación en la fuente se produce a consecuencia de utilizar TBE como biocida en los sistemas de refrigeración, la fabricación de pulpa de madera, el tratamiento de los cueros, los procesos de conservación de la madera y el tratamiento de los productos textiles.

Debido a sus propiedades fisicoquímicas, los compuestos de TBE se concentran en la microcapa superficial y en los sedimentos. La degradación abiótica no parece ser un mecanismo importante de eliminación del TBE en condiciones ambientales. Aunque el OTBE es biodegradable en la columna de agua, este proceso no es suficientemente rápido para impedir la aparición de concentraciones elevadas de TBE en algunos sitios. En la mayor parte de los organismos acuáticos se produce bioacumulación pero la degradación metabólica es un proceso más eficaz en los mamíferos de laboratorio.

El TBE es sumamente peligroso para algunos organismos acuáticos por ser tóxico incluso a concentraciones muy bajas en el agua. Tales concentraciones se han señalado en diversos lugares. En los estudios sobre el terreno se han observado efectos adversos sobre invertebrados, especialmente moluscos, a los que no se pretendía atacar, y esos efectos resultan suficientemente graves para interferir en la reproducción y provocar un descenso de la población. En algunos sitios ha sido posible anular los efectos adversos en la producción comercial de mariscos restringuiendo el empleo de pinturas antiincrustantes, con lo que también se ha logrado suprimir el efecto de imposex en las poblaciones de gasterópodos. Los efectos en las piscifactorías hacen pensar que no conviene utilizar pinturas que contengan TBE en las redes de contención.

Para el medio terrestre, el riesgo general parece ser bajo. La madera tratada con TBE podría ser peligrosa para los organismos terrestres que viven en estrecho contacto con ella.

El aumento de las concentraciones de TBE en la microcapa superficial puede ser peligroso para los organismos del litoral, las especies neustónicas (inclusive invertebrados bénticos y larvas de peces) y las aves salvajes y marinas que se alimentan en la superficie del agua. La acumulación y la baja biodegradación del TBE en los sedimentos puede representar un peligro para los organismos acuáticos cuando esos sedimentos contaminados se movilizan por procesos naturales u operaciones de dragado.

RECOMENDACIONES

1. **Recomendaciones para proteger la salud humana y la higiene del medio**

    a) Hay que instar a los países Miembros que todavía no hayan reglamentado el uso de compuestos de TBE a que lo hagan.

    b) Es necesario evaluar y, si procede reglamentar, el ingreso en el medio ambiente de estaño orgánico procedente de fuentes distintas de las pinturas antiincrustantes. Por ejemplo, convendría evaluar el riesgo potencial que entraña la aplicación al suelo de lodos de alcantarillado contaminados con TBE.

    c) Habrá que mejorar los métodos utilizables para aplicar, eliminar y evacuar en condiciones de seguridad las pinturas de estaño orgánico.

2. **Investigaciones necesarias**

    a) Habrá que mejorar los métodos de detección y análisis a fin de poder determinar con rapidez y precisión los compuestos de butilestaño presentes en concentraciones de pg/litro. Una de las razones que justifican esa recomendación es que ciertos efectos biológicos (por ejemplo, el imposex en los gasterópodos) pueden producirse con concentraciones inferiores a los actuales límites de detección.

    b) Esnecesario estudiar los mecanismos que concentran en vez de dispersar el TBE y que retrasan la degradación, prestando especial atención a los fundamentos químicos de ese compuesto y a su interaccción con las moléculas biológicas. Se necesitan más estudios sobre la absorción del TBE en todos los niveles tróficos.

    c) Habrá que estudiar la toxicidad del TBE en los organismos acuáticos. Estos estudios deberán versar, si procede, sobre el metabolismo, los efectos endocrinos y la toxicidad inmunológica.

    d) Habrá que buscar otras especies sensibles (en particular de agua dulce) que sirvan de bioindicador en otros grupos.

e) Habrá que confirmar la validez de los modelos utilizados para evaluar la inmunotoxicidad en los mamíferos y definir con más precisión los niveles sin efecto de los parámetros pertinentes.

f) Convendría emprender un estudio de toxicidad crónica en una segunda especie de mamífero.

g) Convendría emprender un estudio de tumorigenicidad en una segunda especie de mamífero.

h) Hay que obtener datos mediante métodos de especiación sobre los niveles de residuos de butilestaño en los peces y mariscos destinados al consumo humano.

www.ingramcontent.com/pod-product-compliance
Ingram Content Group UK Ltd.
Pitfield, Milton Keynes, MK11 3LW, UK
UKHW021314180426